Fetal Medicine /1

EDITED BY

CHARLES H. RODECK

BSc, MB, BS, FRCOG
Professor of Obstetrics and Gynaecology
Royal Postgraduate Medical School
Institute of Obstetrics and Gynaecology
Queen Charlotte's Maternity Hospital
University of London

BLACKWELL SCIENTIFIC PUBLICATIONS

OXFORD LONDON EDINBURGH

BOSTON MELBOURNE

© 1989 by
Blackwell Scientific Publications
Editorial offices:
Osney Mead, Oxford OX2 OEL
  (*Orders*: Tel. 0865 240201)
8 John Street, London WC1N 2ES
23 Ainslie Place, Edinburgh EH3 6AJ
3 Cambridge Center, Suite 208
  Cambridge, Massachusetts 02142, USA
107 Barry Street, Carlton
  Victoria 3053, Australia

First published 1989

Set by Setrite Ltd, Hong Kong,
printed by The Alden Press, Oxford,
and bound at The Green Street Bindery,
Oxford

DISTRIBUTORS
USA
  Year Book Medical Publishers
  200 North LaSalle Street,
  Chicago, Illinois 60601
  (*Orders*: Tel. 312 726−9733)

Canada
  The C.V. Mosby Company
  5240 Finch Avenue East
  Scarborough, Ontario
  (*Orders*: Tel. 416−298−1588)

Australia
  Blackwell Scientific Publications
  (Australia) Pty Ltd
  107 Barry Street
  Carlton, Victoria 3053
  (*Orders*: Tel. (03) 347 0300)

British Library
Cataloguing in Publication Data

Fetal medicine —1−
  1. Man. Fetuses. Diseases
  618.3'2

  ISBN 0−632−01972−7

Contents

List of Contributors

R.L. Berkowitz MD, *Department of Obstetrics Gynecology and Reproductive Science, Mount Sinai School of Medicine, 1 Gustave L. Levy Place, New York, USA*

J.E. Bleasdale PhD, *Department of Cell Biology, The Upjohn Company, Kalamazoo, Michigan, USA*

G.C. Di Renzo MD, *Institute for Gynaecology and Obstetrics, Policlinico Monteluce, University of Perugia, Perugia, Italy*

A.W. Flake MD, *Fetal Treatment Program, Department of Surgery, Division of Pediatric Surgery, University of California at San Francisco, California, USA*

S.G. Gabbe MD, *Department of Obstetrics and Gynecology, The Ohio State University College of Medicine, Columbus, Ohio, USA*

M.R. Harrison MD, *Fetal Treatment Program, Department of Surgery, Division of Pediatric Surgery, University of California at San Francisco, California, USA*

N. Kochenour MD, *Division of Maternal–Fetal Medicine, Department of Obstetrics and Gynecology, University of Utah Medical Center, Salt Lake City, Utah, USA*

M.B. Landon MD, *Department of Obstetrics and Gynecology, Division of Maternal–Fetal Medicine, The Ohio State University College of Medicine, Columbus, Ohio, USA*

L. Lynch MD, *Department of Obstetrics Gynecology and Reproductive Science, Mount Sinai School of Medicine, 1 Gustave L. Levy Place, New York, USA*

I.R. McFadyen FRCOG, *University Department of Obstetrics and Gynaecology, 3rd Floor, UCD Building, Royal Liverpool Hospital, Prescott Street, Liverpool L7 8XP, UK*

K. Mehalek MD, *Department of Obstetrics Gynecology and Reproductive Science, Mount Sinai School of Medicine, 1 Gustave L. Levy Place, New York, USA*

J.F. Mowbray MB, BChir, FRCP, *Department of Experimental Pathology, St Mary's Hospital Medical School, London W2 1PG, UK*

K.H. Nicolaides BSc, MB, BS, MRCOG, *Harris-Birthright Research Centre for Fetal Medicine, King's College Hospital, Denmark Hill, London SE5 9RS, UK*

A. Reuss, *Department of Obstetrics and Gynaecology, Academic Hospital Rotterdam Dijkzigt, Erasmus University Rotterdam, Netherlands*

C.H. Rodeck BSc, MB, BS, FRCOG, *Institute of Obstetrics and Gynaecology, University of London, Queen Charlotte's Maternity Hospital, Goldhawk Road, London W6 OXG, UK*

M.J. Seller BSc, PhD, DSc, *The United Medical and Dental Schools of Guy's and St Thomas's Hospitals, Paediatric Research Unit, Guy's Hospital, London SE1 9RT, UK*

P.W. Soothill BSc, MB, BS, MD, *Bristol Maternity Hospital, Bristol BS2 8EG, UK*

P.A. Stewart, *Department of Obstetrics and Gynaecology, Academic Hospital Rotterdam Dijkzigt, Erasmus University Rotterdam, Netherlands*

D.J. Weatherall MA, MD, FRCP, FRS, *MRC Molecular Haematology Unit, Nuffield Department of Clinical Medicine, University of Oxford, John Radcliffe Hospital, Oxford OX3 9DU, UK*

J.W. Wladimiroff, *Department of Obstetrics and Gynaecology, Academic Hospital Rotterdam Dijkzigt, Erasmus University Rotterdam, Netherlands*

Preface

The last two decades have seen enormous scientific and technological advances in a variety of disciplines which have been applied to the study of fetal physiology and pathology, both in humans and laboratory animals. They include biophysical, biochemical, immunological and molecular biological methods, ultrasonic imaging and invasive techniques for fetal sampling. The use of these methods, the large body of knowledge gained by them, and the development of diagnostic and therapeutic possibilities has led to the emergence of fetal medicine as a discipline in its own right.

The fetus, then, is the central theme of this series of biennial reviews, of which this volume is the first. The fetus yields its secrets reluctantly and facts are gained with difficulty. All the more important, therefore, that information on different aspects of intrauterine life is brought together and that the rigid compartmentalization of the older disciplines is avoided. The variety of subjects in this volume reflects a catholic approach which we hope will prove stimulating to the reader.

My grateful thanks are due to my colleagues who have distilled their unrivalled experience and knowledge into reviews of great distinction, and to our publishers for their patience and support in the initiation of this venture.

C.H. RODECK

1

Vitamins and Neural Tube Defects

M.J. SELLER

The current interest in vitamins and neural tube defects (NTD) stems from a report in 1980 by Smithells and colleagues of a highly significant reduction in recurrence of NTD apparently achieved by maternal periconceptional vitamin supplementation. Suddenly, in the face of an increasingly successful programme of secondary prevention of these abnormalities through maternal serum and amniotic fluid alphafetoprotein assay, the most important prospect of primary prevention presented itself. Prenatal diagnosis and termination of pregnancy have been accepted by most people as a form of management for such disorders with very serious consequences. But it was always hoped that they would be only temporary expedients, even if long-term ones, until such times as research provided ways of preventing the abnormalities from happening in the first place. Now there was the prospect that this long-sought goal might possibly have been achieved for NTD.

Although generally well received, there were a few sceptics, even though the work was subsequently repeated (Smithells *et al.* 1983a). Basically the uncertainty was because the study, although planned as a double-blind placebo trial, had not been conducted in that way, since ethical approval for such a method was withheld. The results were therefore judged by some to be due to patient selection bias (Lancet Editorial 1980). Nevertheless, intense interest in the subject was generated and several independent studies along the same lines are now under way.

This chapter first considers the nature of NTD, normal embryogenesis of the neural tube and mode of nutrition of the early embryo, and then examines some of the evidence which comes from studies in both experimental animals and man relating to teratology and to a connection between deficiencies of maternal nutritional factors and NTD.

The natural history of neural tube defects

NTD are a related group of disorders of development of the brain and spinal cord and the surrounding mesodermal structures. However, they are morphologically heterogeneous. In total craniorachischisis, the whole of the neural tube is affected, but more commonly, there is a localized lesion at some point, producing such varied abnormalities as anencephaly or spina bifida or encephalocoele. NTD are also heterogeneous aetiologically. Relatively rarely, the cause is known. They may be chromosomal — NTD are associated with trisomy 18 and triploidy, or genetic — NTD are part of certain autosomal recessive disorders such as Meckel syndrome, or occasionally mechanical, as in the amniogenous malformation. Most often, however, NTD are not associated with any obvious factors and the precise cause or causes are unknown. These are referred to as the multifactorial type and are the most common form of NTD, comprising around 90−95% of the total, and are the subject of this work.

Multifactorial NTD

Multifactorial NTD can be divided into two major groups — those where the defect in the neural tube is the only abnormality present in the individual (disregarding secondary sequelae such as hydrocephaly and talipes), and those which are associated with defects in other body systems. The former, or 'isolated NTD' account for 80% or more of the total (Khoury *et al.* 1982). These workers found that the two groups had different epidemiological characteristics and so proposed that they are therefore different aetiologically. However, Seller & Kalousek (1986) analysed in detail the association of the other defects with the NTD and found a clustering according to site of the NTD lesion, rather than a random distribution within the different morphological types of NTD, and, further, that this clustering conformed to a definite pattern. They concluded that the NTD with other defects were actually related to the isolated NTD group and were simply those where the disruption in development was more far-reaching as a result of a greater primary lesion.

An important point to note, however, is that, in over 80% of cases, the NTD is an isolated, and often quite local, defect; it is the only abnormality in the body, the rest having developed quite normally. It is only in a minority of cases of NTD that there are multiple malformations affecting other body systems. This fact is highly relevant when considering the lessons learned from teratological experiments in animals.

Formation of the neural tube

In man, neural tube formation (described in textbooks of embryology, for instance, Sadler 1985, and also in more specialized sources, for example, Lemire *et al.* 1975) has its observable beginnings around the 18th−19th day after conception when the embryo is at the late presomite stage. The central part of the ectoderm of the embryonic disc is induced to thicken and differentiate into the neural plate by the underlying paraxial mesoderm. The main morphogenetic event is neurulation, when, as the embryonic disc elongates, a longitudinal groove appears on its dorsal surface in the midline, and the lateral edges of the neural plate rise up forming the neural folds, which in turn arch over and gradually meet in the dorsal midline. Initial fusion of the contralateral folds occurs around day 21 in the region of the fourth to the sixth somites, which corresponds to the future lower cervical region. Thereafter, with the embryo rapidly elongating further and increasing in size, fusion occurs from this point concurrently in both the cephalic and caudal directions, so producing a hollow tube. Neurulation is completed when the extreme ends, the neuropores, are sealed, and this is accomplished at the anterior end around days 24−25, and posteriorly around days 26−27. The posterior neuropore corresponds to the future upper lumbar region (Lemire *et al.* 1975), and the lower lumbar and sacral regions of the neural tube arise subsequently by another process, called canalization. Cells are added to the caudal end of the neural tube from the undifferentiated caudal cell mass. Vacuoles develop between them, and gradually coalesce and connect up with the central canal previously formed by neurulation (Lemire, 1969). This process continues until day 48.

Although there are still proponents for the original idea of Morgagni (1769) that NTD arise because a normally closed neural tube later ruptures (Gardner 1973), most hold the view that NTD occur because the neural tube somehow fails to close.

Obviously, neural tube formation is associated with intense cell proliferation. Not only is the neural plate enlarging, but, as the neural folds form and elevate, the underlying mesoderm is expanding, and the gut and notochord are elongating too. There is therefore an excessive demand for precursors and co-factors for the biosynthesis of the macromolecules needed for this growth process, and these necessarily have to be supplied by the mother. The idea that the cause of NTD might be a nutritional deficiency has come mainly from observations on maternal blood vitamin levels, but it must be remembered that the maternal blood is relatively far removed from the crucial site in the embryo, the cells of, and around, the neural plate, which are somehow not able to carry out normal morphogenesis. Nutrients have to be transported and delivered to this area, and the embryonic cells themselves have to have an efficient uptake system and perfectly functioning synthetic machinery.

Nutrition of the embryo

Fetal nutrition is a well studied subject, and conventionally what is discussed is the working of the definitive chorioallantoic placenta. It is known that this established placenta contains vitamins, and that it probably acts as a storage site for some, such as vitamins B, D and E. Further, there is placental transfer of vitamins, with active transport rather than simple diffusion being implicated because concentration gradients exist. For example, vitamin A levels are lower in fetal than maternal blood, while vitamin D levels are higher (Hamilton *et al.* 1976). But such knowledge is largely irrelevant when considering the genesis of NTD, for, at that time, the mature chorioallantoic placenta does not exist.

Initially, nutrition of the embryo is by way of the histiotroph. The conceptus implants in the maternal endometrium through the invasive action of its trophoblast. Spaces occur in the outermost layer, the syncytiotrophoblast, and in the adjacent decidua, wherein gathers a rich mixture, the histiotroph, derived from secretions of the uterine glands, blood from damaged maternal capillaries, and degenerating decidual cells. The trophoblast takes up soluble proteins from this fluid by endocytosis, and cell fragments by pinocytosis. Intracellular digestion by catabolic enzymes occurs within vacuoles and then the resulting simple nutrients diffuse across the yolk sac and extraembryonic coelom to the embryonic disc. This is the sole source of embryonic nutrition until about days 21−22.

From day 14, finger-like projections grow out from the trophoblast, acquire a mesodermal core and then a capillary network and become chorionic villi. Meanwhile, early in the third week, blood vessel formation begins in the mesoderm of the yolk sac, and primitive blood cells and plasma arise from the endothelium of these vessels. Within the embryo, paired heart tubes connect up with these vessels, and around days 21−22 blood circulation, intermittent at first, begins. With circulating blood now bathing the maternal side of the villi too in enlarged intervillous spaces, the second, and definitive, form of nutrition, haemotrophic nutrition, is initiated. In this method, nutrients from the maternal blood have to cross a barrier within the villi, comprising a layer of trophoblastic cells, mesenchyme and fetal capillary endothelium, before reaching the fetal blood, in which they are then carried via the umbilical vessels and embryonic circulation to the cells of the embryo. Histiotrophic nutrition does not cease when haemotrophic nutrition begins; the two forms are utilized concurrently for some time (Beck *et al.* 1985).

Thus, at the time of formation of the neural tube, embryonic nutrition is predominantly histiotrophic, with haemotrophic nutrition additionally coming into play during the later stages. The supply of vital nutrients for neurulation is therefore dependent on efficient endocytosis, pinocytosis and intracellular digestion, and also on the proper development of chorionic villi, the fetal circulation and the maternal perfusing system. Haemotrophic nutrition becomes necessary when diffusion through the embryonic system is insufficient to meet the nutritional needs of the embryo. Since this becomes functional right in the middle of neurulation, it is possible that, if there were some slight delay in its establishment, this could deprive the embryo of adequate nutrition at a time which is vital to formation of the neural tube. It is relatively easy to envisage both genetic and environmental factors acting to influence this process.

Little detail is known about these nutritional mechanisms in human embryos, but insights come from experiments in animals. In the rat, histiotrophic nutrition occurs through the yolk sac, and it has been found that this membrane concentrates vitamin B_{12} (Padykula *et al.* 1966). Further, rabbit yolk sac cells have an energy-dependent mechanism for vitamin B_{12} uptake (Deren *et al.* 1966), and the rabbit uterus secretes vitamin B_{12} into the lumen in concentrations far in excess of that in maternal serum (Jacobson & Lutwak-Mann 1956). In rats, histiotrophic nutrition can be directly influenced by the maternal administration of exogenous agents. Trypan blue inhibits yolk sac endocytosis (Williams *et al.* 1976) and leucopeptin inhibits intracellular digestion (Beck & Lowy 1982). Significantly, in rat embryos both trypan blue and leucopeptin induce NTD and other abnormalities. The inverted yolk sac of rodents differs from the membrane arrangement in primates. However, these rodent experiments are significant because they show that nutrition of the early embryo can be impaired, and that such impairment is associated with the development of abnormalities. They also indicate ways in which embryos can be deprived of nutrients other than through a frank deficiency of the maternal source. Inhibition of transport or nutritional mechanisms at the embryo–maternal interface, either by a teratogen or by a constitutional enzyme or other deficiency, must be a possibility.

Lessons learned from animal teratology experiments

Much has been learned about the teratogenic action of environmental factors from experiments in animals. A cardinal principle is that environmental influences are capable of producing developmental malformations only for a short and specific time during intrauterine life. That critical period is organogenesis, and, prior to and following this, the developmental abnormalities are not produced, although modifications or disruptions of development can occur subsequently. Each individual organ is susceptible to modification by a teratogen only for the brief time immediately before and during its formation. This is its own critical period, and for the neural tube in man presumably approximates to the 16th or 17th day to the 26th day of life.

Another teratogenic principle is that, since, during embryonic development, the different organs begin to develop at different times, and also since they develop at different rates, if the teratogenic insult comes as a single pulse, it will be deleterious to some organs and not to others, so some degree of specificity is possible. However, experiments with numerous teratogens show that they virtually never produce a single specific malformation; instead, they produce a particular pattern of defects (Schardein 1985). The reason is that, at any one time, more than one organ is undergoing development. Thus, in rats, day 7 of gestation is the time of maximum vulnerability of the central nervous system to hypervitaminosis A, and NTD are produced by a single injection of excess vitamin A, but defects of the eye, palate and face also occur. This fact has implications if it is considered that NTD in man arise as a result of some form of teratogenic action, because it must be reconciled with the observation mentioned previously, that over 80% of human NTD occur as an isolated single malformation in the body.

On the other hand, there are rare occasions in experimental animals where a single defect may be produced. In the curly-tail mouse, an animal model of human NTD to be mentioned in more detail later, where there is a definite genetic cause to the NTD, it is possible to increase the penetrance of the gene with environmental agents. Vitamin A is one of these and, as in the rat experiments mentioned above, produces other abnormalities too. Mitomycin C, however, produces an increase of NTD specifically, and no other type of abnormality (Seller & Perkins 1986).

Another pertinent finding in animal experiments is that NTD can be produced with numerous unrelated agents; they are not associated with one substance or even a particular group of substances. This suggests that, even if a vitamin deficiency were finally proven as a cause of NTD in humans, it is unlikely to be the sole cause.

Yet another teratological consideration particularly apposite in the present context is that of synergism, where one substance affects the teratogenic action of another. In mice, maternal pyridoxine deficiency increases the incidence of cortisone-induced cleft palate (Miller 1972). On the other hand, in rats, nicotinamide reduces the teratogenicity of thiadiazole (Beaudoin 1973), and B group vitamins protect against the teratogenic effect of vitamin A (Woollam & Millen 1960). So the possibility exists that, if there is a vitamin effect in human NTD, rather than acting directly on the embryo, it might be similarly indirect.

Aetiology of human NTD

As far as the aetiology of human NTD is concerned, epidemiological studies show that both genetic and environmental factors are implicated. It is generally accepted that a series of genetic factors, together with precipitating environmental factors, create a degree of liability in an individual, which, if sufficiently great, results in an NTD occurring (Carter 1974). Practically, it is not possible to alter the genotype, but it has always been felt that there is potential for prevention of NTD if the environmental factors could be changed. Thus, the identity of the environmental components has long been sought. Since teratogens commonly produce NTD in experimental animals, there has been an exhaustive search for a food component which might similarly be teratogenic to the central nervous system of man. Through epidemiological studies, the list of suspects has become very long. Although associations were noted between NTD offspring and such things as maternal tinned meat consumption in pregnancy (Knox 1972), or excessive tea drinking (Fedrick 1974), or blighted potato eating (Renwick 1972), none could be established as a proven cause of NTD. Concurrently, however, there was a gradual awareness that certain nutritional deficiencies might also be associated with NTD.

Human studies on nutritional deficiency and NTD

Probably the most severe form of nutritional deprivation is that encountered during times of famine. Studies on women exposed in the first trimester of pregnancy to the Dutch famine in 1944–45 show that the incidence of stillbirths, neonatal deaths and congenital malformations in the offspring was increased, amongst which the number of NTD was twice that expected (Stein *et al.* 1975). However, studies of other populations which faced similar deprivation suggest that general malnutrition during pregnancy is less likely to produce specific congenital malformations; rather, it is more generally deleterious, and miscarriage, stillbirth, premature delivery and neonatal death are the common sequelae (Warkany 1951).

Indirect evidence that a general nutritional deficiency might contribute to the cause of NTD comes from the fact that, in the United Kingdom, NTD are more commonly associated with the lower socioeconomic classes (Carter 1974). Smithells *et al.* (1977) have demonstrated a connection between food intake and social class. They assessed the mean daily nutrient intakes, by weighed dietary records, of 195 women in the first trimester of pregnancy and found that social classes III, IV and V had significantly lower intakes of all component nutrients analysed than classes I and II.

There have been a number of studies on nutrition of mothers of NTD offspring. Coffey and Jessop (1958) performed a case-control study of women after delivery, and found evidence of greater defective nutrition in mothers of anencephalics compared with controls. This was based on clinical examination, serum protein and haemoglobin levels. But such observations are far removed from the time of neural tube formation in the early first trimester.

Analysis of the diet of women who have produced NTD children has yielded some information, but it is fraught with problems of accurate recall and possible bias. Richards (1969) performed a retrospective case-control study, and found in mothers of NTD offspring a significant excess of diets in the first trimester which were unbalanced. Laurence and his colleagues (1980) asked women who had had an NTD child to recall what their diet was in the first trimester of that pregnancy. According to food content, the diet was judged good, fair or poor, and it was found that only 10% of the women had a good diet, while 53% had had a poor diet. Some of these women were then given dietary counselling and 71% of them improved their eating habits. In subsequent pregnancies, the recurrence rate for NTD was 3% in the counselled group, and 7% in women who had not been counselled, but all the recurrences occurred in women whose diet was classified as poor. In a second study, Laurence and his colleagues (1984) dispensed with recall of dietary habits and instead studied the diet at the time of interview. 41% of women who had had an NTD child were classed as being on a poor diet, compared with 26% of their sisters without NTD children and 6% of the wives of university teachers. Then all the NTD women were given dietary counselling. In subsequent pregnancies there were five recurrences of NTD, but again they all occurred in the women who remained on a poor diet. Thus, this work would seem to have demonstrated an association between a poor diet and the occurrence of NTD, and also that dietary counselling is beneficial. However, it is criticized because, amongst other things, so much subjectivity is involved (Kirke 1983).

In support of poor nutrition as a major contributor to the cause of NTD, Al-Awadi *et al.* (1984) cite the dramatically falling prevalence of anencephaly in Kuwait. They attribute this exclusively to an improved diet, for the country does not have prenatal diagnosis or termination of pregnancy, and it is well documented in official statistics that there has been a coincident increase in the per capita food consumption, together with a marked improvement in the quality of the food.

Apparently arguing against poor nutrition as a cause, however, is the well-known fact that NTD are not common in Africa and Asia, where malnutrition is rife. Further, there are overt discrepancies. In India, for instance, the incidence of NTD is much higher in the Punjabi people, who are well nourished, than in other population groups elsewhere in the subcontinent (Talwalkar 1981). In South Africa, the NTD prevalence amongst Whites is 1 in 300, in Coloureds it is 1 in 1250, and in Blacks it is 1 in 2000, yet white South Africans are claimed to be the best fed people in the world (Cornell *et al.* 1983).

One answer to this is that the cause of NTD is multifactorial, and environmental factors do not work without the appropriate genetic factors. Negroes and Mongols presumably lack the genetic component, while it is present in Caucasians. Another possible factor could be that the diet of the Third World is largely vegetarian, often consisting of leaves and roots, which, although obviously lacking protein and energy-rich components, may well be abundant in folic acid and vitamins.

Animal studies on nutritional deficiency and NTD

In experimental animals, chronic generalized dietary restriction does not produce overt developmental abnormalities. In rats, small, immature young result (Berg 1965) and this retarded development persists into adult life (Dickerson & Hughes 1972). There is also a high incidence of intrauterine fetal death (Saitoh & Takahashi 1973). These, therefore, are similar findings to those in man. However, in mice, total fasting for 24 hours is teratogenic if performed in the organogenetic period. Cleft palate, skeletal and CNS abnormalities, including exencephaly, are produced (Runner & Miller 1956; Kalter 1960).

Evidence for vitamin deficiency as a cause of NTD in animals

More specifically, deficiencies of individual vitamins are known to be teratogenic in animals. A lack of all vitamins tends to have a profound effect on the developing embryo and, even if malformations do not occur, there is often growth retardation or significant pregnancy wastage.

Deficiencies of five major vitamins — A, B_{12}, D, nicotinic acid and riboflavin — do not seem to produce NTD in a variety of species, although other abnormalities do occur. In rabbits, vitamin A deficiency gives rise to hydrocephaly due to over-production of cerebrospinal fluid by the choroid plexus (Millen & Woollam 1958). In pigs, it produces eye and kidney defects, cleft lip and palate and accessory ears (Hale 1933), and, in rats, urogenital and eye anomalies (Roux *et al.* 1962). A lack of vitamin B_{12} produces hydrocephaly and cleft lip in the rat (Woodard & Newberne 1966). A deficiency of vitamin D gives skeletal abnormalities (Warkany 1943), of riboflavin, skeletal and digital anomalies and cleft palate (Warkany & Schraffenberger 1943), and of nicotinic acid, ocular, urogenital and skeletal anomalies and cleft lip and palate (Chamberlain & Nelson 1963). Deficiencies of vitamin K, choline, biotin and essential fatty acids also do not produce NTD, neither does a diet lacking vitamin C. However, all animals except the guinea-pig and primates synthesize their own supplies of vitamin C (Kalter & Warkany 1959).

There are only four vitamins a lack of which is associated with the production of NTD. However, these CNS abnormalities do not occur alone but are amongst a spectrum of defects produced. The vitamins are folic acid (to be dealt with in a separate section), pantothenic acid, B_6 and E. Deficiency of pantothenic acid produces exencephaly, eye and limb defects and urogenital anomalies (Giroud *et al.* 1957), of vitamin B_6, exencephaly, cleft palate, omphalocoele and micrognathia (Davis *et al.* 1970), and of vitamin E, exencephaly, cleft lip, syndactyly, umbilical hernia and scoliosis in rats (Cheng *et al.* 1960) but no abnormalities in mice (Hook *et al.* 1974).

All the above experiments have been done *in vivo*, and involve maternal dietary deprivation of the substance under study for some time, to ensure depletion of maternal body reserves. Often it is difficult to strike a balance between providing sufficient for the mother to survive, while still ensuring a suitable lack for the experiment. Such problems can be obviated by conducting the experiments on embryos cultured *in vitro*. This method has a number of other advantages. It means that the environment in which the embryos are developing can be more easily and accurately controlled, and also that the effect of a substance directly on the embryo can be studied, rather than, as *in vivo*, after passage through the mother. Cockcroft (1979) has cultured rat embryos *in vitro* from the head fold stage until the formation of the 26th somite, that is, through the whole phase of neural tube formation, and systematically removed, one by one, eight individual nutrients from the culture medium. He observed virtually normal development, and no abnormalities, in the absence of nicotinic acid, vitamin B_6, vitamin B_1 and choline. A lack of folic acid led to a slight, but not significant, decrease in growth rate, but no abnormalities. Deficiency of pantothenic acid led to growth retardation and generalized dysmorphism. However, it was only a lack of inositol which resulted in NTD, in 38% of the embryos.

Thus, the case for a deficiency of a vitamin, or vitamins, as a cause of NTD is not strongly borne out from experiments on animals. *In vivo*, a lack of only four individual vitamins results in NTD amongst other abnormalities, but none produce NTD as an isolated anomaly. *In vitro*, it is only a lack of inositol, hardly even regarded as a vitamin, which results in NTD.

Evidence from human studies that a vitamin deficiency could be a cause of NTD

Smithells *et al.* (1976) measured the levels of certain blood vitamins in the first trimester of pregnancy in an unselected group of over 900 women. Two main facts emerged. Firstly, social classes III, IV and V had significantly lower levels of red blood cell folate, white cell vitamin C, red cell riboflavin and serum vitamin A, and slightly lower serum folate levels, than classes I and II. This relates well to the previous observation by these workers that the lower classes consumed fewer nutrients and that they were nutritionally deprived. Secondly, the six women who were carrying fetuses with NTD had significantly lower red blood cell folate and white blood cell vitamin C levels, and also lower riboflavin and serum folate levels, than women whose fetuses were normal. Mothers of fetuses with congenital heart defects had normal levels of these vitamins. Subsequently, Schorah *et al.* (1980) found decreased vitamin B_{12} levels in first-trimester blood of mothers of anencephalics.

Leck *et al.* (1983) have also performed a prospective dietary and blood vitamin study on pregnant women. They found that three of the four women who had malformed offspring, two of which had NTD, had markedly low serum and red cell folates in early pregnancy. They too found a social class effect, with classes III, IV and V having lower levels of serum vitamin A and folate and red cell folate than the two higher classes.

Smithells *et al.* (1976) proposed that a deficiency of one or more vitamins might be one of the causes of NTD, and organized a clinical trial in which women were supplemented with multivitamins in the periconceptional period. This intervention study was performed in women who were at an above-average risk of having children with NTD by virtue of the fact that they had previously had affected children. The recurrence rate of NTD is around 3–5%. Such women, when planning another pregnancy, were asked to take the vitamins for at least 28 days prior to conception and for the first 8 weeks of that subsequent pregnancy. Pregnative Forte F (Bencard) was used — a multivitamin, iron and folic acid preparation involving physiological doses, not megadoses.

The first cohort of women so treated had a significantly lower recurrence of NTD (0·6%) than contemporaneous untreated women (5·0%) (Smithells *et al.* 1980). This result was repeated in a second cohort, in which the recurrence was 0·9% compared with 5·1% in untreated women (Smithells *et al.* 1983a). Another group (Holmes-Siedle 1983), using the same regime, independently produced similar promising results. Various other workers within the UK, convinced of the benefits, started supplementing their own patients, and the recent cumulated total of all known fully supplemented patients (1080) showed that the recurrence for NTD has remained below 1% (0·92%) (Seller 1985).

On the face of it, NTD do seem to have been prevented, so this work would seem to suggest that at least one of the environmental causes of NTD could well be a subclinical vitamin deficiency in some form, which can be made good by maternal supplementation.

However, the results have been criticized on several counts, the underlying fact being the non-randomized nature of the control group, which it is felt might have led to possible bias. The study was designed as a double-blind controlled trial, and the placebo and vitamin tablets, appropriately coded, were already in the two centres involved at the outset of the trial. However, both hospital research ethical committees independently rejected that protocol, advising that the vitamins should not be withheld from any woman. So, the design had to be changed, and the study was finally run in the following way. All women with a previous NTD child known to the organizing centre were informed of the trial by letter, and invited to participate. All those who accepted were given vitamin supplementation. When each of these reported back that she was pregnant, which was around the 8th–10th week of gestation, a control for her was selected from the clinic amniocentesis register. They were matched firstly for NTD risk, and then, as far as possible, for date of conception, and locality of residence. When selected, the controls had not yet had any prenatal testing, so there was no possibility of choosing those more likely to be carrying an NTD baby. It was hoped that they were similar to the supplemented group. They had not had the opportunity of entering the study, simply because they were not known to the clinic until they requested an amniocentesis. This experimental design is obviously far less satisfactory than the original one, but it was the best that could be worked out under the circumstances.

The critics claim that bias has been introduced into the results, firstly because, in the event, the unsupplemented group contained more women from a high-risk area (Stone 1980) and from a lower social class than the supplemented group (Wald & Polani 1984). Secondly, Oakley *et al.* (1983) pointed out that, during the course of the study, the birth prevalence of NTD, and therefore probably the recurrence risk, was declining, so that, if the results were compared with what they believed was the true recurrence risk, they would not be significant. Thirdly, the supplemented women were self-selected whilst the controls were not, so that the former were self-motivated and self-disciplined, and thus more likely *per se* to have a better outcome of pregnancy (Lancet Editorial 1980).

The work has been defended both independently (James 1981; Renwick 1982) and by the investigators themselves. Whilst acknowledging certain shortcomings, they have answered the criticisms directly (Smithells *et al.* 1983b, 1985), and also more indirectly, by making a statistical analysis of the data in their first two studies, assessing the influence of various risk factors (the number of previous NTD, area of residence, immediately prior pregnancy and pregnancy interval) on the observed recurrence rate of NTD. None of the risk factors contributed any significant differential risk between the supplemented and un-supplemented women (Wild *et al.* 1986). It is true to say, however, that the issue will never be resolved until the results of a properly conducted trial are known. Two such are presently under way.

As yet, there are no other studies with multivitamins published in connection with NTD, but in the United States, where consumption of vitamins is a widespread general phenomenon, Mulinare *et al.* (1981) have compared the preconceptional and/or first-trimester vitamin exposure between women who had NTD offspring and those who had children with other abnormalities. There was a statistically significant protective effect against NTD for vitamin usage in white, but not black, women, and a most pronounced protective effect in white women of the lower classes.

Vitamin supplementation had actually been attempted earlier for another congenital abnormality. Conway (1958), Douglas (1958), Peer *et al.* (1964) and Briggs (1976) all reported that vitamin and folate supplementation in the first trimester reduced the recurrence of cleft lip with or without cleft palate. The numbers involved were small, consequently none reached a level of statistical significance, but all the studies showed the same beneficial trend. Intriguingly, Peer *et al.* (1964) based their work on, amongst other things, the observations of Strauss (1914) that jaguars in a zoo were born with cleft palate until the maternal diet was changed to include fresh meat, and the fact that 99% of the lion cubs at Regent's Park Zoo had cleft palates until maternal dietary improvement was effected (Pickerill 1914; Veevers in Peer *et al.* 1964).

More recently, Tolarova (1982) has performed vitamin supplementation studies in women at risk for children with cleft lip. The recurrence was 1·2%, compared with 7·4% in the controls. Thus, these lines of evidence suggest that cleft lip and/or cleft palate could possibly be prevented by multivitamin treatment, hinting at a relatively non-specific effect of such therapy. However, in the NTD vitamin study (Smithells *et al.* 1980, 1983b; Seller 1985), cleft lip and palate have figured amongst the 32 malformations other than NTD encountered in the 1080 children whose mothers were fully supplemented (Seller 1985). Further, omphalocoele and congenital heart defects have also occurred in this group of children. All these abnormalities, including NTD, are regarded as forming part of a related group of schisis defects which involve faulty midline closure (Czeizel 1981). The fact that NTD alone among them seem to be markedly altered in the Smithells study led Seller (1987) to suggest that this could be an indication of some degree of specificity of the vitamin therapy for NTD. Another line of evidence indicating that NTD is different from other midline defects is that in the blood vitamin study of Smithells *et al.* (1976) mentioned previously, on which the intervention study was based, low maternal vitamin levels were associated only with NTD pregnancies and not with those where the babies had congenital heart defects. Also, over the last decade, in England and Wales, the birth prevalence of NTD has declined markedly while that of other congenital malformations has remained stable (OPCS 1986).

Pregnavite Forte F, the multivitamin preparation used in the supplementation study, has 11 major components, and it is not known whether all, several or only one of them is the effective ingredient. If it were to be just one, the most favoured candidate is folic acid, for it has long been a prime suspect in connection with NTD.

Evidence from humans that folate deficiency is the cause of NTD

The most oft quoted piece of evidence that folate deficiency is the cause of human NTD is the abortifacient, aminopterin. This is a folic acid antagonist, and it is said to produce NTD. There is no doubt that this drug is highly toxic to the embryo; intrauterine death is the usual result, and surviving embryos are often severely malformed. Among a variety of congenital defects, there are actually only two NTD reported (Thiersch 1952, 1960), but of all the cases of maternal treatment documented in the literature (Thiersch 1952, 1960; Warkany 1960; Shaw & Steinbach 1968; review by Milunsky *et al.* 1968) only one patient received the aminopterin early enough in pregnancy to influence the formation of the neural tube. She was treated on days 17, 18 and 19 after conception and she did indeed deliver a female anencephalic (Thiersch 1960). All other patients were treated around, or after, day 50. The second NTD, said to be a meningoencephalocoele with facial anomalies (Thiersch 1952) is shown in a photograph in a later paper (Thiersch 1960) and quite clearly appears to be a case of cervical cystic hygromata rather than NTD. The mother received the aminopterin when the embryo was aged 49−50 days.

Other lines of evidence implicating folic acid deficiency as a cause of NTD include the observation of Hibbard & Smithells (1965) that folate deficiency at the end of pregnancy, as measured by a positive formiminoglutamic acid excretion test, occurred in 65% of mothers of malformed infants, and 69% of those with CNS abnormalities, but only 17% of mothers of normal infants. In the later blood vitamin study of Smithells *et al.* (1976) mentioned previously, there were lower than normal first-trimester RBC and serum folate levels in women carrying NTD fetuses. In contradistinction, however, Scott *et al.* (1970) found no difference in serum folate levels at delivery between women who had given birth to a congenitally abnormal baby and those whose baby was normal. Hall (1972), in a prospective study, similarly could find no difference at the time of booking between the two groups. Two other studies found normal serum folate levels in mothers of NTD offspring (Emery *et al.* 1969; Molloy *et al.* 1985). The discrepancy could be explained by the fact that, in all these, serum rather than red cell folate was measured. The latter is regarded as being a more reliable indicator of folate status.

Drugs which interfere with folate metabolism, such as those used in the treatment of epilepsy, are associated with an increased incidence of congenital malformations, including NTD (Speidal & Meadow 1972). Three women who had had gastric bypass operations, a procedure which is known to result in both folate and vitamin B_{12} deficiency, produced NTD offspring (Haddow *et al.* 1986). On the other hand, NTD do not seem to occur more often in women with severe megaloblastic anaemia, where there is always a folate deficiency. Fraser & Watt (1964) found a high proportion of the children of such women had serious birth defects, although not NTD, while several other studies failed to find a marked increase in any defect (Giles 1966; Varadi *et al.* 1966; Pritchard *et al.* 1970). Schorah (1983) has suggested that folate deficiency alone may not produce NTD in the absence of other, as yet undefined, factors. These could be either genetic or dietary anomalies.

Laurence and his colleagues (1981) mounted an intervention study in women at risk for NTD, using folate alone. As in the Pregnavite trial, women were supplemented periconceptionally, but, unlike that study, this work was performed as a randomized controlled trial, with untreated women receiving placebos. There was a lower recurrence of NTD in the supplemented women (two out of 60) compared with the placebo group (four out of 51), but this was not statistically significant. It is possible that at least one of the two recurrences in the folate group occurred in a woman who, in fact, had not taken her tablets.

Folate deficiency in animals

Folate deficiency can be produced in rats, either chronically, by dietary deprivation coupled with an inhibitor to suppress intestinal synthesis, or acutely, with a folate antagonist such as aminopterin. It should be noted that these are 'artificial' rather than 'natural' methods, and the agents used may have effects other than simply depriving the animals of folate. Both chronic and acute deprivation result in a high incidence, and a whole range, of congenital defects. Exencephaly occurs, but does not figure especially prominently. In chronic deficiency, the abnormalities occur long before there are any detrimental signs in the mother (Nelson 1960). Acute deficiency on days 7 and 8 of gestation results in exencephaly. It is observed to produce arrest in embryonic development especially in the cranial region, and to reduce the mitotic rate in the cells of the neural tube (Johnson *et al.* 1963). Folate deficiency is also associated with an effect on some of the enzymes of the yolk sac. The appearance of some of the isozymes of glucose-6-phosphate dehydrogenase and alkaline phosphatase is delayed (Johnson & Spinuzzi 1968), whilst other transient isozymes persist longer than usual. Further, the effect is specific, for other enzymes remain completely unaffected (Johnson & Spinuzzi 1966).

It is known that folic acid plays a key role in several cellular metabolic processes, as well as in cell proliferation. It is therefore recognized that embryonic requirements for folate will be high, and it has always been assumed that any lack, even a minor deficiency, will be extremely detrimental. The observations on the effects of folate deficiency on the rat embryos and certain enzymes of the yolk sac suggest that the ramifications of folate deficiency could be more manifold, not only having a direct effect on the cells of the embryo, especially of the neural tube, but also impairing enzyme systems in the organ of early embryonic nutrition.

A folate intervention study, similar to that of Laurence *et al.* (1981) in man, has been performed by Moffa & White (1983) in a strain of hamsters genetically predisposed to NTD. The report is brief, but it appears that periconceptional supplementation with folic acid reduces the number of NTD in the offspring, while a folate-deficient diet increases the number of NTD. On the other hand, Graham & Ferm (1985) found that maternal folate treatment in other hamsters did not protect against heat-induced NTD. This may again indicate that different mechanisms can produce NTD, although altered folate metabolism has been observed in hyperthermic patients (Osifo *et al.* 1981).

Animal models of NTD

There are a number of other models of human NTD. The curly-tail mouse is one, and has been used particularly to study the extent to which maternally administered exogenous agents will influence the embryogenesis of NTD. Homozygous mice for the recessive curly-tail gene show a penetrance of around 60%. Roughly 10−20% of the mice have spina bifida cystica, 40−50% a curly tail and 1% exencephaly (Grüneberg 1954; Embury *et al.* 1979). The lesions at the caudal end of the neural tube are directly related to delayed closure of the posterior neuropore (Grüneberg 1954; Copp *et al.* 1982; Copp 1985). Unlike experimentally induced NTD in rodents using teratogens, where, as previously mentioned, other defects are usually produced as well, the NTD of curly-tail mice are an isolated defect. In this respect, therefore, they resemble the majority of human NTD. This, and other features, such as the fact that the NTD occur more commonly in females than males, makes them a good model for human NTD.

The incidence of NTD in the curly-tail mice can be manipulated with relative ease by administration of various substances to the mother during early pregnancy, indicating interaction of environmental factors with the genetic predisposition. This is the principle proposed in the aetiology of human NTD. The incidence in the mice may be either increased or decreased according to the time of treatment in embryogenesis (Seller *et al.* 1979). Primary prevention has been especially investigated. Although a number of agents achieve this, there is some specificity. Vitamin A alone amongst the vitamins is effective (Seller *et al.* 1979 and unpublished data). Folic acid neither increases nor decreases the NTD (Seller & Adinolfi 1981 and unpublished data). Most effective at preventing the NTD are inhibitors of DNA synthesis — hydroxyurea (Seller & Perkins 1983), mitomycin C (Seller & Perkins 1986), 5-fluorouracil (Seller 1983) and cytosine arabinoside (unpublished). By contrast, cycloheximide and triamcinolone, inhibitors of protein and RNA synthesis respectively, have no effect (Seller 1983). These findings led me (Seller 1983) to hypothesize some form of subtle metabolic block, possibly in DNA synthesis, as the underlying cause of the NTD of the mice. Copp has recently (1987), however, found a reduction in extracellular hyaluronate restricted to the caudal neuropore region, and localized it even further to the basement membranes around the noto-chord, overlying the dorsal surface of the hind-gut and underlying the neuroepithelium. From this observation he suggests there is a primary defect of hyaluronate synthesis in these sites which is directly associated with the development of posterior NTD in curly-tail mice.

In another mouse mutant, Splotch, delayed closure of the posterior neuropore has also been shown to be associated with the development of spina bifida (Dempsey & Trasler 1983; Kapron-Bras & Trasler 1984), and maternally administered vitamin A has the same effect on incidence, including the protective effect, as in the curly-tail mice (Kapron-Bras & Trasler 1985).

It would seem therefore, from experiments in the hamster and two different mouse models of NTD, that primary prevention of a large proportion of NTD by maternal therapy is practically possible. So, in principle, it is perfectly possible in man too.

Summary and conclusion

NTD are probably associated with the greatest volume of literature of all the congenital defects afflicting man, and any review could not possibly be comprehensive. What has been attempted in this chapter is, in the light of a report that maternal supplementation with multivitamins seems to have prevented some human NTD, to examine whether this could be supported by evidence from other collateral studies. Inevitably such an examination will be biased to some extent, especially with respect to what the author thinks is important evidence.

It was first felt important to consider the NTD themselves, and the fact that 80% or more of those under consideration are a localized, and the sole, lesion in an otherwise normal body. Teratological experiments in animals show that rarely is such a situation produced in response to an environmental teratogen, even if the exposure is brief and transitory as a single pulse. Instead, defects in more than one body system are produced. Generalized nutritional deficiencies in animals tend to produce pregnancy wastage rather than congenital malformations. In humans, similarly, there is no compelling evidence that NTD are associated with times of deprivation. Deficiencies of a restricted number of specific individual vitamins do produce NTD in animals, but again the findings are that the NTD is not the sole defect, but simply one of several which arise. In man, there is only circumstantial evidence of a connection between vitamin deficiency and NTD. It is actually of much the same order as certain other possible environmental influences, such as hyperthermia and zinc deficiency, which have not been discussed here.

Logically, since many vitamins and folic acid are key factors in cell metabolism and proliferation, a good theoretical case can be made for a deficiency of one or several being detrimental to the developing embryo. However, it is harder to explain how such a situation could produce such a specific defect, localized (usually) to one part of one organ. Surely, a generalized lack of a substance affecting generalized biochemical reactions should produce generalized defects. Some time ago, I suggested (Seller 1983) that the cause of the NTD of the curly-tail mice, and, by extrapolation, in humans also, might be a local metabolic block in the embryo. Copp (1987) now has positive evidence in the curly-tail mouse that its true nature could be a local defect of hyaluronate synthesis. A similar local biochemical defect within the embryo producing the NTD of man would be an explanation which accords well with the observations of a morphologically local defect. It would not rule out vitamins or folic acid being involved for they are vital to many biosynthetic processes, but the error would be located in the embryo rather than the mother.

Whatever the circumstantial evidence, it does seem that periconceptional vitamin therapy has effected primary prevention of some NTD in man. However, it has not prevented all recurrences of NTD. In the animal models too, where primary prevention has been achieved, NTD are never totally eliminated. Seller & Nevin (1984) showed that, in man, vitamin treatment has a better effect in Northern Ireland, an area of high birth prevalence, than in south-east England, which has a lower birth prevalence. This is consistent with the possibility implicit in the theory of multifactorial inheritance that the NTD of the former type of area have a greater environmental component than the latter and so are more easily influenced by environmental manipulation. The declining prevalence of NTD observed in the UK over the last ten years (OPCS 1986) is attributed by some to an improved diet of the population as a whole. If this is so, then in the forthcoming years the residual NTD will be those more genetic in origin and thus less likely to be prevented by vitamin therapy. It is possible, therefore, that there will be an apparent decline in effectiveness of the treatment. However, this does not diminish the probability that vitamin therapy helps those NTD which have a strong environmental component. As a matter of future policy, the most judicious use of such treatment might be to restrict it to areas of highest risk.

References

Al-Awadi S.A., Farag T.I., Teebi A.S. & Naguie K.K. (1984) Anencephaly: disappearing in Kuwait? *Lancet*, **ii**, 701−2.

Beaudoin A.R. (1973) Teratogenic activity of 2-amino-1, 3, 4-thiadiazole hydrochloride in Wistar rats and the protection afforded by nicotinamide. *Teratology*, **7**, 65−71.

Beck F. & Lowy A. (1982) The effect of cathepsin inhibitor on rat embryos grown *in vitro*. *J. Embryol. Exp. Morphol.*, **71**, 1−9.

Beck F., Moffat D.B. & Davies D.P. (1985) *Human Embryology*. Blackwell Scientific Publications, Oxford.

Berg B.N. (1956) Dietary restriction and reproduction in the rat. *J. Nutr.*, **87**, 344−8.

Briggs R.M. (1976) Vitamin supplementation as a possible factor in the incidence of cleft lip/palate deformities in humans. *Clin. Plast. Surg.*, **3**, 647−52.

Carter C.O. (1974) Clues to the aetiology of neural tube malformations. *Dev. Med. Child Neurol.*, **16**, Supplement 32, 3−15.

Chamberlain J.G. & Nelson M.M. (1963) Congenital abnormalities in the rat resulting from single injections of 6-aminonicotinamide during pregnancy. *J. Exp. Zool.*, **153**, 285−99.

Cheng D.W., Bairnson T.A., Rao A.N. & Subbammal S. (1960) Effect of variations of rations on the incidence of teratogen in vitamin E deficient rats. *J. Nutr.*, **71**, 54−60.

Cockcroft D.L. (1979) Nutrient requirements of rat embryos undergoing organogenesis *in vitro*. *J. Reprod. Fertil.*, **57**, 505−10.

Coffey V.P. & Jessop W.J.E. (1958) A three year study of anencephaly in Dublin. *Ir. J. Med. Sci.*, **393**, 391−413.

Conway H. (1958) Effect of supplemental vitamin therapy on the limitation of incidence of cleft lip and cleft palate in humans. *Plast. Reconstr. Surg.*, **22**, 450−3.

Copp A.J. (1985) Relationship between timing of posterior neuropore closure and development of spinal neural tube defects in mutant (curly-tail) and normal mouse embryos in culture. *J. Embryol. Exp. Morphol.*, **88**, 39−54.

Copp A.J. (1987) Report. *New Scientist*, **1542**, 34.

Copp A.J., Seller M.J. & Polani P.E. (1982) Neural tube development in mutant (curly-tail) and normal mouse embryos: the timing of posterior neuropore closure *in vivo* and *in vitro*. *J. Embryol. Exp. Morphol.*, **69**, 151−67.

Cornell J., Nelson M.M. & Beighton P. (1983) Neural tube defects in the Cape Town Area, 1975−1980. *S. Afr. Med. J.*, **64**, 83−4.

Czeizel A. (1981) Schisis association. *Am. J. Med. Genet.*, **10**, 25−35.

Davies J.A. (1980) Multivitamin prophylaxis against neural tube defects. *Lancet*, **i**, 1302.

Davis S.D., Nelson T. & Shepard T.H. (1970) Teratogenicity of vitamin B_6 deficiency: omphalocoele, skeletal and neural defects and splenic hypoplasia. *Science*, **169**, 1329−30.

Dempsey E.E. & Trasler D.G. (1983) Early morphological abnormalities in Splotch mouse embryos and predisposition to gene- and retinoic acid-induced neural tube defects. *Teratology*, **28**, 461−72.

Deren J.J., Padykula H.A. & Wilson T.H. (1966) Development of structure and function in the mammalian yolk sac. II Vitamin B_{12} uptake by rabbit yolk sacs. *Dev. Biol.*, **13**, 349−69.

Dickerson J.W.T. & Hughes P.C.R. (1972) Growth of the rat skeleton after severe nutritional intrauterine and postnatal retardation. *Resuscitation*, **1**, 163−70.

Douglas B. (1958) The role of environmental factors in the etiology of 'so-called' congenital malformations. II Approaches in humans; study of various extragenital factors; 'theory of compensatory nutrients'; development of regime for first trimester. *Plast. Reconstr. Surg.*, **22**, 214–29.

Embury S., Seller M.J., Adinolfi M. & Polani P.E. (1979) Neural tube defects in curly-tail mice. I Incidence, expression and similarity to the human condition. *Proc. R. Soc. Lond. [Biol.]*, **206**, 85–94.

Emery A.E.H., Timson J. & Watson-Williams E.J. (1969) Pathogenesis of spina bifida. *Lancet*, **ii**, 909–10.

Fedrick J. (1974) Anencephalus and maternal tea drinking: evidence for a possible association. *Proc. R. Soc. Med.*, **67**, 356–60.

Fraser J.L. & Watt H.J. (1964) Megaloblastic anaemia in pregnancy and the puerperium. *Am. J. Obstet. Gynecol.*, **89**, 532–4.

Gardner W.J. (1973) *The Dysraphic States.* Excerpta Medica, Amsterdam.

Giles C. (1966) An account of 335 cases of megaloblastic anaemia of pregnancy and the puerperium. *J. Clin. Pathol.*, **19**, 1–11.

Giroud A., Démas A., Prost H. & Lefebvres J. (1957) Malformations encéphaliques par carence en acide pantothénique et leur interprétation. *Acta Anat.*, **29**, 209–27.

Graham J.M. & Ferm V.H. (1985) Heat and alcohol-induced neural tube defects: interactions with folate in a Golden Hamster model. *Paediatr. Res.*, **19**, 247–51.

Grüneberg H. (1954) Genetical studies on the skeleton of the mouse. VIII Curly-tail. *J. Genet.*, **52**, 52–67.

Haddow J.E., Hill L.E., Kloza E.M. & Thanhauser D. (1986) Neural tube defects after gastric bypass. *Lancet*, **i**, 1330.

Hale F. (1933) Pigs born without eyeballs. *J. Hered.*, **24**, 105–6.

Hall M.H. (1972) Folic acid deficiency and congenital malformation. *J. Obstet. Gynaecol.*, **79**, 159–61.

Hamilton W.J., Boyd J.D. & Mossman H.W. (1976) *Human Embryology.* Macmillan, London.

Hibbard E.D. & Smithells R.W. (1965) Folic acid metabolism and human embryopathy. *Lancet*, **i**, 1254.

Holmes-Siedle M. (1983) Vitamin supplementation and neural tube defects. *Lancet*, **ii**, 41.

Hook E.B., Healy K.M., Niles A.M. & Skalko R.G. (1974) Vitamin E: a teratogen or antiteratogen? *Lancet*, **i**, 809.

Jacobson W. & Lutwak-Mann C. (1956) The vitamin B_{12} content of the early rabbit embryo. *J. Endocrinol.*, **14**, 19–20.

James W.H. (1981) Recurrence rates for neural tube defects and vitamin supplementation. *J. Med. Genet.*, **18**, 249–51.

Johnson E.M. & Spinuzzi R. (1966) Enzymic differentiation of rat yolk-sac placenta as affected by a teratogenic agent. *J. Embryol. Exp. Morphol.*, **16**, 271–88.

Johnson E.M. & Spinuzzi R. (1968) Differentiation of alkaline phosphate and glucose-6-phosphate dehydrogenase in rat yolk-sac. *J. Embryol. Exp. Morphol.*, **19**, 137–43.

Johnson E.M., Nelson M.M. & Monie I.W. (1963) Effects of transitory pteroylglutamic acid (PGA) deficiency on embryonic and placental development in the rat. *Anat. Rec.*, **146**, 215–24.

Kalter H. (1960) Teratogenic action of a hypocaloric diet and small doses of cortisone. *Proc. Soc. Exp. Biol. Med.*, **104**, 518–20.

Kalter H. & Warkany J. (1959) Experimental production of congenital malformations in mammals by metabolic procedures. *Physiol. Rev.*, **39**, 69–115.

Kapron-Bras C.M. & Trasler D.G. (1984) Gene teratogen interaction and its morphological basis in retinoic acid induced mouse spina bifida. *Teratology*, **30**, 143–50.

Kapron-Bras C.M. & Trasler D.G. (1985) Reduction in the frequency of neural tube defects in splotch mice by retinoic acid. *Teratology*, **32**, 87–92.

Khoury M.J., Erickson J.D. & James L.M. (1982) Etiologic heterogeneity of neural tube defects: clues from epidemiology. *Am. J. Epidemiol.*, **115**, 538–48.

Kirke P. (1983) Discussion. In *Prevention of Spina Bifida and Other Neural Tube Defects* (Ed. by J. Dobbing), pp. 117–18. Academic Press, London.

Knox E.C. (1972) Anencephalus and dietary intakes. *Br. J. Prev. Soc. Med.*, **26**, 219–23.

Lancet Editorial (1980) Vitamins, neural-tube defects and ethical committees. *Lancet*, **i**, 1061–2.

Laurence K.M. (1984) Causes of neural tube malformations and their prevention by dietary improvement and preconceptional supplementation with folic acid and multivitamins. In *Recent Vitamin Research* (Ed. by M.H. Briggs), pp. 177–201. CRC Press, Boca Raton, Florida.

Laurence K.M., James N., Miller M., Tennant G. & Campbell H. (1980) Increased risk of recurrence of neural tube defects to mothers on poor diets and the possible benefits of dietary counselling. *Br. Med. J.*, **281**, 1542–4.

Laurence K.M., James N., Miller M., Tennant G. & Campbell H. (1981) Double blind randomised controlled trial of folate treatment before conception to prevent recurrence of neural-tube defects. *Br. Med. J.*, **282**, 1509–11.

Leck I., Iles C.A., Sharman I.M., Toe T. & Wadsworth G.R. (1983) Maternal diet and nutrition during early pregnancy and after delivery in North London. In *Prevention of Spina Bifida and Other Neural Tube Defects* (Ed. by J. Dobbing), pp. 197–218. Academic Press, London.

Lemire R.J. (1969) Variations in development of the caudal neural tube in human embryos (horizons XIV–XXI). *Teratology*, **2**, 361–70.

Lemire R.J., Loeser J.D., Leech R.W. & Alvord E.C. (1975) *Normal and Abnormal Development of the Human Nervous System*, pp. 71–83. Harper, New York.

Millen J.W. & Woollam D.H.M. (1958) Vitamins and cerebrospinal fluid. In *Ciba Foundation Symposium on the Cerebrospinal Fluid* (Ed. by G.E.W. Wolstenholme & C.M. O'Conner), pp. 168–85. Little, Brown, Boston.

Miller T.J. (1972) Cleft palate formation: a role for pyridoxine in the closure of the secondary palate in mice. *Teratology*, **6**, 351–6.

Milunsky A., Graef J.W. & Gaynor M.F. (1968) Methotrexate-induced congenital malformations. *J. Pediatr.*, **72**, 790–5.

Moffa A.M. & White J.A. (1983) The effect of periconceptional supplementation of folic acid on the incidence of open neural tube defects in Golden Hamster embryos. *Teratology*, **27**, 64A.

Molloy A.M., Kirke P., Hillary I., Weir D.E. & Scott J.M. (1985) Maternal serum folate and vitamin B_{12} concentrations in pregnancies associated with neural tube defects. *Arch. Dis. Child.*, **60**, 660–5.

Morgagni J.B. (1769) *The Seats and Causes of Disease Investigated by Anatomy* (English translation: Benjamin Alexander). A. Miller and T. Cadell, London.

Mulinare J., Cordero J.F. & Erickson J.D. (1981) Vitamin use and the occurrence of neural tube defects (NTDs). *Teratology*, **23**, 54A.

Nelson M.N. (1960) Teratogenic effects of pteroylglutamic acid deficiency in the rat. In *Congenital Malformations. A Ciba Foundation Symposium* (Ed. by G.E.W. Wolstenholme & C.M. O'Conner), pp. 134–51. Churchill, London.

Oakley G.P., Adams M.J. & James L.M. (1983) Vitamins and neural tube defects. *Lancet*, **ii**, 798–9.

OPCS Monitor MB3 86/2 (1986). *Congenital Malformations 1985*. Office of Population Censuses and Surveys, Her Majesty's Stationery Office, London.

Osifo B.O.A., Lukanmbi F.A. & Familusi J.B. (1981) Increase in body temperature and folic acid metabolism. *Acta Vitaminol. Enzymol.*, **3**, 177–81.

Padykula H.A., Deren J.J. & Wilson T.H. (1966) Development of structure and function in the mammalian yolk sac. I Developmental morphology and vitamin B_{12} uptake of the rat yolk sac. *Dev. Biol.*, **13**, 311–48.

Peer L.A., Bernhard W.G. & Gordon H.W. (1964) Vitamin deficiency as a cause for birth deformities. *Academy of Medicine, New Jersey, Bulletin*, **10**, 140–4.

Pickerill H.P. (1914) The anatomy and physiology of cleft palate and a new method of treatment. *Transactions of the Sixth International Dental Congress, London,* 453–69.

Pritchard J.A., Scott D.E., Whalley P.J. & Haling R.F.P. (1970) Infants of mothers with megaloblastic anaemia due to folate deficiency. *JAMA,* **211**, 1982–4.

Renwick J.H. (1972) Hypothesis: anencephaly and spina bifida are usually preventable by avoidance of a specific but unidentified substance present in certain potato tubers. *Br. J. Prev. Soc. Med.,* **26**, 67–88.

Renwick J.H. (1982) Food and malformation. *The Practitioner,* **226**, 1947–53.

Richards I.D.G. (1969) Congenital malformations and environmental influences in pregnancy. *Br. J. Prev. Soc. Med.,* **23**, 218–25.

Roux, C., Fournier P., Dupuis Y. & Dupuis R. (1962) About teratogenic vitamin A deficiency. *Biol. Neonate,* **4**, 371–8.

Runner M.N. & Miller J.R. (1956) Congenital deformity in the mouse as a consequence of fasting. *Anat. Rec.,* **124**, 437–8.

Sadler T.W. (1985) *Langman's Medical Embryology,* 5th edn. Williams & Wilkins, Baltimore.

Saitoh M. & Takahashi S. (1973) Changes of embryonic wastage during pregnancy in rats fed low and high energy diets. *J. Nutr.,* **103**, 1652–7.

Schardein J.L. (1985) *Chemically Induced Birth Defects.* Marcel Dekker, New York & Basel.

Schorah C.J. (1983) Discussion. In *Prevention of Spina Bifida and Other Neural Tube Defects* (Ed. by J. Dobbing), p. 111. Academic Press, London.

Schorah C.J., Smithells R.W. & Scott J. (1980) Vitamin B_{12} and anencephaly. *Lancet,* **i**, 880.

Scott D.E., Whalley P.J. & Pritchard J.A. (1970) Maternal folate deficiency and pregnancy wastage. *Obstet. Gynecol.,* **36**, 26–8.

Seller M.J. (1983) The cause of neural tube defects: some experiments and a hypothesis. *J. Med. Genet.,* **20**, 164–8.

Seller M.J. (1985) Periconceptional vitamin supplementation to prevent recurrence of neural tube defects. *Lancet,* **i**, 1392–3.

Seller M.J. (1987) Nutritionally induced congenital defects. *Proc. Nutr. Soc.,* **46**, 227–35.

Seller M.J. & Adinolfi M. (1981) The curly-tail mouse: an experimental model for human neural tube defects. *Life Sci.,* **29**, 1607–15.

Seller M.J. & Kalousek D.K. (1986) Neural tube defects: heterogeneity and homogeneity. *Am J. Med. Gen.,* Supplement 2: The Developmental Field Concept, Part 2, 77–87.

Seller M.J. & Nevin N.C. (1984) Periconceptional vitamin supplementation and the prevention of neural tube defects in south-east England and Northern Ireland. *J. Med. Genet.,* **21**, 325–30.

Seller M.J. & Perkins K.J. (1983) Effect of hydroxyurea on neural tube defects in the curly-tail mouse. *J. Craniofac. Genet. Dev. Biol.,* **3**, 11–17.

Seller M.J. & Perkins K.J. (1986) Effect of mitomycin C on the neural tube defects of the curly-tail mouse. *Teratology,* **33**, 305–9.

Seller M.J., Embury S., Polani P.E. & Adinolfi M. (1979) Neural tube defects in curly-tail mice. II Effects of maternal administration of vitamin A. *Proc. R. Soc. Lond. [Biol.],* **206**, 95–107.

Shaw E.B. & Steinbach H.L. (1968) Aminopterin-induced fetal malformation: survival of infant after attempted abortion. *Am. J. Dis. Child.,* **115**, 477–82.

Smithells R.W., Sheppard S. & Schorah C.J. (1976) Vitamin deficiencies and neural tube defects. *Arch. Dis. Child.,* **51**, 944–50.

Smithells R.W., Ankers C., Carver M.E., Lennon D., Schorah C.J. & Sheppard S. (1977) Maternal nutrition in early pregnancy. *Br. J. Nutr.,* **38**, 497–506.

Smithells R.W., Sheppard S., Schorah C.J. et al. (1980) Possible prevention of neural tube defects by periconceptional vitamin supplementation. *Lancet,* **i**, 339–40.

Smithells R.W., Nevin N.C., Seller M.J. et al. (1983a) Further experience of vitamin supplementation for the prevention of neural tube defect recurrences. *Lancet,* **i**, 1027–31.

Smithells R.W., Seller M.J., Harris R. (1983b) Vitamins and neural tube defects. *Lancet*, **ii**, 799.

Smithells R.W., Sheppard S., Wild J. *et al.* (1985) Neural tube defects and vitamins: the need for a randomised clinical trial. *Br. J. Obstet. Gynaecol.*, **92**, 185–6.

Speidal B.D. & Meadow S.R. (1972) Maternal epilepsy and abnormalities of the fetus and newborn. *Lancet*, **ii**, 839.

Stein Z., Susser M., Saenger G. & Marolla F. (1975) *Famine and Human Development: the Dutch Hunger Winter of 1944/1945*. Oxford University Press, London.

Stone D.H. (1980) Possible prevention of neural tube defects by periconceptional vitamin supplementation. *Lancet*, **i**, 647.

Strauss O.A. (1914) The predisposing causes of cleft palate and harelip. *Transactions of the Sixth International Dental Congress, London*, 470–1.

Talwalkar V.C. (1981) Caution on preventing neural tube defects. *Lancet*, **ii**, 917–18.

Thiersch J.B. (1952) Therapeutic abortions with a folic acid antagonist. 4-aminopteroyl-glutamic acid (4-amino PGA) administered by the oral route. *Am. J. Obstet. Gynecol.*, **63**, 1298–304.

Thiersch J.B. (1960) Discussion. In *Congenital Malformations. A Ciba Foundation Symposium*, (Ed. by G.E.W. Wolstenholme & C.M. O'Conner), pp. 152–4. Churchill, London.

Tolarova M. (1982) Periconceptional supplementation with vitamins and folic acid to prevent recurrence of cleft lip. *Lancet*, **ii**, 217.

Varadi S., Abbot D. & Elwis A. (1966) Correlation of peripheral white cells and bone marrow changes with folate levels in pregnancy and their clinical significance. *J. Clin. Pathol.*, **19**, 33–6.

Wald N.J. & Polani P.E. (1984) Neural tube defects and vitamins: the need for a randomised clinical trial. *Br. J. Obstet. Gynaecol.*, **91**, 516–23.

Warkany J. (1951) Congenital anomalies. *Pediatrics*, **7**, 607–10.

Warkany J. (1960) Discussion. In *Congenital Malformations. A Ciba Foundation Symposium* (Ed. by G.E.W. Wolstenholme & C.M. O'Conner), p. 154. Churchill, London.

Warkany J. (1943) Effect of maternal rachitogenic diet on skeletal development of young rat. *Am. J. Dis. Child.*, **66**, 511–16.

Warkany J. & Schraffenberger E. (1943) Congenital malformations induced in rats by maternal nutritional deficiency. V Effects of purified diet lacking riboflavin. *Proc. Soc. Exp. Biol. Med.*, **54**, 92–4.

Wild J., Read A.P., Sheppard S. *et al.* (1986) Recurrent neural tube defects, risk factors and vitamins. *Arch. Dis. Child.*, **61**, 440–4.

Williams K.E., Roberts G., Kidston E.M., Beck F. & Lloyd J.B. (1976) Inhibition of pinocytosis in the rat yolk sac by trypan blue. *Teratology*, **14**, 343–54.

Woodard J.C. & Newberne P.M. (1966) Relation of vitamin B_{12} and one-carbon metabolism to hydrocephalus in the rat. *J. Nutr.*, **88**, 375–81.

Woollam D.H.M. & Millen J.W. (1960) The modification of the activity of certain agents exerting a deleterious effect on the development of the mammalian embryo. In *Congenital Malformations. A Ciba Foundation Symposium* (Ed. by G.E.W. Wolstenholme & C.M. O'Conner), pp. 158–72, Churchill, London.

2

Early Fetal Loss

I.R. McFADYEN

Early pregnancy loss has been documented with increasing accuracy in the past two decades. This has been made possible by the introduction of sensitive assays for chorionic gonadotrophin, by developing analyses of fetal and placental tissues, and by the use of ultrasound early in pregnancy. Until the early 1970s 10–20% of pregnancies were thought to abort spontaneously. Now it appears likely that 40–50% of conceptions do not reach 28 weeks. Some of these losses are due to ectopic implantations (generally thought to be around 0·8% but possibly more than this due to unrecognized ectopic pregnancies which present as lower abdominal pain close to the time of menstruation), or to hydatidiform moles. The majority, however, are spontaneous abortions. Many of these are not consciously recognized as pregnancies by the mother before they abort.

The advent of readily available ultrasound has illuminated the natural history of early pregnancy loss. While the number of spontaneous abortions at any time after the first missed period can be assessed reasonably accurately, the proportion of all conceptions which are alive at that time cannot be determined clinically. Maternal signs and symptoms are not an accurate guide, neither are most hormonal assays. Yet, to determine whether or not treatment is appropriate at that time, or to assess the efficacy of a treatment or the risks of any diagnostic intervention, it is necessary to know which pregnancies are then alive.

In this chapter the natural history of spontaneous abortion will be reviewed, as will associations with spontaneous abortion, and possible causes and mechanisms.

Natural history

Spontaneous abortion tends to be under-reported. There are a number of reasons for this. The mother may forget the event because she did not consider it to be important, or suppress its memory because it was so traumatic. Previous abortions may be concealed because they were pre-marital or procured. A very early pregnancy loss may present as a period delayed by only a few days and so not be recognized by the mother as a conception, particularly if she had no symptoms or normally has an irregular cycle. Prospective surveys are more accurate, especially if hor-monal methods are used to diagnose pregnancy, but follow-up may not be complete.

Examination of the available data suggests that 15% of fertilized ova do not implant and 27% abort spontaneously during the implantational and previllous stages in the second week (Hertig *et al.* 1959). Measure-ment of the β subunit of hCG in maternal blood has also revealed the extent of loss so early in pregnancy, frequently before the mother is aware that she has conceived. The results of several extensive investi-gations are, however, not in total agreement (Table 2.1). While the rate of abortion was found by the first three groups to be 11·8−13·7%, it was 23·5−24·9% in the final two investigations. Even more discrepant is the number of clinical pregnancies resulting from those diagnosed by the presence of βhCG: in these five investigations it ranged from 43% to 92%. While βhCG may be secreted by the non-pregnant pituitary (Suginami & Kawoi 1982) or unaccompanied by αhCG in some preg-nancies (Hay 1985), technical differences in measurement of the hor-mone or differences in age or other factors among the populations reviewed may also account for some of the variation in these results (Good *et al.* 1977; Sharp *et al.* 1986). There does not appear to be a consistent difference between those in whom the hormone levels were

Table 2.1. Some investigations into pregnancy loss

	βhCG in	Pregnancies		
		Biochemical only	Clinical	Aborted
Miller *et al.* 1980	urine	50	102	14
Edmonds *et al.* 1982	urine	67	51	6
Whittaker *et al.* 1983	blood	7	85	11
Australian IVF 1985	blood	43	188	50*
Wilcox *et al.* 1985	urine	4	17	4

* plus 13 ectopics

Although the proportion of clinical pregnancies which aborted is 12−25%, those concep-tions which were diagnosed from the presence of hCG alone show a wider range of loss, 8−57%. Some of the losses (particularly in women being treated for infertility) may have been unrecognized ectopic pregnancies but there is no single factor which accounts for the discrepant observations.

measured in blood or in urine, or whether the women investigated were being treated for infertility or had discontinued contraception because they wished to conceive. There is agreement, however, that not all conceptions develop into clinical pregnancies: the 57% loss found by Edmonds *et al.* (1982) is the only one higher than the 42% assessed from the data of Hertig *et al.* (1959), and the 33% of Miller *et al.* (1980) comes closest, while in the remainder it is 8−19%. Whatever the reasons for these differences there is no doubt that many fertilized ova are lost without the mother realizing that she has conceived.

Of the pregnancies which do progress beyond this stage 7−10% later abort, the majority in the first trimester at 9−10 weeks (Tietze *et al.* 1950; Stevenson *et al.* 1959; Berry 1980; Wilcox *et al.* 1981). Pregnancy loss in the second trimester is very much lower than in the first. Among 500 abacteriuric women it was 1·6% between 13 and 28 weeks (Kincaid-Smith & Bullen 1965); among 24 497 unselected pregnancies it was 1·28% (Stromme & Haywa 1963); and in a group of mothers awaiting counselling for amniocentesis it was 1·2% between 12 and 16 weeks (Golbus *et al.* 1979). Another 1519 scheduled for prenatal diagnosis had an abortion rate of 4% between 12 and 16 weeks, but if they were first seen at 6−7 weeks 20% had spontaneously aborted by 16 weeks (Lippman *et al.* 1984). In a group of controls for a study of amniocentesis the rate was 1% between 16 and 28 weeks (Sant-Cassia *et al.* 1984) (Fig. 2.1).

Many women who abort are aware that their symptoms of pregnancy have abated days or weeks before they abort. Thorough examination of the material recovered often confirms that the fetus had been dead for some time, being small and frequently macerated (Singh & Carr 1967; Brotherton & Craft 1972). The advent of ultrasound has helped to clarify the relationship between fetal death and abortion and several investigations have been reported. Although these were carried out on different populations in various countries, with both large and small numbers of subjects, their broad conclusions are similar. One from an English district general hospital surveyed 3091 women with apparently normal pregnancies who had an ultrasound examination at 7−12 weeks (McFadyen 1984, 1985; McFadyen & Brassil 1988). Forty of these were not pregnant: their next period might then have been considered an abortion and thus falsely an early pregnancy loss. Five pregnancies were terminated because of significant fetal anomaly and 11 for other reasons. Forty-nine were twin pregnancies and will be considered later. Twenty-one moved out of the district (6 before 16 weeks). Abortion occurred in 172

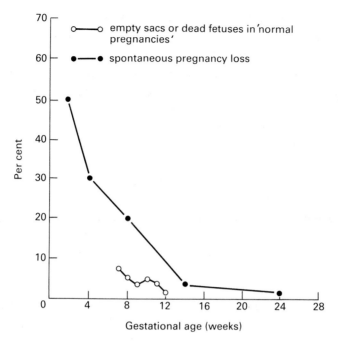

Fig. 2.1. Pregnancy losses decline from 50% before implantation to 1% at 16–28 weeks. The proportion of empty sacs and dead fetuses in pregnancies which are clinically normal also decreases with increasing gestational age.

(5·7%) of the 3042 singleton pregnancies: a lower rate than in some series, possibly because many abortions may have occurred before the mothers could book and because those who had threatened to abort were excluded. Those booking scans revealed that, although there had not been any clinical abnormality, 172 (5·7%) of the pregnancies were not viable: 98 (87·5%) had an empty gestation sac, and in 14 (12·5%) a fetus was present but was dead. Another 60 (2·11% of the live pregnancies) aborted spontaneously 1–18 weeks after the initial ultrasound: 5 of these followed amniocentesis. Both the non-viable pregnancies and the later abortions were related to gestational and maternal age. A dead fetus or an empty sac was found in 6·1% of those examined at 7 weeks, and this incidence fell week by week to 2·1% at 12 weeks, empty sacs being 5–8 times as frequent as dead fetuses. Later spontaneous abortion occurred in 6·1% of those seen at 7 weeks, falling to 1·1% at 12 weeks. The relationship with maternal age was not quite so regular. The minimum rate of later abortion was 0·7% and this occurred in 25-year-old mothers. It then rose regularly with increasing maternal age until it reached 9·6% in those of 40 or more. Non-viable pregnancies showed the same pattern: 2·7% at 25, rising to 15·4% at 40 or more. Younger than 20, however, also had an increased rate of non-viable pregnancies (4%) and of later abortion (1·3%). The spontaneous abortion rate in mothers who had live pregnancies at 9−12 weeks (the gestational age relevant to chorionic villus sampling) was 0·7% among mothers aged 24−26, 4% at 37−39 and 9·1% at 43 or more.

Other series of ultrasound examinations have been carried out in the United Kingdom, continental Europe and North America. Only one has been on a similar population of unselected mothers. In this, 2144 were examined during the first 10 weeks of pregnancy (Gilmore & McNay 1985): 8·3% had non-viable pregnancies at this time, and 2·04% of those with live fetuses subsequently aborted. Elsewhere 920 mothers were scanned at 7−12 weeks; 124 were lost to follow-up: 2·14% of the remaining 796 aborted by 20 weeks (Wilson *et al.* 1984). Another 274 scans were carried out before the end of the tenth week (Christiaens & Stoutenbeek 1984): 3·3% of these aborted before 16 weeks but this high rate may be explained by selection since the rate in the hospital population was 2·1% and those referred by general practitioners (presumably because of problems in the pregnancy) was 10·5%. Of 225 women scanned at 8 weeks and found to have a live normal fetus (Simpson 1984), 0.9% died at 8−12 weeks and 2·7% after 12 weeks. Among 42 women aged 39−45 a dead fetus was found in 9·52% at 7−11 weeks although a beating heart had been seen 6−11 days earlier (Gustavii 1984). In a group of 1068 women randomly selected who were scanned at 14 weeks or earlier and found to have a normal live fetus, 1·5% aborted before 16 weeks and 1·2% after this (Liu *et al.* 1987): of those who had threatened to abort before they were examined, 38% spontaneously aborted.

From these studies it appears that, among live fetuses found in pregnancies which have been normal until 7−12 weeks, the abortion rate is about 2·1%. The rate of non-viable pregnancies depends on the gestational age at which the scan is done, the reason for which the scan is requested, and the maternal age: it varies between 2% and 30%. The highest rate reported was in 190 women who were considered for termination of their pregnancies and scanned at 6−12 weeks (Lippman *et al.* 1984). The overall rate of non-viable pregnancy was 12·6%, but this fell from 30% at 6−7 weeks to 3·8% at 12 weeks. The reasons for requesting termination may well be relevant to this high rate and this suggests that further whole population studies are required.

Associations with spontaneous abortion

Fetal abnormality

Anatomical and chromosomal anomalies of the fetus are positively associated with abortion. Structural abnormalities are present in 10−70%
of these fetuses (Mikamo 1970), the wide range being due to differences
in the stage of pregnancy at which they are obtained. The earlier the
abortion the more likely is there to be major anomaly (Poland & Yven
1978). Among seven pre-implantation embryos found by chance at
hysterectomy, four were anatomically abnormal, and of 21 found at day
12−17 six were abnormal (Hcrtig *et al.* 1959). In one study of 2020
spontaneous abortions from which a fetus was recovered (Poland *et al.*
1981), 84% of those less than 30 mm were abnormal and 26% of those
30−180 mm. In another of 2620 abortions (Creasy & Alberman 1976)
there was no fetus or sac in 62%, but where a fetus was found 65%
were abnormal. The rate was much lower in 395 mid-trimester abortions,
being only 3% (Stromme & Haywa 1963). In another group of 47 who
were aborted in the middle trimester, however, the rate was 23% and
most studies incline to this higher figure (Wingate 1968). The abnormalities most likely to be found at any gestational age are those of the
central nervous system. Multiple anomalies are present in about 40% of
those with any major abnormality.

Chromosome anomalies are found in both anatomically normal and
abnormal fetuses, but more commonly in the latter (Poland *et al.* 1981);
and the earlier in pregnancy the loss occurs the more likely are there to
be chromosome anomalies. Among 23 pre-ovulatory oocytes obtained
from infertile women 14 had abnormal chromosomes (Wramsby *et al.*
1987). In fetuses of less than 30 mm which were anatomically abnormal,
chromosome anomalies were found in 67% whereas among the structurally normal the rate was 25%: in fetuses of 30−180 mm the chromosomes were anomalous in 22% of those anatomically abnormal but in
only 2% of the normal (Poland *et al.* 1981). The state of the chromosomes
can be assessed in many pregnancies even if no fetus is found since the
placental or membranous chromosome complement reflects that of the
fetus in almost all cases (Carr 1963), although occasionally there is an
abnormality in the placenta which is not present in the fetus (Markert &
Petters 1978). Where the fetus is absent but the sac is intact, the rate of
chromosome anomalies is 40−60%: if the fetus is present but only as
disorganized tissue the rate is at least as high (Thiede & Salm 1964;

Thiede & Metcalfe 1966; Singh & Carr 1967; Geisler & Kleinebrecht 1978; Kajii *et al.* 1980; Poland *et al.* 1981). Overall the rate of chromosome anomaly in spontaneously aborted material is 60–80% at 6 weeks or earlier, 50% at 8–11 weeks, 40% at 12–15 weeks, 20% at 16–19 weeks, and 5–10% later than this, which is the rate commonly found in perinatal deaths (Thiede & Metcalfe 1966; Machin 1974; Boue *et al.* 1975; Creasy *et al.* 1976; Warburton *et al.* 1980). In therapeutically terminated pregnancies it is 7.3% (Yamamoto *et al.* 1975).

The chromosome abnormalities found most frequently in spontaneous abortions are the trisomies. They account for 50% of the anomalies, 45 XO 19%, triploidy 16%, and tetraploidy 6% (Boue *et al.* 1975; Creasy *et al.* 1976; Geisler & Kleinebrecht 1978; Warburton *et al.* 1979; Hassold *et al.* 1980; Kajii *et al.* 1980). Most XO conceptions are aborted. It is likely that 40–50% of Down's fetuses also are lost, as are other autosomal trisomies (Polani 1969;.Creasy & Crolla 1974); Ferguson-Smith 1983) many of these losses occurring in the second trimester. The abortion rate of trisomy 21 singleton fetuses diagnosed by amniocentesis but for whom therapeutic termination was refused was 21%, but only 2·7% for those with a less abnormal genotype (Hook 1978): in trisomy 18 it may be as high as 70%. The mechanism for elimination of chromosome anomaly is efficient. So is that for the anatomically abnormal. Even in areas which have a high prevalence of anencephaly and other abnormalities of the central nervous system, these are found 10 times more frequently in abortions than later in pregnancy (MacHenry *et al.* 1979).

There are ethnic as well as geographical differences in the rate of anomalies found. Whites abort more growth-disorganized fetuses than North American Indians, but Orientals abort more than either (Poland *et al.* 1981). In Britain neural tube defects are most common in those of Celtic origin (Carter & Evans 1973) and in India they are more common in Sikhs (Verma 1978). Even within a limited geographical area with an ethnically amorphous population, however, there may be differences in the proportion of these fetuses which are aborted (Roberts & Lloyd 1973). Also, while intermarriage between close relatives may increase the rate of abnormal conceptions, it does not necessarily raise the abortion rate (Asha Bai *et al.* 1981). The stage of pregnancy at which abortions occur shows ethnic variation too. North American Indians and Negroes abort later than do Whites (Naylor 1967; Poland *et al.* 1981). Such comparisons between ethnic groups is complicated not only by differences in diet and social customs, but also by the availability of medical care or willingness to seek it, and by differences in the notification of abortions. For these and other reasons the causes of ethnic differences in abortion rates remain obscure.

Metabolic abnormalities may account for a number of abortions. They may be inherited or sporadic. No extensive study of affected families is available, and, because the possibilities also are extensive, knowledge about their sporadic appearance is likely to be slow to accumulate. It is probable that these disorders account for some abortions of undetermined origin.

Maternal age and gravidity

Fetal anomalies tend to increase with maternal age, but this is not absolute: a chromosome complement of 45 XO is most likely to be found in the fetuses of teenage mothers (Kajii & Ohama 1979; Warburton *et al.* 1980). It is generally true, however: 60% of abortions from 20-year-old mothers do not have chromosome anomalies, whereas in 40-year-olds this is true of only 15% (Leridon 1973). Trisomies due to non-disjunction increase with maternal age, but 45 XO is not due to non-disjunction, and XYY, autosomal or sex mosaics are not age-related because their non-disjunction occurs after fertilization (Ferguson-Smith 1983). It may be that it is not the age of the mother which is relevant but the number of years before her menopause (Brook *et al.* 1984), but whatever the reason the risk of chromosomal anomalies is least at 19–20, and is raised in both younger and older women (Fig. 2.2).

The rising risk of abortion with increasing age is due to more than ageing of the ova. As she gets older the mother is more likely to be hypertensive or have other medical problems predisposing to abortion. She is also more likely to have had other pregnancies. Age and gravidity may have a combined effect in increasing the abortion rate (Stevenson *et al.* 1959; Warburton & Fraser 1964; Naylor 1967) or age alone may be relevant (Kline *et al.* 1978; Resseguie 1974). Most investigators have found that the abortion rate is lowest in women aged 20–25 and raised both in the younger and older groups (Fig. 2.3). While the greatest rise is in those of 35 years or older, an early menarche also increases the risk (Liestol 1980; Casagrande *et al.* 1982). Generally the risk is least in second and third pregnancies but this is related to the outcome of the previous pregnancy or pregnancies: if they include one or more abortions the risk of any subsequent pregnancy aborting is increased (Naylor &

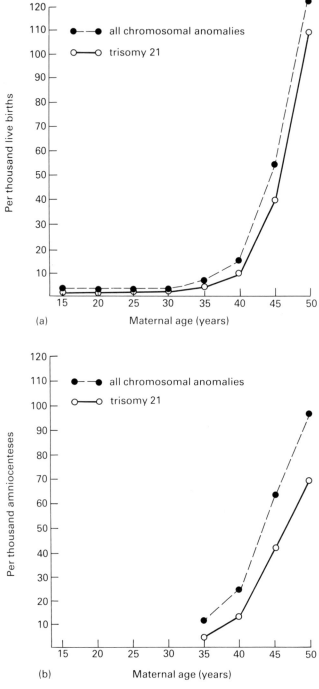

Fig. 2.2. Not only Down's but total chromosome anomalies increase with maternal age, particularly after 35 (a). Their incidence, however, depends on the gestational age at which they are found. Since 30% of Down's spontaneously abort or are stillborn (and possibly a greater proportion of other trisomies), the incidence at amniocentesis (b) is greater than in the live-born (after Hook 1978 and Ferguson-Smith 1983).

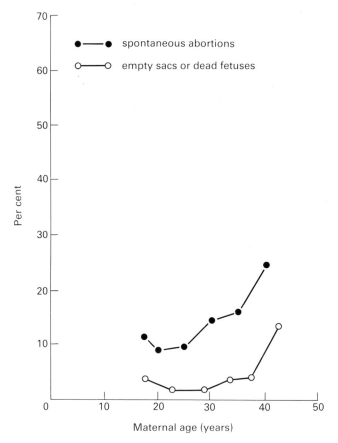

Fig. 2.3. The rates of spontaneous abortion, and of empty sacs and dead fetuses, are least in women aged 20−25. Younger women have higher rates but the highest are found in older age groups, particularly those of 40 or more.

Warburton 1979). The interval between pregnancies also is relevant: if it is less than 3−6 months abortion is more likely than with longer delays (Srisuphan & Bracken 1986).

Smoking

Maternal smoking increases the risk of spontaneous abortion and this is dose-related (Zabriskie 1963; Butler *et al.* 1972). The abortion rate in smokers is 1·7−2 times that of non-smokers (Kline *et al.* 1977b; Himmelberger *et al.* 1978). These are more likely to be mid-trimester (Kullander & Kallen 1971) and to be chromosomally normal (Boue *et al.* 1975; Warburton *et al.* 1979) than in non-smokers. Relevant associations with smoking are that the age of the menopause is reduced in both active (Baron 1984) and passive (Everson *et al.* 1986) smokers. Fetal health is reduced by passive smoking so this may increase the abortion rate directly or by altering the interval until the menopause. The association with smoking is not simple since this itself is related to social class, ethnicity, alcohol intake, and other factors which themselves may be related to abortion.

Caffeine

Caffeine intake and spontaneous abortion are related. Consumption of more than 150 mg of caffeine a day in tea, coffee, cola or medication is associated with an increase in abortion rate late in the first trimester or in the second trimester to almost double that of women who took no caffeine (Srisuphan & Bracken 1986). In another study 16 women consumed more than 600 mg caffeine daily: 8 of them aborted (Weathersbee *et al.* 1977). These mothers were studied in North America but the results are relevant elsewhere, especially where there is also a high consumption of chocolate. While the relationship may be cause and effect, it may in part be associated with the personality which requires caffeine stimulation or (like smoking) with the use of other drugs.

Alcohol and other drugs of addiction

Alcohol intake also increases the abortion rate (Harlap & Shiono 1980; Kline *et al.* 1980), particularly late abortion (Kullander & Kallen 1971; Harlap & Shiono 1980). It may well act directly on the ovum or on the fetus (Kline *et al.* 1977b), but it also interacts with the effects of social class, smoking and other drugs of addiction. Heroin and other 'harder' drugs are associated with chromosome and other anomalies. Their effects on pregnancy may, however, be related to how they are used: whether they are ingested, inhaled or injected. So complex are their interactions with other facets of life style that their precise place in the incidence of abortion cannot be defined.

Therapeutic drugs

The rate of spontaneous abortion is raised with many therapeutic drugs, but sometimes this may be due to the illness for which the therapy is given. Nevertheless there are possible direct effects. Antimetabolites, folic acid antagonists and similar drugs are teratogenic and do have a significant effect: among women treated with aminopterin the abortion rate is 70% (Wilson 1973). Treatment of the father may have a similar effect as these drugs may affect the spermatozoa.

Surgery during pregnancy may precipitate abortion, but it is difficult to separate the effects of the intervention from the indication for it. Pregnant anaesthetists or nurses working in theatre have a slightly increased risk, possibly due to the effect of nitrous oxide in their environment (Vessey & Nunn 1980): exposure of dental nurses to nitrous oxide doubles the risk (Cohen *et al.* 1979). Ethylene oxide in sterilizing departments has also been implicated as an environmental factor (Hemminki *et al.* 1982).

Oral contraceptive use does not increase the risk of abortion in conceptions which occur after they have been discontinued (Rothman 1977). Conception with an IUCD in the uterus does, however, considerably increase the probability of mid-trimester abortion (Foreman *et al.* 1981).

Maternal illness

It is possible that any acute illness may increase the risk of abortion because of the systemic upset or the treatment given. Many acute infections are well documented: some are less so. Rubella and mumps do increase the rate (Siegel *et al.* 1966), influenza probably does so (Naib *et al.* 1970). These viral illnesses caused by organisms which cross the placenta may be directly embryotoxic or produce their effects indirectly by the fetal anomalies which they create.

Chronic infection has long been implicated. Untreated syphilis is very likely to lead to mid-trimester abortion. So is untreated bacteriuria (Kincaid-Smith & Bullen 1965). *Chlamydia trachomatis,* mycoplasmas and other organisms commonly found in aborted material are probably incidental and not causative (Munday *et al.* 1984). It is also possible, however, that an infection is an index of the mother's immune status, which may determine whether or not she aborts.

Chronic non-infective disease is also relevant. While endometriosis has recently been shown not to be related to spontaneous abortion (Fitzsimmons *et al.* 1987), the traditional but sometimes questioned association with diabetes mellitus has been confirmed. Mild insulin-dependent diabetes is not associated with an increased rate of abortion but in severe cases this may rise to 40% (Miodovnik *et al.* 1984). Poor control before conception or early in pregnancy increases the risk (Miodovnik *et al.* 1985). Chronic nephritis is associated with an increase in abortion as is systemic lupus erythematosus some of whose victims have in their circulations the lupus anticoagulant. Despite its name this autoantibody promotes thrombosis, probably by inhibiting prostacyclin production and increasing thromboxane release from damaged platelets, and so increasing the probability of abortion (Lubbe & Liggins 1985). Of all the women with lupus anticoagulant only 40% have SLE: it is found in rheumatoid arthritis and other chronic diseases, but also in women who have no discoverable disease. If it is associated with recurrent abortions, the trend is for them to be progressively earlier. They can be prevented by treatment with prednisolone and aspirin.

Multiple pregnancy

Multiple pregnancies have a higher abortion rate than singleton. The loss may be of one or both fetuses, and it is likely that 30–50% of twin conceptions which are found on ultrasound examination will lose one or both fetuses (Robinson 1977; Livingston & Poland 1980). They may be aborted or die *in utero* and disappear (Kurjak & Latin 1979). Part of the explanation for this is likely to be that the rate of fetal anomalies in twins is more than twice the rate in singletons (Hendricks 1966).

Iatros

Iatrogenic abortion is a consequence of diagnostic intervention or of treatment. Amniocentesis in most centres carries an additional 0·5–1% risk of abortion (Simpson *et al.* 1976; Working Party 1978) and that of fetoscopy is about 5%. Chorionic villus sampling and cord needling have been introduced too recently for their risk to be precisely assessed.

Mechanisms and pathology

While the many associations with spontaneous abortion are well recognized and documented, the mechanisms which actually produce death of the fetus or its expulsion are not. Cervical incompetence may disturb the normal balance of intrauterine pressure, as could a septum in the uterus or a submucous fibroid. Congenital anomalies of the uterus are, however, also associated with vascular insufficiency in the organ (Burchell *et al.* 1978; Andrews & Jones 1982), which could lead to poor placentation. Intrauterine contraceptive devices predispose to intrauterine infection, but equally their presence could stimulate contractions or their mineral content could affect myometrial physiology.

Failure of physiological processes or pathological changes may be found in the maternal placental bed, in the placenta itself, or in the fetus. Many abortuses, however, do not contain a fetus, or it is present as a disorganized mass of tissue, both situations which are associated with chromosome anomalies (Poland *et al.* 1981). If one is present, the fetus is frequently smaller than expected for its gestational age. The slower growth of trisomic cells (Paton *et al.* 1974) would explain many of these, but XO cells divide more frequently than normal (Barlow 1972): possibly such anomalous behaviour disrupts the normal pattern of growth and leads to fetal death. Intracellular metabolic disorganization could also produce fetal death. Unless there was a history of metabolic disease this would not be suspected, and in many spontaneous abortions it would be a mutation without other evidence of its presence.

Such observations explain why fetal death so often precedes abortion but they do not reveal why the abortion occurs. Placental death may release hormonal inhibition of the myometrium, but the excretion of hCG and other placental proteins sometimes remain high up to the time of abortion. Persistently low or falling maternal levels of these hormones may be due to poor implantation, while normal levels might be due to maternal rejection of the pregnancy because the fetus is abnormal or for some other reason (Chartier *et al.* 1979; Schweditsch *et al.* 1979; Edmonds *et al.* 1982; Ahmed & Klopper 1984). The maternal levels of PAPP-A may, however, be low for weeks before an abortion while the fetus is alive (Westergaard *et al.* 1985). While many data are known, the deductions from them frequently remain hypothetical and other associations do not have even tenuous data to explain their mechanisms, but some pathological processes have been established.

Maternal adaptation to the pregnancy is not physiological in many who abort; normal trophoblastic invasion of the decidua and its arteries has not taken place even if the fetus is chromosomally normal (Khong *et al.* 1987). Abnormalities are found also in the placenta (Abaci & Aterman 1968; Honore *et al.* 1976; Rushton 1984). Hypoplastic or oedematous villi are associated with empty sacs or disorganized fetuses, and subchorionic haematoma is not uncommon. Normal fetuses, however, are not associated with abnormal villi. Those with lysosomal or other storage diseases may show typical changes in the placenta (Powell *et al.* 1976).

Immune mechanisms and their associations with spontaneous abortion are discussed in Chapter 3. It is relevant to mention here, however, that smoking may impair humoral responses to pregnancy (Rocklin *et al.* 1976), and the recent observation that it reduces the activity of killer cells (Hersey *et al.* 1983). An autoimmune disease associated with spontaneous abortion as well as other complications of pregnancy is systemic lupus erythematosus. While its mechanism may be the passage of maternal antibodies across the placenta (Smolen & Steinberg 1981) or the cross reaction of lymphocytotoxic antibodies with trophoblast (Bresnihan *et al.* 1979), the effect of lupus anticoagulant is also relevant: its association with thrombosis in placental bed vessels is well established (Abramowsky *et al.* 1980; De Wolf *et al.* 1982).

Recurrent abortion

Three or more spontaneous abortions in sequence occur in 0·4—0·8% of recognized pregnancies, which is more often than would be expected by chance (Stray-Pedersen & Lorentzen-Styr 1979). This suggests that in many cases there are persistent predisposing factors, so it is not surprising that after two consecutive abortions the risk of a third pregnancy aborting is 45—50% (Leridon 1973; Poland *et al.* 1977). If the mother has also delivered viable babies the risk is reduced to about 30% (Poland *et al.* 1977). It is, therefore, worth investigating couples who recurrently abort since some can be treated successfully and others may require early antenatal diagnosis. The larger the number of abortions in the sequence, the more likely is there to be a discoverable cause (Stray-Pedersen & Stray-Pedersen 1984).

Significant chromosome anomalies are found in 6—10% of couples who recurrently abort, but if, in addition, they have had a malformed infant the rate rises to 23% (Tho *et al.* 1979; Sant-Cassia & Cooke 1981; Davis *et al.* 1982). Also common in women who recurrently abort are abnormalities of the uterine body and cervix. They are found in 10—15% (Tho *et al.* 1979; Bottini *et al.* 1983; Stray-Pederson & Stray-Pedersen 1984). Anomalies of the body tend to be associated with first-trimester and cervical incompetence with second-trimester abortions but both may be present in the same uterus (Craig 1974). In those with a unicornuate uterus the abortion rate may be over 50% (Fedele *et al.* 1987).

While syphilis or malaria may contribute to recurrent abortions, the relevance of other organisms is still uncertain. It may vary in different geographical areas but as relevant is the anatomical area from which they are recovered. Many, such as *Ureaplasma urealyticum*, are normal inhabitants of the lower genital tract and so are likely to be found in much aborted material, but the finding of this and *Toxoplasma gondii* in endometrial biopsies from asymptomatic recurrent aborters suggests that they could be relevant (Stray-Pedersen & Stray-Pedersen 1984); however, it does not currently appear likely that many organisms are important aetiologically.

Endocrine dysfunction and other maternal disease have been implicated in spontaneous abortion but their relevance is difficult to assess since, among those that do not have an anatomical, chromosomal or other discoverable cause, the caring physician appears to be the best possible treatment, with a success rate of 80% (Stray-Pedersen & Stray-Pedersen 1984).

Where now?

Awareness that half or more of all conceptions may be lost is relevant to the treatment of infertility and to the assessment of risk or benefit which may be associated with diagnostic or therapeutic intervention. Recognition of factors related to spontaneous abortion does not necessarily explain their mode of action. Increased understanding of these mechanisms might lead to specific treatment in some cases. This is most likely to be true for recurrent aborters since the basic pathology is constant. Even now, this group repays intensive investigation since many are found to have lesions or problems for which there are remedies.

References

Abaci F. & Aterman K. (1968) Changes of the placenta and embryo in early spontaneous abortion. *Am. J. Obstet. Gynecol.*, **102**, 252–63.

Abramowsky C.R., Vegas M.E., Swinehart G. & Gyves M.T. (1980) Decidual vasculopathy of the placenta in lupus erythematosus. *New Engl. J. Med.*, **303**, 668–72.

Ahmed A.G. & Klopper A. (1984) Detection of subclinical abortion by assay of pregnancy specific $\beta 1$ glycoprotein. *Br. Med. J.*, **288**, 113.

Andrews M.C. & Jones H.W. (1982) Impaired reproductive performance of the unicornuate uterus: intrauterine growth retardation, infertility, and recurrent abortion in five cases. *Am. J. Obstet. Gynecol.*, **144**, 173–5.

Asha Bai P.V., John T.J. & Subramaniam V.R. (1981) Reproductive wastage and developmental disorders in relation to consanguinity in South India. *Trop. Geogr. Med.*, **33**, 275–80.

Australian IVF Collaborative Group (1985) High incidence of preterm births and early losses in pregnancy after *in vitro* fertilisation. *Br. Med. J.*, **291**, 1160–3.

Barlow P.W. (1972) Differential cell division in human X-chromosome mosaics. *Hum. Genet.*, **14**, 122–7.

Baron J.A. (1984) Smoking and estrogen-related disease. *Am. J. Epidemiol.*, **119**, 9–22.

Berry C. (1980) The examination of embryonic and fetal material in diagnostic histopathology laboratories. *J. Clin. Pathol.*, **33**, 317–26.

Bottini E., Coromaldi L., Carapella E. *et al.* (1983) Intrauterine death: an approach to the analysis of genetic heterogeneity. *J. Med. Genet.*, **20**, 196–8.

Boue J., Boue A. & Lazar P. (1975) Retrospective and prospective epidemiological studies of 1500 karyotyped spontaneous human abortions. *Teratology*, **12**, 11–26.

Bresnihan B., Griger R.R., Oliver M. *et al.* (1979) Immunological mechanism for spontaneous abortion in systemic lupus erythematosus. *Lancet*, **ii**, 1205–7.

Brook J.D., Gosden R.G. & Chandley A.C. (1984) Maternal ageing and aneuploid embryos — evidence from the mouse that biological and not chronological age is the important factor. *Hum. Genet.*, **66**, 41–5.

Brotherton J. & Craft I.L. (1972) A clinical and pathologic survey of 91 cases of spontaneous abortion. *Fertil. Steril.*, **23**, 298–9.

Burchell R.C., Creed F., Rasoulpour M. & Whitcomb M. (1978) Vascular anatomy of the human uterus and pregnancy wastage. *Br. J. Obstet. Gynaecol.*, **85**, 698–706.

Butler M.R., Goldstein H. & Ross E.M. (1972) Cigarette smoking in pregnancy: its influence on birthweight and perinatal mortality. *Br. Med. J.*, **2**, 127–30.

Carr D.H. (1963) Chromosome studies in abortuses and stillborn infants. *Lancet*, **ii**, 603–6.

Carter C.O. & Evans K. (1973) Spina bifida and anencephalus in Greater London. *J. Med. Genet.*, **10**, 209–34.

Casagrande J.T., Pike M.C. & Henderson B.E. (1982) Menarcheal age and spontaneous abortion: a causal connection? *Am. J. Epidemiol.*, **115**, 481–3.

Chartier M., Roger M., Barrat J. & Michelon B. (1979) Measurement of plasma human chorionic gonadotrophin (hCG) and β-hCG activities in the late luteal phase: evidence of the occurrence of spontaneous menstrual abortions in infertile women. *Fertil. Steril.*, **31**, 134–7.

Christiaens G.C.M.L. & Stoutenbeek P.H. (1984) Spontaneous abortions in proven intact pregnancies. *Lancet*, **ii**, 571–2.

Cohen E.N., Brown B.E., Wee M. *et al.* 1979. Anesthetic health hazards in the dental operator. *Anesthesiology*, **51**, S254.

Craig C.J.T. (1974) Congenital abnormalities of the uterus and fetal wastage. *Obstet. Gynecol. Surv.*, **29**, 612–14.

Creasy M.R. & Alberman E.D. (1976) Congenital malformations of the central nervous system in spontaneous abortions. *J. Med. Genet.*, **13**, 9–16.

Creasy M.R. & Crolla J.A. (1974) Prenatal mortality of trisomy 21 (Down's syndrome). *Lancet*, **i**, 473–4.

Creasy M.R., Crolla J.A. & Alberman E.D. (1976) A cytogenetic study of human spontaneous abortions using banding techniques. *Hum. Genetik.*, **31**, 177–96.

Davis J.R., Weinstein L., Veomett I.C. *et al.* 1982. Balanced translocation karyotypes in patients with repetitive abortion. *Am. J. Obstet. Gynecol.*, **144**, 229–33.

De Wolf F., Carreras L.O., Moerman P. *et al.* (1982) Decidual vasculopathy and extensive placental infarction in a patient with repeated thromboembolic accidents, recurrent fetal loss, and a lupus anticoagulant. *Am. J. Obstet. Gynecol.*, **142**, 829–34.

Edmonds D.K., Lindsay K.S., Miller J.F. *et al.* (1982) Early embryonic mortality in women. *Fertil. Steril.*, **38**, 447–53.

Everson R.B., Sandler D.P., Wilcox A.J. *et al.* (1986) Effect of passive exposure to smoking on age at natural menopause. *Br. Med. J.*, **293**, 792.

Fedele L., Zamberletti D., Vercellini P. *et al.* (1987) Reproductive performance of women with unicornuate uterus. *Fertil. Steril.*, **47**, 416–19.

Ferguson-Smith M.A. (1983) Prenatal chromosome analysis and its impact on the birth incidence of chromosome disorders. *Br. Med. Bull.*, **39**, 355–64.

Fitzsimmons J., Stahl R., Gocial B. & Shapiro S.S. (1987) Spontaneous abortion and endometrios. *Fertil. Steril.*, **47**, 696–8.

Foreman H., Stadd B.U. & Schlesselman S. (1981) Intrauterine device usage and fetal loss. *Obstet. Gynecol.*, **58**, 669−77.

Geisler M. & Kleinebrecht J. (1978) Cytogenetic and histologic analyses of spontaneous abortions. *Hum. Genet.*, **45**, 239−51.

Gilmore D.H. & McNay M.B. (1985) Spontaneous fetal loss rate in early pregnancy. *Lancet*, **i**, 107.

Golbus S.M., Loughman W.D., Epstein C.J. *et al.* 1979. Prenatal genetic diagnosis in 300 amniocenteses. *New Engl. J. Med.*, **300**, 157−63.

Good A., Uribe M.R., Ryan R.J. & Kempers R.D. (1977) Molecular forms of HCG in serum, urine and placental extracts. *Fertil. Steril.*, **28**, 846−50.

Gustavii B. (1984) Chorionic biopsy and miscarriage in first trimester. *Lancet*, **i**, 562.

Harlap S. & Shiono P.H. (1980) Alcohol, smoking and incidence of spontaneous abortions in the first and second trimester. *Lancet*, **ii**, 173−6.

Hassold T., Chen N., Funkhouser J. *et al.* (1980) A cytogenetic study of 1000 spontaneous abortions. *Ann. Hum. Gen.*, **44**, 151−78.

Hay D.L. (1985) Discordant and variable production of hCG and its free alpha and beta subunits in early pregnancy. *J. Clin. Endocrinol. Metab.*, **61**, 1195−200.

Hemminki K., Mutanen P., Saloniemi I. *et al.* (1982) Spontaneous abortions in hospital staff engaged in sterilising instruments with chemical agents. *Br. Med. J.*, **285**, 1461−3.

Hendricks C.H. (1966) Twinning in relation to birthweight, mortality, and congenital anomalies. *Obstet. Gynecol.*, **27**, 47−53.

Hersey P., Prendergast D. & Edwards A. (1983) Effects of cigarette smoking on the immune system. Follow-up studies in normal subjects after cessation of smoking. *Med. J. Aust.*, **2**, 425−9.

Hertig A.T., Rock J., Adams E.C. & Menkin M.C. (1959) Thirty-four fertilized human ova, good, bad, and indifferent, recovered from 210 women of known fertility. A study of biologic wastage in early human pregnancy. *Pediatrics*, **23**, 202−11.

Himmelberger D.U., Brown B.W. & Cohen E.N. (1978) Cigarette smoking during pregnancy and the occurrence of spontaneous abortion and congenital abnormality. *Am. J. Epidemiol.*, **108**, 470−9.

Honore L.M., Dill F.J. & Poland B.J. (1976) Placental morphology in spontaneous human abortuses with normal and abnormal karyotypes. *Teratology*, **14**, 151−66.

Hook E.B. (1978) Spontaneous deaths of fetuses with chromosomal abnormalities diagnosed prenatally. *New Engl. J. Med.*, **299**, 1036−8.

Kajii T. & Ohama K. (1979) Inverse maternal age effect in monosomy K. *Hum. Genet.*, **51**, 147−51.

Kajii T., Ferrier A., Niikawa N. *et al.* (1980) Anatomic and chromosomal anomalies in 639 spontaneous abortions. *Hum. Genet.*, **55**, 87−98.

Khong T.Y., Liddell H.S. & Robertson W.B. (1987) Defective haemochorial placentation as a cause of miscarriage: a preliminary study. *Br. J. Obstet. Gynaecol.*, **94**, 649−55.

Kincaid-Smith P. & Bullen M. (1965) Bacteriuria in pregnancy. *Lancet*, **i**, 395−9.

Kline J., Stein Z., Strobino B. *et al.* (1977a) Surveillance of spontaneous abortions. *Am. J. Epidemiol.*, **106**, 345−50.

Kline J., Stein Z.A., Susser M. & Warburton D. (1977b) Smoking: a risk factor for spontaneous abortion. *New Engl. J. Med.*, **297**, 793−6.

Kline J., Shrout P.E., Stein Z.A. *et al.* (1978) An epidemiological study of the role of gravidity in spontaneous abortion. *Early Hum. Dev.*, **1**, 345−56.

Kline J., Stein Z., Susser M. & Warburton D. (1980) In *Human Embryonic and Fetal Death* (Ed. by I.H. Porter & E.B. Hook), pp. 225−40. Academic Press, London & New York.

Kullander S. & Kallen B. (1971) A prospective study of smoking and pregnancy. *Acta Obstet. Gynecol. Scand.*, **50**, 83−94.

Kurjak A. & Latin V. (1979) Ultrasound diagnosis of fetal abnormalities in multiple pregnancy. *Acta Obstet. Gynecol. Scand.*, **58**, 153−61.

Leridon H. (1973) Démographie des échecs de la reproduction. In *Les accidents chromosomiques de la reproduction* (Ed. by A. Bone & C. Thibault), pp. 13–27. Inserm, Paris.

Leridon H. (1976) Facts and artifacts in the study of intrauterine mortality: a reconsideration from pregnancy histories. *Pop. Stud.*, **30**, 319–35.

Liestol K. (1980) Menarcheal age and spontaneous abortion: a causal connection? *Am. J. Epidemiol.*, **111**, 753–8.

Lippman A., Vekemans M.J.J. & Perry T.B. (1984) Fetal mortality at the time of chorionic villus sampling. *Hum. Genet.*, **68**, 337–9.

Liu D.T.Y., Jeavons B., Preston C. & Pearson D. (1987) A prospective study of spontaneous miscarriage in ultrasonically normal pregnancies and its relevance to chorionic villus sampling. Personal communication.

Livingston J.E. & Poland B.T., (1980) A study of spontaneously aborted twins. *Teratology*, **21**, 139–48.

Lubbe W.F. & Liggins G.C. (1985) Lupus anticoagulant and pregnancy. *Am. J. Obstet. Gynecol.*, **153**, 322–7.

McFadyen I.R. (1984) Medical Research Council meeting to discuss the evaluation of the safety of chorion biopsy techniques. 30 March, London.

McFadyen I.R. (1985) Missed abortion and later spontaneous abortion, in pregnancies clinically normal at 7–12 weeks. *Europ. J. Obstet. Gynecol., Reprod. Biol.*, **20**, 381–4.

McFadyen I.R. & Brassil M.J. (1988) Empty sacs, dead fetuses, and later spontaneous abortions in pregnancies clinically normal at 6–12 weeks. Submitted for publication.

MacHenry J.C.R.M., Nevin M.C. & Merrett J.D. (1979) Comparison of central nervous system malformations in spontaneous abortions in Northern Ireland and south-east England. *Br. Med. J.*, **1**, 1395–7.

Machin G.A. (1974) Chromosome abnormality and perinatal death. *Lancet*, **i**, 549–51.

Markert C.L. & Petters R.M. (1978) Manufactured hexaparental mice show that adults are derived from three embryonic cells. *Science*, **202**, 56–8.

Mikamo K. (1970) Anatomic and chromosomal anomalies in spontaneous abortion. *Am. J. Obstet. Gynecol.*, **106**, 243–54.

Miller J.F., Williamson E., Glue J. *et al.* (1980) Fetal loss after implantation: a prospective study. *Lancet*, **ii**, 554–6.

Miodovnik M., Lavin J.P., Knowles H.C. *et al.* (1984) Spontaneous abortion among insulin-dependent diabetic women. *Am. J. Obstet. Gynecol.*, **150**, 372–6.

Miodovnik M., Skellman C., Holroyde J.C. *et al.* (1985) Elevated maternal glycohemoglobin in early pregnancy and spontaneous abortion among insulin-dependent diabetic women. *Am. J. Obstet. Gynecol.*, **153**, 439–42.

Munday P.E., Porter R., Falder P.F. *et al.* (1984) Spontaneous abortion — an infectious aetiology? *Br. J. Obstet. Gynaecol.*, **91**, 1177–80.

Naib Z.M., Nahmias A.J., Josey W.E. & Wheeler J.H. (1970) Association of maternal genital herpetic infection with spontaneous abortion. *Obstet. Gynecol.*, **35**, 260–3.

Naylor A.F. (1967) Ethnoracial comparisons of intraclass correlations and mean gestation times in spontaneous abortion and perinatal death. *Am. J. Obstet. Gynecol.*, **97**, 931–5.

Naylor A.F. & Warburton D. (1979) Sequential analysis of spontaneous abortion. ii. Collaborative study data show that gravidity determines a very substantial risk. *Fertil. Steril.*, **31**, 282–6.

Paton G.R., Silver M.F. & Allison A.C. (1974) Comparison of cell cycle time in normal and trisomic cells. *Hum. Genet.*, **23**, 173–82.

Poland B.J. & Yven B.H. (1978) Embryonic development in consecutive specimens from recurrent spontaneous abortions. *Am. J. Obstet. Gynecol.*, **130**, 512–15.

Poland B.J., Miller J.R., Jones D.C. & Trimble B.K. (1977) Reproductive counselling in patients who have had a spontaneous abortion. *Am. J. Obstet. Gynecol.*, **127**, 685–91.

Poland B.J., Miller J.R., Harris M. & Livingston J. (1981) Spontaneous abortion. A study of 1961 women and their conceptuses. *Acta Obstet. Gynecol. Scand. Suppl.*, **102**, 1–32.

Polani P.E. (1969) Autosomal imbalance and its syndromes, excluding Down's. *Br. Med. Bull.*, **25**, 81−93.

Powell H.C., Benirschke K., Favara B.E. & Pflueger O.H. (1976) Foamy changes of placental cells in fetal storage disorders. *Virchows Arch.*, **369**, 191−6.

Resseguie L.J. (1974) Pregnancy wastage and age of mother among the Amish. *Hum. Biol.*, **46**, 633−9.

Roberts C.J. & Lloyd S. (1973) Area differences in spontaneous abortion rates in South Wales and their relation to neural tube defect incidence. *Br. Med. J.*, **4**, 20−2.

Robinson H. (1977) Sonar evidence of early pregnancy failure in patients with twin conceptions. *Br. J. Obstet. Gynaecol.*, **84**, 22−5.

Rocklin R.E., Kitzmiller J.E., Carpenter C. B. *et al.* (1976) Maternal fetal relation. Absence of an immunologic blocking factor from the serum of women with chronic abortions. *New Engl. J. Med.*, **295**, 1209−13.

Rothman K.J. (1977) Fetal loss twinning and birth weight after oral contraceptive use. *New Engl. J. Med.*, **297**, 468−71.

Rushton D.I. (1984) The classification and mechanisms of spontaneous abortion. *Perspect. Pediatr. Path.*, **8**, 269−87.

Sant-Cassia L.J. & Cooke P. (1981) Chromosomal analysis of couples with repeated spontaneous abortions. *Br. J. Obstet. Gynaecol.*, **88**, 52−8.

Sant-Cassia L.J., MacPherson M.B.A. & Tyack A.J. (1984) Mid trimester amniocentesis: is it safe? A single centre controlled prospective study of 517 consecutive amniocenteses. *Br. J. Obstet. Gynaecol.*, **91**, 736−44.

Schweditsch M., Dubin N.H., Jones G.S. & Wentz A.C. (1979) Hormonal considerations in early normal pregnancy and blighted ovum syndrome. *Fertil. Steril.*, **31**, 252−7.

Sharp N.C., Anthony S., Miller J.F. & Masson G.M. (1986) Early conceptual loss in subfertile patients. *Br. J. Obstet. Gynaecol.*, **93**, 1072−7.

Siegel M., Fuerst H.T. & Peress N.S. (1966) Comparative fetal mortality in maternal virus diseases. A prospective study on rubella, measles, mumps, chicken pox and hepatitis. *New Engl. J. Med.*, **274**, 768−71.

Simpson J.L. (1984) Low fetal loss rate after normal ultrasound at eight weeks gestation: implications for chorionic villus sampling (CVS). The diabetes in early pregnancy project NICHD. *Am. J. Hum. Genet.*, **36**, 1975.

Simpson N.E., Dallaire L., Miller J.R. *et al.* (1976) Prenatal diagnosis of genetic disease in Canada: report of a collaborative study. *Canada Med. Assoc. J.*, **115**, 739−45.

Singh R.P. & Carr D.H. (1967) Anatomic findings in human abortions of known chromosomal constitution. *Am. J. Obstet. Gynecol.*, **29**, 806−18.

Smolen J.S. & Steinberg A.D. (1981) Systemic lupus erythematosus and pregnancy: clinical, immunological, and theoretical aspects. *Reprod. Immun.*, **70**, 283−302.

Srisuphan W. & Bracken M.B. (1986) Caffeine consumption during pregnancy and association with late spontaneous abortion. *Am. J. Obstet. Gynecol.*, **154**, 14−20.

Stevenson A.C., Dudgeon M.Y. & McClure H.I. (1959) Observations on the results of pregnancies in women resident in Belfast. ii. Abortions, hydatidiform moles and ectopic pregnancies. *Ann. Hum. Genet.*, **23**, 395−414.

Stray-Pedersen B. & Lorentzen−Styr A.M. (1979) The prevalence of *Toxoplasma* antibodies among 11 736 women in Norway. *Scand. J. Infect. Dis.*, **ii**, 159−65.

Stray-Pedersen B. & Stray-Pedersen S. (1984) Etiologic factors and subsequent reproductive performance in 195 couples with a prior history of habitual abortion. *Am. J. Obstet. Gynecol.*, **148**, 140−6.

Stromme W.B. & Haywa E.W. (1963) Intrauterine death in the second trimester. *Am. J. Obstet. Gynecol.*, **85**, 223−33.

Suginami H. & Kawoi A. (1982) Immunohistochemical localisation of an hCG-like substance in the human pituitary gland. *J. Clin. Endocrinol. Metab.*, **55**, 1161−6.

Thiede H.A. & Metcalfe S. (1966) Chromosomes and human pregnancy wastage. *Am. J. Obstet. Gynecol.*, **96**, 1132−8.

Thiede H.A. & Salm S.B. (1964) Chromosome studies of human spontaneous abortions. *Am. J. Obstet. Gynecol.*, **90**, 205−15.

Tho P.T., Byrd J.R. & McDonough P.G. (1979) Etiologies and subsequent reproductive performance of 100 couples with recurrent abortion. *Fertil. Steril.*, **32**, 389.

Tietze C., Guttmacher A.F. & Rubin S. (1950) Unintentional abortion in 1497 planned pregnancies. *J. Am. Med. Assoc.*, **142**, 1348−50.

Verma J.C. (1978) High frequency of neural-tube defects in North India. *Lancet*, **ii**, 879−80.

Vessey M.P. & Nunn J.F. (1980) Occupational hazards of anaesthesia. *Brit. Med. J.*, **281**, 696−8.

Warburton D. & Fraser F.C. (1964) Spontaneous abortion risks in man. *Am. J. Hum. Genet.*, **16**, 1.

Warburton D., Susser M., Stein Z. & Kline J. (1979) Genetic and epidemiologic investigation of spontaneous abortion: relevance to clinical practice. *Birth Defects*, **15**, 127−36.

Warburton D., Kline J., Stein Z. & Susser M. (1980) Monosomy X: a chromosomal anomaly associated with young maternal age. *Lancet*, **i**, 167−9.

Weathersbee P.S., Olsen L.K. & Lodge J.R. (1977) Caffeine and pregnancy: a retrospective survey. *Postgrad. Med. J.*, **62**, 3, 64−9.

Westergaard J.G., Teisner B., Sinosich M.J. *et al.* (1985) Does ultrasound examination render biochemical tests obsolete in the prediction of early pregnancy failure? *Br. J. Obstet. Gynaecol.*, **92**, 77−83.

Whittaker P.G., Taylor A. & Lind T. (1983) Unsuspected pregnancy loss in healthy women. *Lancet*, **i**, 1126−7.

Wilcox A.J., Treloar A.E. & Sandler D.P. (1981) Spontaneous abortion over time: comparing the occurrences in two cohorts of women a generation apart. *Am. J. Epidemiol.*, **114**, 548−53.

Wilcox A.J., Weinberg C.R., Wehmann R.E. *et al.* (1985) Measuring early pregnancy loss: laboratory and field methods. *Fertil. Steril.*, **44**, 366−74.

Wilson J.G. (1973) Present status of drugs as teratogens in man. *Teratology*, **7**, 3−15.

Wilson R.D., Kendrick V., Wittmann B.K. & McGillivray B.C. (1984) Risk of spontaneous abortion in ultrasonically normal pregnancies. *Lancet*, **i**, 920−1.

Wingate M.B. (1968) Anatomic studies in mid trimester abortions. *Am. J. Obstet. Gynecol.*, **102**, 901−2.

Working Party on Amniocentesis (1978) An assessment of the hazards of amniocentesis. *Br. J. Obstet. Gynaecol.*, **85**, Suppl. 2.

Wramsby H., Frega K. & Liedholm P. (1987) Chromosome analysis of human oocytes recovered from preovulatory follicles in stimulated cycles. *New Engl. J. Med.*, **316**, 121−4.

Yamamoto M., Fujimon R., Ito T. *et al.* (1975) Chromosome studies in 500 induced abortions. *Hum. Genet.*, **29**, 9−14.

Zabriskie J.R. (1963) Effect of cigarette smoking during pregnancy. Study of 2000 cases. *Obstet. Gynecol.*, **21**, 405−11.

3

Immunization with Paternal Cells in the Treatment of Recurrent Abortion

J.F. MOWBRAY

Introduction

It has become clear that some couples have recurrent abortions because of an inability of the woman to prevent herself from rejecting the fetoplacental unit as a foreign tissue, by virtue of paternal antigens present on the cell surfaces of the conceptus. Normal women make a set of antibodies of which there are at least four types, each of which can prevent one of the pathways by which such attack can occur. A large group of recurrently aborting women do not have any of these anti-bodies, but they can be produced by immunization with paternal lymphocytes, or cells from multiple unrelated donors. The efficiency of this immunization in preventing abortion has led to its acceptance as an important therapeutic advance in the treatment of a difficult clinical group. Our controlled clinical trial (Mowbray et al. 1985) showed that the effect was immunological and not psychological, and most of the groups taking up this kind of treatment have done so since that trial.

Three groups of workers — Beer and his group (1981), Page Faulk and Taylor (Taylor et al. 1985) and ourselves (Mowbray et al. 1983) — all started immunization treatment of recurrent spontaneous abortion at about the same time. Since then there has been a considerable expansion of interest, and in 1987 there are some 25 active groups throughout the world.

The advent of AIDS has reduced the use of immunization of women with multiple unrelated, third-party blood donors as advocated by Faulk, although at least one other group using this method is still active (Unander et al. 1985). As most groups have used paternal cell immuniz-ation, particularly since the publication of our controlled clinical trial, I shall concentrate mostly on this form of immunization.

There are clearly several causes of repeated abortion, as there are of single abortion. None of the immunologists involved in this area have ever suggested that immunological treatment was appropriate for all recurrently aborting couples, although some obstetricians have looked on it as a panacea which might work in abortion of any cause. Because it is necessary to select the couples which are suitable for treatment by immunization, before considering the methods of treatment, and the results obtained, we should first consider selection of patients, and their investigation. Again I shall limit most of the description of this to the selection procedures which we use. With only a few exceptions, our methods of selection are the same as those used in most centres.

Selection of patients

The aim of investigation of recurrently aborting couples, as of any condition, should be to identify the problem and, if possible, its cause. Only then will we obtain a homogeneous group of patients which may be expected to respond to a particular therapy, in this case, immunization with paternal cells. To investigate rationally we must consider the differential diagnosis of recurrent abortion. Since it is very difficult to do investigations in this area which point positively to a particular cause, we are largely left with tests of exclusion.

As a physician, I viewed the causes of single or recurrent abortion commonly listed with some scepticism. I thought that, if there was an immunological cause, it would be in a small group, which would have to be carefully picked out if any benefit of immunization was to be demonstrated. However, judging by the very effective results in the large number we have chosen to treat (Mowbray 1986), it would appear that I was wrong in thinking that this group was a small proportion of all couples with recurrent abortion. Table 3.1 shows the frequency of the main causes of *recurrent* abortion in over 1500 couples seen in the Recurrent Miscarriage Clinic at the Samaritan Hospital, London.

The basis of investigation of the patients is to assign them to the different aetiological groups, in particular to identify those with a possible genetic cause, and the group (about 2·5%) who have the syndrome associated with antiphospholipid antibodies, lupus anticoagulant, or collagenoses (Lubbe & Liggins 1985). It might be thought unusual that I have not specifically listed abnormalities of the uterine cavity but, if they occur, they are found under 'other causes'. In our considerable experience of aborting women with bicornuate uterus of all degrees, the evidence that repair alone was associated with successful pregnancies is very poor. Although continuing to abort after surgery, they have not aborted

Table 3.1. Probable distribution of causes of recurrent abortion

Aetiological factor	Frequency in recurrent abortion (%)
Immunological	75
Genetic	10
Non-repeating genetic (trisomy, etc.)	10
Antiphospholipid antibody syndrome	2·5
Other	2·5
Total	100·0

after immunization. In seven pregnancies after immunization in women with uncorrected bicornuate uterus, only one aborted a subsequent pregnancy. Although implantation on a thin septum, with a poor blood supply, may result in abortion, there is no reason why implantation should always occur at such a site. It may be, therefore, that it is a cause of occasional abortion in a woman having several successful pregnancies. If so, this woman would have been excluded from treatment on other grounds, *vide infra*, even if she had been unfortunate enough to have implanted on a thin septum at least three times.

The basic separation occurs in the history: any woman who has had three or more abortions with the present partner, and not more than one successful pregnancy with the same partner, is potentially one with an immunological cause. Patients with more than one live child with this partner are likely to have an as yet undefined recessive genetic cause. A postulated recessive genetic fault leading to abortion will cause loss in 25% of pregnancies, and a woman who has had more than one successful pregnancy could be in this group. In addition, if either husband or wife has had another partnership which has produced more than one abortion, we would consider it likely that a genetic factor is carried by that partner. A similar history could also be obtained in women with anatomical causes. Thus couples, either of whom have had a previous partnership producing abortions, are excluded from the treatment group because they are less likely to have an immunological cause.

The group of women with antiphospholipid antibodies associated with repeated pregnancy loss are characterized by abortions occurring after 18 weeks, severe fetal growth retardation, large placental infarcts visible to the naked eye, and often venous thromboses occurring during or between pregnancies. In collaboration with Dr N. Harris at St Thomas's Hospital London, we have screened sera of 400 recurrently aborting women for anticardiolipin antibody, with an incidence, as previously stated, of 2·5%. Women with high levels of antibody have the syndrome of late abortion, placental infarction, etc., and it seems that the clinical history, rather than the antibody, could be used for screening. The antibody may not be detectable outside pregnancy, and is more of a confirmative investigation than a screening procedure. It is obviously desirable to identify these patients in whom a diagnosis of cervical incompetence is often made, since treatment with heparin, steroids or aspirin may be very effective.

Cervical incompetence is not a common cause of repeated abortion, if it exists at all. Having seen a very large number of women who have aborted despite Shirodkar suture, but who have not aborted when treated appropriately, I feel that premature rupture of membranes for mechanical reasons is a most uncommon cause of repeated pregnancy loss.

Investigations

Investigations can be divided into those for selecting couples with immunological causes of abortion, as discussed above, and those for the immunization process. Of the latter it is obviously necessary to screen the husband for the same infections as those checked for blood donors. We only measure HBsAg (Australia antigen) and HIV antibody, but some groups, who consider cytomegalovirus (CMV) a hazard during immunization in pregnancy, have included anti-CMV in their screen. The relevance of this antibody to the exclusion of donors is not clear.

It is obviously necessary to know the blood groups of husband and wife before immunization in order to ensure that rhesus-negative women with rhesus-positive men get anti-D antibody to cover the small number of red cells which contaminate the lymphocytes of the husband which are used for immunization. We have seen two women not so treated and, although the numbers of red cells they received were in both cases less than 2×10^4, they made anti-D antibodies in the next pregnancy, fortunately without serious problems resulting. As many women only find out their blood groups when attending antenatal clinics, and most abortions occur before booking, many recurrently aborting women do not know their rhesus blood group. Neither of these women had therefore had anti-D antibody with their previous abortions, and this may have resulted in prior sensitization to the red cells accompanying the lymphocyte immunization. The use of 500 iu of anti-D antibody in nearly two hundred other rhesus-negative women treated has been completely successful in preventing any other example of rhesus antibody response to the immunization.

Other investigations have been carried out sporadically by other groups, and by us for purely clinical research reasons. These include HLA typing, which was, in early publications (Beer *et al.* 1981; Faulk & McIntyre 1983), thought to be important in identifying immunological abortion. This was based on the belief that sharing of HLA antigens between husband and wife would lead to inability to make protective anti-HLA antibodies. A recent multicentre study of about 1000 couples confirms the results of studies of smaller numbers, namely that, although some slight increase in sharing of HLA class I and class II antigens is present, it is insufficient in itself to explain the phenomenon of recurrent abortion (Reznikoff-Etiévant 1986). In addition, it is known that trophoblast cells do not have the normal class I or class II HLA antigens on their surfaces, and it is to these cells that the immunological attack is directed (Johnson & Stern 1987). The minor degree of sharing found is probably a consequence of gene similarities at other loci in linkage disequilibrium with the standard HLA loci, and it is these gene products which are important.

Methods of immunization

Immunization with paternal cells has in general been done as a purified preparation of peripheral blood lymphocytes, contaminated with variable numbers of platelets. The third-party donor white cell infusions of Faulk & Taylor (Taylor *et al.* 1985) have been of unpurified buffy-coat white cells, containing large numbers of red cells and polymorphs, as well as lymphocytes and platelets. Because of the heavy red cell contamination of the latter, the donors have had to be matched for major and minor red cell antigens, which, for more than twenty occasions, represents a formidable task. The use of paternal cells is easier, although requiring concurrent anti-D antibody administration in about 15% of couples.

The paternal cells used need to be of adequate amount, and administered in such a fashion as to produce a useful antibody response. In our group a single dose of immunization has been the norm, with, in the past two years, additional boost injections given to some women not becoming pregnant early, and not showing cytotoxic antibody conversion after immunization. This fairly economical regime has enabled us to immunize a large number of women. The regimes used by Dr Reznikoff-Etiévant in Paris and of Drs Alexandre and Gottlieb in Brussels, where in both cases multiple doses are given, considerably increase the work undertaken per patient. Nevertheless, were we to start again, it is possible that we would also have used multiple immunization routinely and not just confined it to the women who did not show seroconversion after immunization. It became apparent that this small group of women contained most of the treatment failures, i.e. those that had a further abortion. However, this outcome was largely averted by giving a small boost dose of cells from 50 ml of blood at the start of the next pregnancy. Our standard initial dose of cells is that derived from about 400 ml of blood, a yield of $200-550 \times 10^6$ lymphocytes. In a single immunization, the threshold dose is about 110×10^8 cells (Mowbray 1986), although a smaller dose seems to suffice in other centres using multiple immunization. It is unlikely that a single-dose regime of cells from less than 100 ml will be very efficient. Such a lower dose has been used by Beer's group (1981), and this may explain their finding that they have not prevented the fetal growth retardation which is a problem before treatment (Beer *et al.* 1987). With larger doses the birthweights of children born in our series are the same as those for the normal population (Table 3.2).

Purification of the paternal cells for immunization has in general been carried out using density gradient centrifugation in Ficoll-Hypaque gradients. As our usage increased we changed from locally manufactured gradient medium to the use of commercial Lymphoprep (Nygaard, Oslo). Citrated blood from the husband taken into Fenwal bags (Travenol Ltd.)

Table 3.2. Distribution of birthweights in pregnancies before and after immunization in recurrent spontaneous abortion

Standard deviation from mean birthweight	Untreated	After immunization
> 2·0 SD above mean weight	2	0
1·5−2·0 SD " " "	1	3
1·0−1·5 SD " " "	1	6
0·5−1·0 SD " " "	17	14
0−0·5 SD " " "	23	12
0−0·5 SD below mean weight	17	26
0·5−1·0 SD " " "	18	17
1·0−1·5 SD " " "	19	9
1·5−2·0 SD " " "	6	4
> 2·0 SD " " "	8	1

is centrifuged at 4C, the buffy coat removed to 50 ml sterile centrifuge tubes (Nunc) and Lymphoprep layered underneath. The tubes are then centrifuged at 4C, the lymphocyte layer harvested, and the cells washed twice by centrifugation, and resuspended in 5 ml saline. The cells are then injected into the wife intravenously (3 ml), intradermally (1 ml) and subcutaneously (1 ml). I have not changed from our original regime, as it was, and still is, quick and simple (Mowbray *et al.* 1985). Other groups have usually given the dose intravenously, except Beer, who has given all the dose intradermally. The third-party donor crude buffy coat of Faulk and Taylor was, of course, given intravenously. It is impossible to separate differences in route of administration, dose and number of doses in deciding on relative efficacy. Our studies of dose are controlled for the other factors and do suggest that a large single dose is needed. The need for additional doses to protect those not showing seroconversion and getting pregnant more than 80 days after immunization also seems well established (Mowbray 1986). Many groups have wanted to start without the trouble and expense of setting up large-volume centrifugation of blood in refrigerated centrifuges, but the dose needed does seem to be larger than that easily accommodated in small centrifuges, or indeed in syringes of blood rather than blood bags.

Results

One of the striking results of all the methods of treatment of recurrently aborting couples, by immunization with paternal cells (Beer *et al.* 1981; Mowbray *et al.* 1985), third-party cells (Taylor *et al.* 1985), syncytiotrophoblast membrane microvesicles (Johnson *et al.* 1987) or intensive one-to-one psychotherapy (Stray-Pedersen & Stray-Pedersen 1987), is that all seem effective, and to roughly the same degree. The only controlled clinical trial which has been completed was reported by us (Mowbray *et al.* 1985), although a controlled trial of trophoblast immunization by P. Johnson is under way in Liverpool.

   We have published results of a large series of couples treated with paternal cell immunization as well as the controlled trial referred to above. The latter showed that immunization was an immunological and not a placebo effect, as immunization with paternal cells was much more effective than giving the woman's own lymphocytes to her, in a double-blind study. With an efficiency of about 80% overall, it was some time before enough failures had been obtained to analyse them usefully. When this was done, it was seen that the women not showing seroconversion did badly if they did not become pregnant within about 80 days (Fig. 3.1). Giving this group a boost injection of about 50×10^6 cells has resulted in the success in this group rising from about 30% to 80%. We have recently also shown (Mowbray 1986) that immunization very early in pregnancy is accompanied by very successful results (Fig. 3.2) and, although difficult to arrange, immunization in the first 6 weeks is best for protecting the pregnancy. This implies that the damage leading to abortion has not occurred irrevocably by then, and that the changes resulting from immunization must be rapidly effective, as the abortions which are prevented would have reached a peak incidence after about 8 weeks of pregnancy.

Children born after immunization

There has been concern that children born after immunization, or indeed other treatments for recurrent abortion, might be developmentally abnormal, or suffer intrauterine growth retardation. In particular this was raised by Beer (Beer *et al.* 1987) after he found 3 infants out of 36 with birthweights below the tenth centile (although this may not differ from the normal distribution). Our results show that, of a large number of children born after immunization, the birthweight distribution is that of the normal population, and the incidence of preterm labour, another feature of children born to repetitively aborting women, is not significantly different from that found in normals. In addition, developmental abnormalities are not of increased frequency compared with the normal population (major birth defect < 2·5% of births).

It should be recognized that the efficiency with which different centres exclude other causes from immunological treatment, and the efficacy of particular immunization protocols, will vary. This may mean that results vary between centres for either of these reasons, and it behoves every centre to keep a continual audit of results. If poorer results are obtained in some centres compared with others, this may be a useful guide to the relative importance of different parts of the procedure by which patients are selected, and then treated. It is my belief (Mowbray 1987) that exclusion of the inappropriate patients from treatment is a major reason for the highly successful programme which I have outlined. Treatment of unselected couples, defined only by recurrent abortion, could lead to unsatisfactory results, in terms of developmentally abnormal children or of low birthweight and preterm labour (Reginald *et al.* 1987).

Cytotoxic antibody after immunization

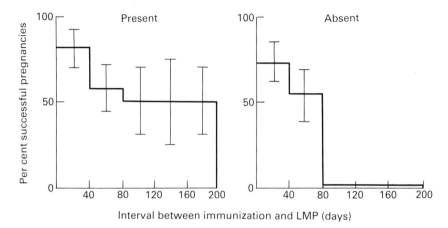

Fig. 3.1. Women without seroconversion after immunization are protected for only 80 days. Production of antipaternal antibody is associated with long-term protection. LMP = last monthly period.

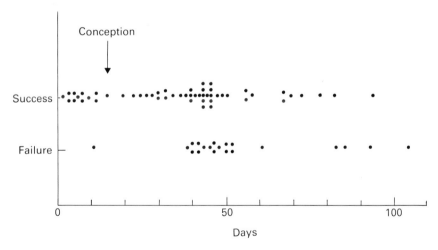

Fig. 3.2. Immunization in the beginning of pregnancy is very effective in preventing further abortion. If given too late in pregnancy, irreversible damage may have already occurred. Each dot is one pregnancy.

References

Beer A.E., Quebbeman J.F., Ayers J.W.T. & Haines R.F. (1981) Major histocompatibility antigens, maternal and paternal immune responses and chronic habitual abortion in humans. *Am. J. Obstet. Gynecol.*, **141**, 987.

Beer A.E., Quebbeman J.F., Hamazaki Y. & Semprini A.E. (1987) Immunotherapy of spontaneous abortion. In *Immunoregulation and Fetal Survival* (Ed. by T.J. Gill & T.G. Wegmann), pp. 286–99. Oxford University Press, New York.

Faulk W.P. & McIntyre J.A. (1983) Trophoblast survival. *Transplantation*, **32**, 1–5.

Johnson P.M. & Stern P.L. (1987) Antigen expression at human maternofetal interfaces. In *Progress in Immunology VI* (Ed. by B. Cinader & R.G. Miller), pp. 1056–69. Academic Press, Orlando.

Johnson P.M., Chia K.V., Hart C.A., Griffith H.B. & Francis W.J.A. (1987) Trophoblast membrane immunization in unexplained recurrent spontaneous abortion. *Am. J. Reprod. Immunol. Microbiol.*, **14**, 11.

Lubbe W.F. & Liggins G.C. (1985) Lupus anticoagulant and pregnancy. *Am. J. Obstet. Gynecol.*, **153**, 322–7.

Mowbray J.F. (1986) Effect of immunisation with paternal cells on recurrent spontaneous abortion. In *Reproductive Immunology* (Ed. by D.A. Clark & B.A. Croy), pp. 269–76. Elsevier, Amsterdam.

Mowbray J.F. (1987) Genetic and immunological factors in human recurrent abortion. *Am. J. Reprod. Immunol. Microbiol.*, **15**, 138–40.

Mowbray J.F., Gibbings C.R., Sidgwick A.S., Ruszkiewicz M. & Beard R.W. (1983) Effects of transfusion in women with recurrent spontaneous abortion. *Transplant. Proc.*, **15**, 896–9.

Mowbray J.F., Gibbings C., Liddell H., Reginald P.W., Underwood J.L. & Beard R.W. (1985) Controlled trial of treatment of recurrent spontaneous abortion by immunisation with paternal cells. *Lancet*, **i**, 941–3.

Reginald P.W., Beard R.W., Chapple J. *et al.* (1987) Outcome of pregnancies progressing beyond 28 weeks of gestation in women with a history of recurrent miscarriage. *Br. J. Obstet. Gynaecol.*, **11**, 643–8.

Reznikoff-Etiévant M.F. (1986) Personal communication.

Stray-Pedersen B. & Stray-Pedersen S. (1984) Etiologic factors and subsequent reproductive performance in 15 couples with a prior history of recurrent abortion. *Am. J. Obstet. Gynecol.*, **148**, 140–6.

Taylor C.G., Faulk W.P. & McIntyre J.A. (1985) Prevention of recurrent spontaneous abortions by leukocyte transfusions. *J. Roy. Soc. Med.*, **78**, 623–37.

Unander M., Lindholm A. & Olding L.B. (1985) Blood transfusions generate/increase previously absent/weak blocking antibody in women with habitual abortion. *Fertil. Steril.*, **44**, 766–71.

4

Fetal Blood Gas and Acid−Base Parameters

P.W. SOOTHILL, K.H. NICOLAIDES & C.H. RODECK

The techniques developed for prenatal diagnosis of inherited disease are now being used to diagnose fetal hypoxia. Should knowledge of the acid−base status of the fetus lead to improved management, the impact on perinatal mortality and morbidity is likely to be even greater than that achieved by prenatal diagnosis and abortion of congenitally abnormal fetuses. This chapter reviews the studies on fetal blood gas and acid−base parameters in normal and pathological pregnancies.

Definitions and measurements

The principles of blood gas and acid−base physiology are based on observations in adults. Investigation of these parameters in fetal blood has assumed that these concepts apply to the fetus.

Fetal respiration

Oxygenation is the process of transporting molecular oxygen from air to the tissues of the body. This involves: (i) oxygen uptake from the environment, (ii) oxygen transport within the organism, and (iii) oxygen consumption. The equivalent steps in the fetus are (i) oxygen transfer across the placenta, (ii) reversible binding of oxygen to fetal haemoglobin and fetal blood flow, and (iii) fetal growth and metabolism.

Energy is derived from the combination of oxygen and glucose to form carbon dioxide and water. Less than 5% of the carbon dioxide produced is transported by blood in solution, because carbonic anhydrase converts carbon dioxide and water into carbonic acid, which rapidly dissociates into bicarbonate and hydrogen ions. If the hydrogen ions were released into a closed system, the carbonic acid dissociation would reach equilibrium at a pH of 4·60 (Huber 1978). Therefore, removal of carbon dioxide and protection against acidosis are just as important as the supply of oxygen. Carbon dioxide is removed by the reverse of the mechanisms described for oxygen delivery but is helped by the rapid diffusion and high solubility and volatility of this gas. In the adult, carbon dioxide is excreted in the lungs while bicarbonate and hydrogen ions are removed by the kidney. In the fetus, both these functions are thought to be carried out by the placenta.

When there is inadequate oxygen supply the Krebs cycle cannot operate and the pyruvate is converted to lactic acid. This enters the blood, leading to systemic acidosis unless it is either metabolized or excreted.

pH

pH (potentia hydrogenii) is $-\log_{10}$ of the hydrogen ion concentration; for example, the pH of water (hydrogen ion concentration 10^{-7} moles l^{-1}) is 7·00. When a glass electrode which contains a solution of known pH is immersed in a solution of unknown pH an electropotential develops on the surface of the glass which is proportional to the difference in the hydrogen ion concentrations of the two solutions.

pO_2 and pCO_2

The partial pressure of a gas is a measure of its concentration relative to other gases in a mixture. The partial pressure of oxygen (pO_2) is measured by the Clark electrode, which consists of a platinum cathode and silver ($Ag/AgCl$) anode in an electrolyte solution surrounded by a semipermeable membrane. A constant potential difference is maintained across the electrode, and oxygen is reduced at the platinum cathode. The resulting current indicates the pO_2. The measurement of partial pressure of carbon dioxide (pCO_2) is by a modified pH electrode. A plastic membrane surrounds a bicarbonate solution in which the pH electrode is immersed. When this unit is placed into a liquid, carbon dioxide can diffuse in but the bicarbonate cannot diffuse out, and the resulting change in the pH of the solution bathing the electrode is measured.

Derived parameters of base

A variety of indices derived from the pH and pCO_2 (e.g. 'actual' bicarbonate = constant $\times pCO_2/pH$) have been used in an attempt to achieve a better indication of whether an acid−base disturbance is of respiratory or metabolic origin. Although estimates of bicarbonate concentration and the base excess are automatically displayed by most blood gas and acid–base machines, they are of questionable value (Harington *et al.* 1982) since the same information can be obtained by examination of the measured parameters from which these indices are derived. For example, if the pH is low but the pCO_2 is normal, then the acidosis is not respiratory but metabolic.

Lactate concentration

Lactate is the main acid produced by anaerobic metabolism. It can be estimated by measurement of NADH production when lactate is converted to pyruvate by lactate dehydrogenase. More recently a modified oxygen electrode has been devised which measures the oxygen consumed when lactate is converted to acetic aldehyde.

Blood oxygen content

Unlike pO_2, oxygen content is the concentration of oxygen (moles or litres) in a volume of blood. It can be determined by extraction and volumetric measurement of oxygen. Alternatively, it can be calculated from the haemoglobin concentration (Hb) and the haemoglobin oxygen saturation percentage (which is derived from the pO_2 and pH using the Hill and Bohr equations):

$$\text{oxygen content} = 1{\cdot}39 \times \text{Hb} \times \% \text{ saturation}$$

The oxygen content automatically displayed on most blood gas and acid–base machines is calculated assuming that the blood is adult (HbA) and so these values must be corrected for the different oxygen affinity of fetal blood (HbF).

Haemoglobin oxygen affinity

A property of haemoglobin is that the amount of oxygen bound is not linearly related to the pO_2. Each type of haemoglobin has a characteristic oxygen dissociation curve which can be modified by environmental factors (Fig. 4.1), such as pH and the concentration of 2,3-diphosphoglycerate (2,3-DPG). For example, when 2,3-DPG rises, in response to anaemia or hypoxia, it binds to and stabilizes the deoxygenated form of haemoglobin, resulting in a shift of the oxygen dissociation curve to the right and therefore release of oxygen to the tissues.

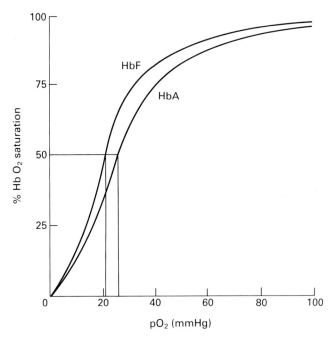

Fig. 4.1. The oxygen dissociation curves of adult (HbA) and fetal (HbF) haemoglobins. The affinity of haemoglobin can be described by its P_{50} (partial pressure of oxygen at which the haemoglobin is 50% saturated). The normal P_{50} for fetal blood is 21 mmHg compared with 27 mmHg for adult. Acidosis or increase in pCO_2 or 2,3-DPG decreases the haemoglobin oxygen affinity (moves the curve to the right).

Although, *in vitro*, both HbA and HbF have the same oxygen dissociation curves, human adult blood has a lower affinity for oxygen than fetal because of its greater binding of 2,3-DPG (Maurer *et al.* 1970). The affinity of haemoglobin can be described by its P_{50} (partial pressure of oxygen at which the haemoglobin is 50% saturated), and normal values for fetal blood are about 21 mmHg whereas those for adult are about 27 mmHg (Fig. 4.1). It has been suggested that the higher affinity of fetal blood helps placental transfer of oxygen. Furthermore, since the greatest amount of oxygen is released for a given fall in pO_2 at the steepest part of the oxygen dissociation curve, fetal haemoglobin releases more oxygen than adult at low levels of pO_2.

Hypoxia

Hypoxia, failure of the normal processes of oxygenation, results in oxygen deficiency in the tissues.

Hypoxic hypoxia (reduced uptake) occurs because the arterial blood oxygen content is reduced as a result of an abnormally low pO_2. In the adult, this occurs at high altitude or as a result of diseases of the lungs.

Anaemic hypoxia (reduced transport) occurs when the arterial blood oxygen content is reduced as a result of a low haemoglobin concentration. Although the pO_2 and haemoglobin oxygen saturation are normal, the blood oxygen content and therefore the amount delivered to the tissues is reduced.

Stagnant or ischaemic hypoxia (reduced transport) occurs when oxygen delivery is reduced as a result of inadequate blood flow to the tissues. The oxygen content of the blood is normal but the amount of oxygen delivered is reduced.

Histotoxic hypoxia (reduced consumption) occurs when there is adequate oxygen supply but the tissue is unable to use it. For example, in cyanide poisoning oxygen uptake stops because there is no consumption.

Hypoxia of any cause leads to a conversion from aerobic to anaerobic metabolism. This produces less energy, but more acid. Compensatory mechanisms for acidosis in the adult include increased renal reabsorption of bicarbonate and excretion of acid and increased pulmonary excretion of carbon dioxide. If the oxygen supply is not restored there is reduced reserve for exercise, followed by compromise at rest and then death.

'Asphyxia'

Asphyxia is the Greek word for 'pulselessness', which can be reversible in a neonate but when diagnosed in the fetus indicates death. However, in both common (Sykes 1979) and specialist (Myers *et al.* 1984) usage, it has come to mean defective oxygenation of blood as a result of impaired respiration. In fetal medicine, the word asphyxia is best replaced by hypoxia.

Fetal temperature

Blood gas measurements require knowledge of the *in vivo* temperature and, since fetal intramuscular temperature is 36·9 °C (Soothill *et al.* 1987a), the 37 °C assumed by most machines is a reasonable approximation.

Data from animal fetuses

Many of the concepts on human fetal blood gas and acid–base status originate from the results of animal studies. The first measurements were made in blood samples taken from the uterine and umbilical cord vessels, exposed by hysterotomy under general anaesthesia. Although transplacental gradients of oxygen, carbon dioxide and pH were demonstrated (Huggett 1927; Barcroft 1946), the anaesthesia and surgery required could have affected the results. A major advance was made when Meschia *et al.* (1965) introduced a method for inserting and maintaining catheters in umbilical cord and uterine vessels. This allowed repeated observations to be made on conscious animals in a steady state. Normal ranges for several species were established and it was possible to study the effect of various experiments on fetal blood gases.

Normal data

The umbilical venous and arterial pO_2, pCO_2, pH, oxygen content and P_{50} of various species are shown in Table 4.1. In all species, the umbilical venous blood pO_2 is less than half the maternal arterial pO_2 and this observation led to the concept of 'Mount Everest *in utero*'. Despite the low pO_2 and rapid growth, the normal fetus does not develop lactic acidosis. This is because fetal blood has a high concentration of a haemoglobin with high oxygen affinity and so the oxygen content is maintained. The higher haemoglobin oxygen affinity in the fetus than the adult may be the result of: (i) an intrinsic property of its haemoglobin, e.g. sheep and goats (Blunt *et al.* 1971) or (ii) lower concentration of 2,3-DPG, e.g. pigs, horses, guinea pigs and rabbits (Baumann *et al.* 1973; Bunn & Kitchen 1973; Bard & Shapiro 1979). The P_{50} of fetal blood is similar to the umbilical arterial pO_2. This means that the fetus operates over the steepest part of the haemoglobin oxygen dissociation curve so that a relatively large amount of oxygen is released from the haemoglobin for a given drop in pO_2 (Fig. 4.1). Furthermore, fetal oxygen consumption of various species ($6.0-8.5$ ml kg^{-1} min^{-1}; Comline & Silver 1974) is higher than the oxygen consumption of adult humans (3.5 ml kg^{-1} min^{-1}) and so the fetus has a large oxygen supply despite the low pO_2 levels.

Although most animal studies have concentrated on fetuses near term, some early studies in sheep suggested that the fetal pO_2 falls with advancing gestational age (Barcroft *et al.* 1940; Barron 1946). Similarly, the fetal haemoglobin oxygen saturation is higher in early than in late gestation (Bell *et al.* 1986).

Table 4.1. Umbilical cord blood pO_2, pCO_2, pH, oxygen content ($[O_2]$) and P_{50} of animal fetuses near term

Units	Umbilical vein				Umbilical artery					Reference
	pO_2 mmHg	pCO_2 mmHg	pH $-\log H^+$	$[O_2]$ mM/l	pO_2 mmHg	pCO_2 mmHg	pH $-\log H^+$	$[O_2]$ mM/l	P_{50}* mmHg	
Rabbit	44			5·1	16			1·3	27	Barron & Battaglia (1955–6)
		48	7·37							Young (1952)
Guinea pig	26	47	7·31						19	Lafeber (1981)
Sheep	34	42	7·40		23	46	7·35		17	Comline & Silver (1970)
		44	7·41	4·9		51	7·36	1·5		Kaiser & Cummings (1957)
	38	39	7·41							Rivard et al. (1969)
Goat	27		7·42	3·6	14	49	7·34	1·4	19	Prystowsky et al. (1960)
		46	7·33	4·1			7·32	1·5		Kaiser & Cummings (1958)
Llama	20		7·20	4·3	7		7·08	0·4	18	Meschia et al. (1960)
Pig	31	46	7·48		21	52	7·43		22	Comline & Silver (1974)
		54	7·37	3·4		61	7·34	1·7		Cummings & Kaiser (1959)
Monkey	33	46	7·32		23	49	7·29		19	Behrman et al. (1970)
	16				12					Battaglia et al. (1965)
Cow	38	44	7·40		26	49	7·37		22	Comline & Silver (1974)
	19	41	7·36		12	48	7·33			Gahlenbeck et al. (1968)
Horse	48	43	7·39		31	50	7·36		31	Comline & Silver (1974)

* Values of P_{50} from Novy & Parer (1969).

Fetal hypoxia

Fetal hypoxia can be produced by reducing oxygenation in several ways.

Reduction in oxygen uptake

Reduction in atmospheric pressure

When chronically catheterized sheep are taken to high altitude, there is an initial fall in umbilical venous blood pO_2 and oxygen content which returns to normal over a period of two weeks (Makowski *et al.* 1968). These changes are also found in the uterine venous but not maternal arterial blood, suggesting that in response to fetal hypoxia the blood flow of the healthy uteroplacental circulation can increase to improve the supply of oxygen to the fetus. A fall in fetal pO_2 can also be produced by reducing atmospheric pressure with hypobaric chambers, and such fetuses improve their oxygen content by polycythaemia (Kaiser & Cummings 1958).

Reduction in the percentage of inspired oxygen

Reduction in the percentage oxygen inspired by the mother lowers the fetal blood pO_2 and oxygen content, producing a rise in pCO_2, lactate and pyruvate and a fall in pH and glucose (Mann 1970; Van Geijn *et al.* 1980). In moderate hypoxia in sheep, there is a compensatory increase in blood flow to most fetal tissues which maintains oxygenation. In severe hypoxia, there is increased flow to the brain and heart at the expense of the less vital organs, such as kidney, digestive tract and carcass; this is associated with systemic lactic acidosis (Peeters *et al.* 1979).

Reduction in uteroplacental blood flow

The blood flow in the uteroplacental circulation can be reduced by occlusion of the maternal aorta (Lafeber 1981), ligation of one of the two uterine arteries (Wigglesworth 1964) or microsphere embolization of the uteroplacental circulation (Creasy *et al.* 1972). All methods can result in fetal hypoxia and growth retardation. However, a 50% reduction in the uteroplacental circulation is necessary before fetal hypoxia is produced (Wilkening & Meschia 1983). When the uteroplacental blood supply is reduced, the arteriovenous oxygen content difference increases, because there is an increase in the extraction of oxygen from maternal blood by the fetus (Clapp 1978). Fetal polycythaemia occurs, presumably to help maintain blood oxygen content (Pickart *et al.* 1976).

Reduction in placental size

When endometrial caruncles are removed before pregnancy in sheep, the number of 'placentae' is reduced and fetal hypoxia, polycythaemia, hypoglycaemia and growth retardation occur (Alexander 1964; Robinson *et al.* 1979).

Reduced oxygen transport

Reduction in umbilical blood flow

Reduction of umbilical blood flow by compression of the umbilical cord does not change the umbilical venous pO_2 in sheep (Itskovitz *et al.* 1983). However, ischaemic fetal hypoxia and a fall in oxygen consumption occurs when the umbilical flow is reduced by 50%. Until then, oxygenation is maintained by increasing the extraction of oxygen from the fetal blood (Clapp 1978). The high affinity of fetal blood provides a reserve of oxygen which can be used when the levels of pO_2 are low.

Another method of reducing umbilical blood flow is by ligation of an umbilical artery. This leads to transient hypoxia and, subsequently, fetal growth retardation (Emmanoulides *et al.* 1968).

Fetal anaemia

Exchange of fetal blood for plasma results in anaemia and decreased oxygen transport to the fetal tissues, because the blood oxygen content is reduced. In moderate anaemia, fetal oxygen consumption is maintained by increased extraction of oxygen from the blood but, when this is overcome, fetal hypoxia occurs (Edelstone *et al.* 1985). As in fetuses with reduced pO_2, fetal blood flow is increased to maintain oxygen delivery until severe anaemia occurs, when blood is redistributed to the brain and heart at the expense of the less vital organs (Fumia *et al.* 1984).

Reduced haemoglobin oxygen affinity

When fetal blood is exchanged for adult, which has a lower oxygen affinity, the haemoglobin oxygen saturation is reduced, despite a rise in umbilical venous pO_2 (Meschia *et al.* 1969). The fetal reticulocyte count rises, suggesting reduced fetal tissue oxygenation (Battaglia *et al.* 1969).

Limitations of animal studies

Despite the knowledge gained by the study of animal fetuses, extrapolation of these results to growth-retarded human fetuses is unwise, because of the differences in the placentae and fetuses of the various species, and the unknown nature of human 'placental insufficiency'. Furthermore, many of these 'models' also result in maternal and placental hypoxia, so that changes in fetal blood may merely reflect those in the mother. For example, uteroplacental blood flow falls in response to maternal hypoxia (Makowski *et al.* 1973), and therefore placental transfer and compensatory mechanisms may have been reduced.

Human data: during labour or at delivery

Capillary blood samples

In the 1960s Saling introduced a method for sampling fetal blood from the presenting part (usually scalp) after cervical dilatation and amniotomy in labour (Saling 1968). Subsequently, the lower limit of the normal range for scalp pH (7·20) was adopted as the cut-off point for the diagnosis of fetal acidosis and emergency delivery (Beard 1974). Using the scalp sampling technique it was shown that the fetal pH was lower than normal in pregnancies with hypertensive proteinuria (Lumley *et al.* 1969). Furthermore, fetuses of high-risk pregnancies, identified using clinical criteria, became acidotic in labour more quickly than those of normal pregnancies (Modanlou *et al.* 1974). These findings suggested either that such fetuses are chronically hypoxic or that they have reduced 'reserve' to the stress of labour.

Normal data

In early labour, the range of mean values of pH, pO_2 and pCO_2 is 7·29–7·34, 20–24 mmHg and 41–45 mmHg respectively (Saling 1963; Beard & Morris 1965; Kubli & Berg 1965; Lumley *et al.* 1969; Beard 1974). The values obtained immediately before delivery (mean pH = 7·28, pO_2 = 17 mmHg and pCO_2 = 51 mmHg; Saling 1968) are approximately half-way between those of umbilical arterial and venous blood after delivery.

Detection of fetal distress in labour

Intermittent fetal scalp blood sampling

This is widely used for the investigation of abnormal fetal heart rate patterns in labour and was found to be a sensitive method of detecting fetal distress (Tejani *et al.* 1976). It reduced the number of unnecessary caesarean section operations done because of false positive cardiotocograph results (Zalar & Quilligan 1979). More recently, Bowen *et al* (1986) found that the use of paired maternal and fetal blood samples improves the accuracy of the test by eliminating the effect of maternal acidosis or hyperventilation. Electrochemical methods of lactate determination are quick and accurate and require less than 100 µl of blood. It has been suggested that this measurement is as good as pH and better than the other blood gas and acid—base measurements in determining fetal condition (Eguiluz *et al.* 1983).

Continuous fetal scalp blood monitoring

A miniaturized glass pH electrode was developed which can be placed subcutaneously (Stamm *et al.* 1976). Initial problems included sterilization, calibration, fixation to the presenting part, and broken tips sometimes remaining in the fetal scalp. Furthermore, there was a poor correlation with intermittent fetal scalp blood measurements. Subsequently, the pH electrode was inserted through the core of an ECG electrode, already attached to the fetal scalp, and much better correlations with intermittent scalp blood results were obtained (Hochberg 1978). Huch *et al.* (1977) used an oxygen electrode attached to the fetal scalp and found a correlation between transcutaneous pO_2 and capillary blood pO_2. Transcutaneous monitoring of pCO_2 in labour has also been tried (Lysikeiwicz *et al.* 1981). Although these techniques have been used to investigate the factors that affect fetal oxygenation in labour, they have not received widespread clinical application.

Limitations of capillary blood samples

Scalp blood may be more acidotic than systemic samples because of the circulatory stasis that accompanies the formation of caput succedaneum (O'Connor *et al.* 1979). Alternatively, the scalp may be one of the last tissues to become acidotic, because of the head-sparing effect of the redistribution of blood in response to hypoxia.

Cord blood samples at delivery

Normal data

A large number of studies have investigated blood gas and acid–base parameters in human cord blood after normal term deliveries, and typical values are shown in Table 4.2.

Blood gas and acid–base measurements have also been made in cord blood samples obtained from second trimester fetuses at the time of hysterotomy abortions. The values for umbilical venous and arterial blood were: pH 7·31 and 7·24, pO_2 50 and 21 mmHg and pCO_2 43 and 55 mmHg respectively (Morris *et al.* 1974). Although the general anaesthesia, maternal preoxygenation and surgical procedure used could have altered the results, they were less hypoxic than those of term fetuses in labour or after normal delivery.

Human fetal blood oxygen affinity has also been studied, and the predominant haemoglobin of fetal blood has a different structure from adult (Brinkman & Jonxis 1935). Although in solution the oxygen affinity of these two haemoglobins is the same, *in vivo* fetal blood has a higher affinity (lower P_{50}) than adult because adult haemoglobin binds 2,3-DPG more strongly than fetal (Bauer *et al.* 1968; deVerdier & Garby 1969). It has been suggested that the higher oxygen affinity of fetal blood may help placental oxygen transfer. The proportion of adult haemoglobin in fetal blood rises with gestational age and so its affinity falls (Bard *et al.* 1970).

Pathophysiology of pregnancy complications

Most complications of pregnancy, including maternal toxaemia and diabetes, premature delivery and meconium staining of the liquor, are

Table 4.2. Human cord blood pO_2, pCO_2, pH and lactate after vaginal or elective caesarean delivery at term

Umbilical vein				Umbilical artery				
pO_2	pCO_2	pH	lactate	pO_2	pCO_2	pH	lactate	Reference
26				12				Quilligan *et al.* (1960)
29	40	7·32	4·1	18	49	7·25	4·6	Rooth & Sjostedt (1962)
24	43	7·30		15	57	7·25		Saling (1968)
	41	7·43				7·39		Crawford (1965)
			2·1					Eguiluz *et al.* (1983)
29	38	7·35		18	49	7·28	2·5	Yeomans *et al.* (1985)

associated with fetal hypoxia at birth (Low *et al.* 1975). Furthermore, 50% of growth-retarded fetuses are hypoxic, hypercapnic, acidotic or hyperlacticaemic at birth (Low *et al.* 1972). Hypoxic fetuses are poly-cythaemic (Finne 1966; Wirth *et al.* 1979) and have a higher proportion of fetal haemoglobin, which results in a higher oxygen affinity (Bard 1974).

Limitations of cord blood samples after delivery

Studies of blood gases in cord blood have been of great importance, both in improving the understanding of fetal physiology and in clinical prac-tice. However, measurements in scalp blood samples have shown that even normal labour alters blood gas and acid—base results and therefore studies after delivery do not necessarily reflect prelabour values. Fur-thermore, the observation that antenatal pregnancy complications pre-dicted fetal acidosis at birth better than complications during labour and delivery implies that fetal hypoxia often occurs before labour (Low *et al.* 1975).

Data from human pregnancies before labour

Hysterophotography

The first attempt to study human fetal oxygenation was by inspection of the colour of the umbilical cord vessels (Westin 1957). Fetuses at 14—18 week's gestation were photographed through a telescope introduced transcervically before elective abortion. Westin found that the fetus *in utero* did not look cyanosed and was much pinker than after delivery and concluded that the second-trimester human fetus was not as hypoxic as suggested by animal or postdelivery studies.

Amniotic fluid

Several investigators measured pH, pO_2 and pCO_2 in samples obtained by amniocentesis (Table 4.3). Although it was hoped that, as a result of diffusion through the fetal skin, amniotic fluid gases would indicate fetal oxygenation, no significant correlation was found with the umbilical arterial blood pO_2 (Sjostedt *et al.* 1961; Quilligan 1962). More recently, however, Koresawa *et al.* (1986) found that the amniotic fluid pO_2 was much higher than previously reported and that the values did correlate with cord blood values at delivery. The differences from the observations

Table 4.3. Human amniotic fluid pO_2, pCO_2 and pH

	pO_2	pCO_2	pH
Vasicka *et al.* (1960)	19		
Vasicka (1966)	9		
Sjostedt *et al.* (1961) a	11	51	7·12
b	7	57	7·04
Quilligan (1962) live	13	47	
dead	9	50	
Romney *et al.* (1962)	26		
Koresawa *et al.* (1986) (third trimester)	67	50	7·13

a = early pregnancy, b = late pregnancy.

made in the 1960s could be the result of improvements in the methods of measurement or differences in the patients sampled, and this area merits further investigation.

Intervillous blood

In the late 1950s and the 1960s, several investigators punctured the placenta, which they localized by abdominal palpation and auscultation, and aspirated blood before the onset of labour (Table 4.4). These studies were criticized because of the large variation in results (Fuchs *et al.* 1963), which may have been due to the 'blind' method of sampling and therefore the uncertainty as to whether the sampled blood was from the placenta, a uterine artery or vein, or even the fetus. These problems have been overcome by the use of an ultrasound-guided technique to obtain blood from placental 'lakes' (Fig. 4.2; Nicolaides *et al.* 1986a). When ultrasound-guided sampling of umbilical cord blood ('cordocentesis') is done through the placenta, both intervillous and fetal blood can be sampled in the same procedure. Similarly, when fetal blood sampling is done transamniotically, the needle can be advanced into a subchorionic 'lake' to sample intervillous blood. Using this technique, the intervillous blood pO_2 was found to fall with advancing gestational age and to be about 10 mmHg higher than the umbilical venous value (Fig. 4.3; Soothill *et al.* 1986b).

Fetal blood

The umbilical cord is usually punctured at its placental insertion and pure fetal blood can be aspirated (Rodeck & Campbell 1979). Initially,

Table 4.4. Human intervillous blood pO_2, pCO_2 and pH at term

	pO_2	pCO_2	pH
Quilligan *et al.* (1960)	23		
Sjostedt *et al.* (1960)	40		
Rooth & Sjostedt (1962)	45	37	7·25
Quilligan & Cibils (1964)	42		
Soothill *et al.* (1986c)	[42]*	33	7·40

* Changes with gestation: value for term.

the needle was guided by fetoscopy (Rodeck & Campbell 1978) but more recently by ultrasound (Daffos *et al.* 1983; Nicolaides *et al.* 1986a). Accurate identification of the vessel sampled is essential for blood gas studies and the best method is by ultrasonic observation of the turbulence produced after the intravascular injection of saline (Nicolaides *et al.* 1986a).

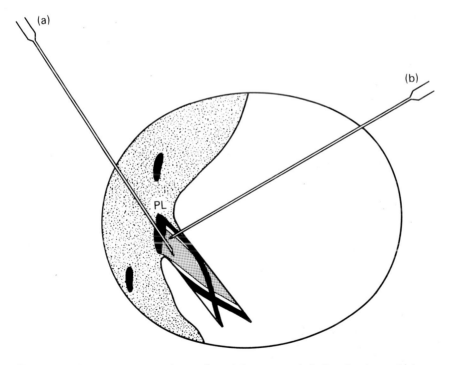

Fig. 4.2. Cordocentesis (a) transplacentally and (b) transamniotically. The placental lakes (PL) can be sampled for intervillous blood in the same procedure.

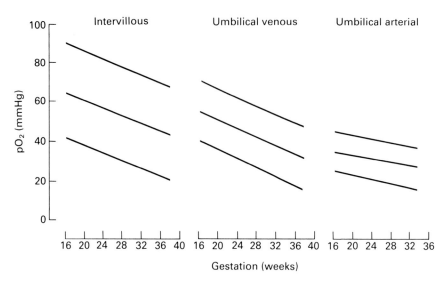

Fig. 4.3. The normal range (individual 95% confidence intervals) of pO_2 in intervillous, umbilical venous and umbilical arterial blood plotted against gestational age (adapted from Soothill *et al.* 1986b).

Normal data

Fetal blood sampling in the second trimester is usually performed for prenatal diagnosis of inherited disease. If the fetus is not affected by the condition under investigation its acid–base status is likely to be normal. Blood samples are also taken from fetuses in the third trimester found to have correctable malformations associated with chromosomal abnormalities (Nicolaides *et al.* 1986b). Many of the structural abnormalities would not affect blood gas and acid–base status (for example, mild hydronephrosis) when the karyotype is found to be normal. Reference ranges of umbilical venous and arterial blood gas and acid–base parameters were established by the study of 200 such cases at 16–38 weeks' gestation (Figs 4.3–4.6; Soothill *et al.* 1986d).

The results near term are similar to, but slightly less hypoxic, hypercapnic, acidotic and hyperlacticaemic than those found in cord blood after normal delivery (Table 4.2). The pO_2 decreases linearly with advancing gestation and this explains the high pO_2 found in second-trimester fetuses (Soothill *et al.* 1986a). Since intervillous blood pO_2 also falls with advancing gestation, the cause of the decrease in pO_2 could be decreased supply or increased consumption of oxygen.

Umbilical venous pCO_2, bicarbonate, base excess and plasma lactate

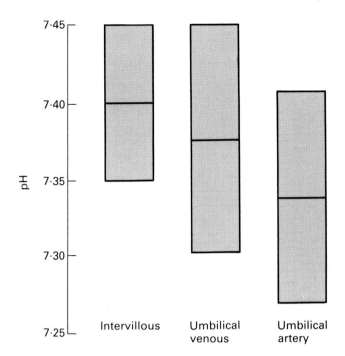

Fig. 4.4. The normal range (individual 95% confidence intervals) for pH in intervillous, umbilical venous and umbilical arterial blood (adapted from Soothill *et al.* 1986b).

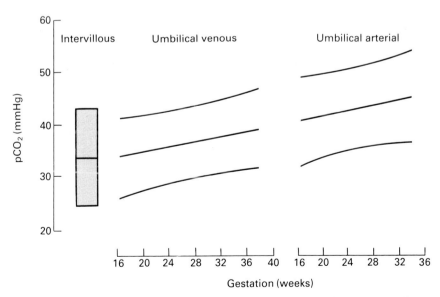

Fig. 4.5. The normal range (individual 95% confidence intervals) for pCO_2 in intervillous, umbilical venous and umbilical arterial blood (adapted from Soothill *et al.* 1986b).

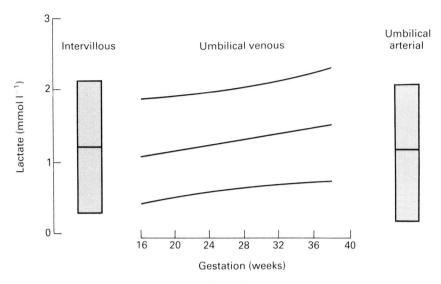

Fig. 4.6. The normal range (individual 95% confidence intervals) for plasma lactate in intervillous, umbilical venous and umbilical arterial blood (adapted from Soothill *et al.* 1986b).

rise with advancing gestation. However, the rise in umbilical venous but not umbilical arterial plasma lactate with gestation may indicate fetal consumption of lactate in normal human third-trimester fetuses, as found in animal studies (Burd *et al.* 1975).

The pO_2, pCO_2, pH and haemoglobin in 'arterial' (umbilical venous in the fetus) blood from the second trimester of pregnancy to the end of the neonatal period are shown in Fig. 4.7. There is an inverse relationship between the haemoglobin concentration and pO_2. This suggests that the human maintains a relatively constant blood oxygen content despite variations in pO_2. This is achieved by compensatory changes in haemoglobin concentration.

Pathophysiology of pregnancy complications

Anaemia

When the haemoglobin concentration falls to less than 70% of normal, the umbilical arterial plasma lactate rises and this is the earliest sign of fetal tissue hypoxia. The fetal blood oxygen content at which this occurs is 2 mmol l^{-1} (Fig. 4.8), which in sheep fetuses leads to redistribution of blood flow to the heart and brain at the expense of the less vital organs

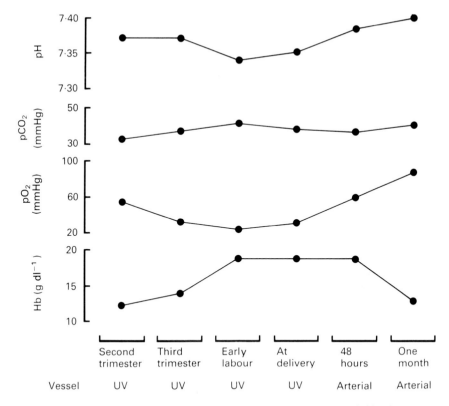

Fig. 4.7. The pH, pCO_2, pO_2 and haemoglobin concentration in 'arterial' blood (UV indicates umbilical vein) of normal humans from the second trimester of pregnancy to the end of the neonatal period. (Data from Soothill *et al.* 1986a, 1986b, Beard 1974, Yeomans *et al.* 1985, Nelson 1973 and Forfar *et al.* 1973).

(see before). It seems likely that a similar mechanism operates in human fetuses. However, the umbilical venous lactate remains normal until the haemoglobin concentration falls to less than 30%, presumably because the extra lactate is cleared from the fetal circulation in a single passage through the placenta (Fig. 4.9; Soothill *et al.* 1987b). Similarly, in severe anaemia, the umbilical arterial blood may be acidotic (Fig. 4.10) and therefore the bicarbonate and base excess are lower. However, no changes in umbilical venous pO_2, pCO_2, pH, bicarbonate or base excess are found (Soothill *et al.* 1987c). This is not surprising because, if the blood supplying an already compromised fetus was acidotic, a spiral of increasing acidosis would rapidly lead to fetal death.

Fetal 2,3-DPG concentration is increased in severe anaemia (Fig. 4.11; Soothill *et al.* 1988a), as in the adult (Torrance *et al.* 1970).

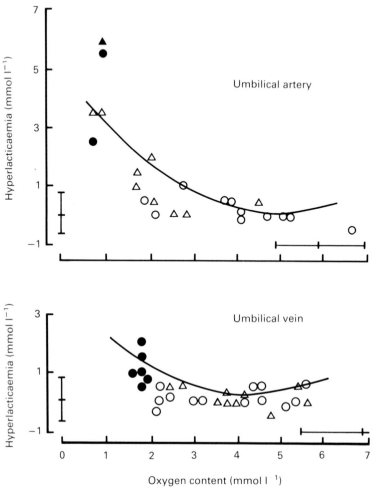

Fig. 4.8. The relationship of fetal hyperlacticaemia (observed plasma lactate minus normal mean for gestational age) to oxygen content in 32 rhesus-affected pregnancies. The normal ranges (mean + 2 SD) for each parameter are shown. The values from first (○) and subsequent (△) transfusions are shown and solid points indicate the values from hydropic fetuses (adapted from Soothill *et al.* 1987b).

Although fetal haemoglobin binds 2,3-DPG only 60% as well as adult, the fetus may adjust its haemoglobin oxygen affinity. In severe anaemia, when there is a low blood oxygen content but normal pO_2, a high 2,3-DPG level would reduce oxygen affinity and help delivery of oxygen to the tissues.

Adult blood (HbA) is used successfully to treat fetal anaemia, due to red cell isoimmunization (Rodeck *et al.* 1984; Nicolaides *et al.* 1987a).

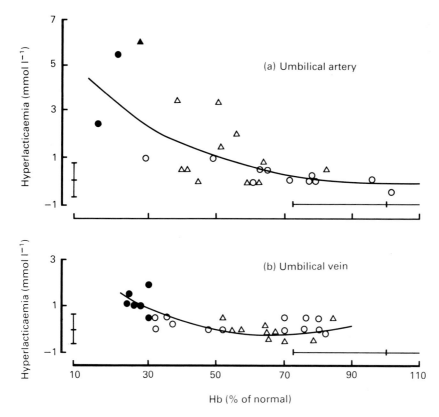

Fig. 4.9. The relationship of hyperlacticaemia (observed plasma lactate minus normal mean for gestational age) to haemoglobin concentration (expressed as a percentage of the normal mean for gestational age) in 32 rhesus-affected pregnancies. The normal ranges (mean + 2 SD) for each parameter are shown. The values before first (O) and subsequent (△) transfusions are shown and solid points indicate the values from hydropic fetuses (adapted from Soothill *et al.* 1987b).

When the blood gases of two groups of fetuses with similar haemoglobin concentrations were compared, umbilical arterial blood was significantly more acidotic and had a higher base deficit when adult rather than fetal blood was in the fetal circulation (Fig. 4.12; Soothill *et al.* 1988b). These findings suggest that fetal oxygenation is worse with HbA than with HbF.

Fetal growth retardation (IUGR)

Small fetuses can be (i) constitutionally small, with no increased perinatal mortality or morbidity, (ii) due to low growth potential ('fetal

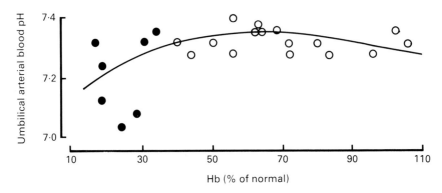

Fig. 4.10. The relationship between haemoglobin concentration (expressed as the percentage of normal for gestational age) and umbilical arterial blood pH ($r = -0.59$, $n = 23$, $P = 0.022$). It was significantly better described by a quadratic equation and the 'best fit' line is shown. Fetuses without hydrops fetalis are represented by open dots ($\bigcirc$), and those with hydrops fetalis by solid dots ($\bullet$) (from Soothill *et al.* 1987c).

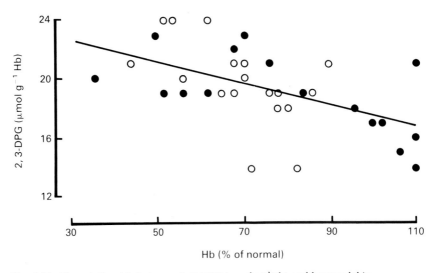

Fig. 4.11. The relationship between 2, 3-DPG (μmol g^{-1}Hb) and haemoglobin concentration (expressed as the percentage of normal for gestational age). Solid dots ($\bullet$) indicate samples obtained before any intrauterine blood transfusion and open dots ($\bigcirc$) indicate those which had received previous transfusions and so contained adult red blood cells (from Soothill *et al.* 1988a).

insufficiency'), the result of genetic disease or environmental damage, and (iii) the result of 'uteroplacental insufficiency', with an increased risk of hypoxia and a 10-fold increase in perinatal mortality.

In a study of 38 growth-retarded fetuses, in which cordocentesis was

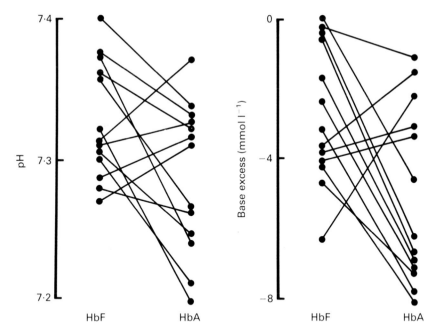

Fig. 4.12. Umbilical arterial pH and base excess in blood samples containing either fetal (HbF) or adult (HbA) haemoglobin, paired for Hb concentration. The samples with HbA are significantly more acidotic and have a higher base deficit than those with HbF (paired $t = -2.37$, $n = 26$, $P = 0.036$ and paired $t = -2.3$, $n = 26$, $P = 0.04$ respectively) (from Soothill *et al.* 1988b).

performed to exclude chromosomal abnormalities, the pO_2 was significantly lower than normal in about one-third (Fig. 4.13; Soothill *et al.* 1987d). The hypoxic IUGR fetuses were also acidotic, hypercapnic and hyperlacticaemic and had a high nucleated red blood cell count. These findings demonstrate that 'birth asphyxia' is not necessarily due to the process of birth and provide direct evidence that neonatal hypoxia and its consequences are often wrongly attributed to mismanaged labour (Illingworth 1979; Paul *et al.* 1986). The study also showed that the 'neonatal' complication of hypoglycaemia in growth retardation starts before labour (Fig. 4.14), and suggests that the reduced glycogen stores of small-for-dates neonates may be the result, rather than the cause, of the hypoglycaemia.

Histopathological studies have shown that in some pregnancies with IUGR there is failure of the normal development of maternal placental bed arteries into low resistance vessels (Brosens *et al.* 1977; Sheppard & Bonnar 1981). It has been suggested that failure of this physiological change to occur reduces nutrient supply to the fetus, resulting in IUGR.

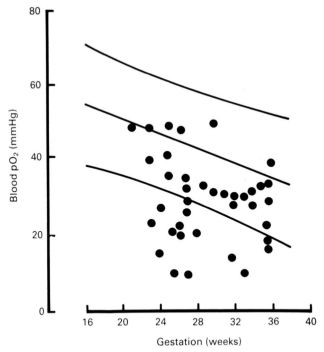

Fig. 4.13. The umbilical venous blood pO$_2$ of 38 growth-retarded fetuses plotted against the normal range (95% individual confidence intervals) for gestational age (adapted from Soothill *et al.* 1987d).

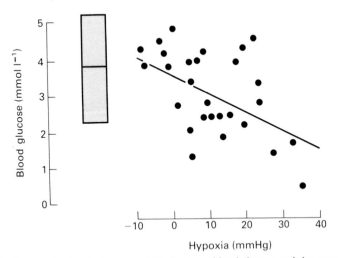

Fig. 4.14. The relationship between umbilical venous blood glucose and the severity of hypoxia (normal mean for gestational age minus observed pO$_2$) in growth-retarded fetuses. The shaded box represents the normal range of blood glucose (mean ± 2 SD). There was a significant negative correlation ($r = -0.58$, $n = 28$, $P < 0.002$) (adapted from Soothill *et al.* 1987d).

The uteroplacental blood velocity resistance index, determined by Doppler ultrasound scanning (Campbell *et al.* 1983), significantly correlated with the parameters of hypoxia in blood from fetuses with IUGR (Fig. 4.15; Soothill *et al.* 1986c). This supports the concept that one of the causes of IUGR is poor maternal blood supply leading to fetal undernutrition.

Evaluation of the non-invasive methods of fetal assessment

The measurement of fetal blood velocity by the Doppler effect on ultra-sound is used to assess fetal condition. Several studies found significant correlations between abnormal fetal blood velocity waveforms and poor perinatal outcome (Jouppila & Kirkinen 1984; Hackett *et al.* 1987). In growth-retarded fetuses the mean velocity of blood in the descending thoracic aorta correlated significantly with fetal blood gas and acid−base measurements (Fig. 4.16; Soothill *et al.* 1986d). These findings provide the first direct evidence that blood velocity measurements can detect fetuses with hypoxia.

We are investigating the relationship between fetal blood gas measurements and the findings of cardiotocography, kick count charts and biophysical profiles.

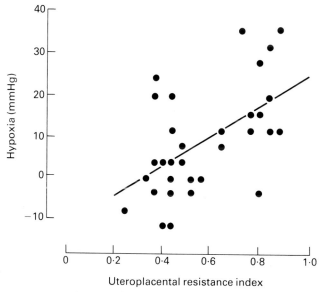

Fig. 4.15. The relationship between umbilical venous blood hypoxia (normal mean for gestational age minus observed pO_2) and the uteroplacental resistance index ($r = 0.55$, $n = 32$, $P < 0.001$) (from Soothill *et al.* 1986c).

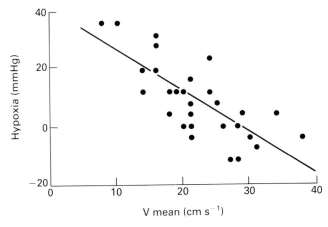

Fig. 4.16. The relationship between umbilical venous blood hypoxia (normal mean for gestational age minus observed pO_2) and the mean velocity (V mean) of blood in the fetal aorta ($r = -0.73$, $n = 29$, $P < 0.0001$) (from Soothill *et al.* 1986d).

Implications for fetal medicine

The example of red cell immunization shows that better understanding of the pathophysiology of a fetal disease can lead to successful antenatal diagnosis, therapy and prevention. Should the same process achieve a similar success in the management of conditions associated with fetal hypoxia, the impact on perinatal mortality and morbidity would be even greater. The benefits must be balanced against the risks of an invasive test but the procedure-related risk of fetal death in the hands of experienced operators is less than 1% (Daffos *et al.* 1985) and this would be lower still when the fetus is mature enough to be delivered in the event of fetal bradycardia or premature labour.

Timing and mode of delivery

In order to determine whether or not timing delivery by prelabour fetal blood gas measurements was useful, we compared the outcome of hypoxic or acidotic growth-retarded fetuses after two methods of management: (i) traditional, without knowledge of the blood gas results, and (ii) emergency delivery (unpublished observation). Hypoxia or acidosis was found in 14 fetuses; with conventional management 5 of 9 died, whereas all 5 delivered by caesarean section because of the blood gas results survived and are developing normally. These preliminary results suggest that timing the delivery of high-risk pregnancies by blood gas assessment may improve prognosis. Furthermore, the prognosis of fetuses with normal blood gas and acid−base results was excellent, and so this investigation may reduce unnecessary antenatal intervention such as maternal hospitalization, intensive fetal monitoring and premature delivery.

None of the hypoxic fetuses in this study had an abnormal karyotype. Occasionally, these abnormalities occur together, and, since chromosome analysis of fetal blood takes 2−3 days, karyotyping within a few hours, such as by direct chromosome preparation of placental biopsy (Nicolaides *et al.* 1986c), may be necessary.

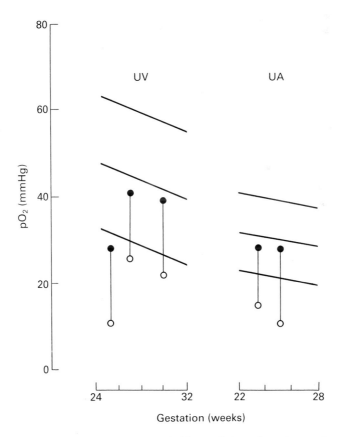

Fig. 4.17. Fetal blood pO_2 in 5 growth-retarded fetuses before (○) and after (●) 10 minutes of maternal hyperoxygenation plotted on the normal range for gestation (mean and individual 95% data intervals shown; UV = umbilical vein, UA = umbilical artery) (from Nicolaides *et al.* 1987b).

Fetal therapy

If a hypoxic or acidotic fetus is too immature for delivery, intrauterine therapy may be considered. For example, administration of oxygen to the mother can improve fetal pO_2 (Fig. 4.17; Nicolaides *et al.* 1987b). This may reduce the damage of hypoxia and allow the pregnancy to continue long enough for the fetus to be viable after delivery. This approach requires further study but the increasing understanding of fetal blood gas and acid−base pathophysiology is stimulating ideas about fetal therapy and allowing their more accurate assessment.

Medicolegal consequences

A very low cord pH at delivery has been used to imply poor labour management. The results reviewed in this chapter show that this is not necessarily the case. However, fetal acidosis at birth may be the result of inadequate prelabour assessment, which may need to include cordo-centesis and blood gas analysis.

Conclusions

The ideas and technologies developed in postnatal medicine can now be applied to the fetus because the uterus no longer prevents access. The derivation of the word obstetrics is 'to stand before' and the implied passive role of the obstetrician may result from the difficulty in fetal diagnosis. The study of fetal blood gases and the prenatal diagnosis of hypoxia illustrate the way in which fetuses will become patients. If over the next 30 years the diseases of the unborn are studied as enthusiasti-cally as those of childhood have been over the last 30 years, the advances in fetal medicine may mirror the great achievements in paediatrics.

References

Alexander G. (1964) Studies on the placenta of the sheep (*Ovis aries* L.): effect of reduction in the number of caruncles. *J. Reprod. Fert.*, **7**, 307−22.

Barcroft J. (1946) *Researches on Pre-natal Life, Vol 1*. Blackwell Scientific Publications, Oxford.

Barcroft J., Kennedy J.A. & Mason M.F. (1940) Oxygen in blood of umbilical vessels of sheep. *J. Physiol.*, **94**, 347−56.

Bard H. (1974) The effect of placental insufficiency on fetal and adult hemoglobin synthesis. *Am. J. Obstet. Gynecol.*, **120**, 67−72.

Bard H. & Shapiro M. (1979) Perinatal changes of 2,3-diphosphoglycerate and oxygen affinity in mammals not having fetal type hemoglobins. *Pediatr. Res.*, **13**, 167−9.

Bard H., Makowski E.L., Meschia G. & Battaglia F.C. (1970) The relative rates of synthesis of hemoglobins A and F in immature red cells of newborn infants. *Pediatrics*, **45**, 766–72.

Barron D.H. (1946) Appendix VII. In *Researches on Pre-natal Life* (Ed. by J. Barcroft), p. 285. Blackwell Scientific Publications, Oxford.

Barron D.H. & Battaglia F.C. (1955–6) The oxygen concentration gradient between the plasmas in the maternal and fetal capillaries of the placenta of the rabbit. *Yale J. Biol. Med.*, **28**, 197–207.

Battaglia F.C., Behrman R.E., Bruns P.D. *et al.* (1965) Gestational changes in arteriovenous differences of oxygen across the uterus of the rhesus monkey. *Am. J. Obstet. Gynecol.*, **93**, 32–43.

Battaglia F.C., Bowes W., McGaughey H.R., Makowski E.L. & Meschia G. (1969) The effect of fetal exchange transfusions with adult blood upon fetal oxygenation. *Pediatr. Res.*, **3**, 60–5.

Bauer C., Ludwig I. & Ludwig M. (1968) Different effects of 2,3-diphosphoglycerate and adenosine triphosphate on the oxygen affinity of adult and fetal human hemoglobin. *Life Sci.*, **7**, 1339–43.

Baumann R., Teischel F., Zoch R., & Bartels H. (1973) Changes in red cell 2,3-diphosphoglycerate concentration as cause of the postnatal decrease of pig blood oxygen affinity. *Resp. Physiol.*, **19**, 153–61.

Beard R.W. (1974) The detection of fetal asphyxia in labor. *Pediatrics*, **53**, 157–69.

Beard R.W. & Morris E.D. (1965) Foetal and maternal acid–base balance during normal labour. *J. Obstet. Gynaec. Br. Cwlth.*, **72**, 496–503.

Behrman R.E., Lees M.H., Peterson E.N., Lannoy C.W. de & Seeds A.E. (1970) Distribution of the circulation in the normal and asphyxiated female primate. *Am. J. Obstet. Gynecol.*, **108**, 956–69.

Bell A.W., Kennaugh J.M., Battaglia F.C., Makowski E.L. & Meschia G. (1986) Metabolic and circulatory studies of fetal lamb at midgestation. *Am. J. Physiol.*, **250**, E538–44.

Blunt M.H., Kitchens J.L., Mayson S.M. & Huisman T.H.J. (1971) Red cell 2,3-DPG and oxygen affinity in newborn goats and sheep. *Proc. Soc. Exp. Biol. Med.*, **138**, 800–3.

Bowen L.W., Kochenour N.K., Rehm N.E. & Woolley F.R. (1986) Maternal–fetal pH difference and fetal scalp pH as indicators of neonatal outcome. *Obstet. Gynecol.*, **67**, 487–95.

Brinkman R. & Jonxis J.H.P. (1935) The occurrence of several different types of haemoglobin in human blood. *J. Physiol.*, **85**, 117.

Brosens I., Dixon H.G. & Robertson W.B. (1977) Fetal growth retardation and the arteries of the placental bed. *Br. J. Obstet. Gynaecol.*, **84**, 656–64.

Bunn H.F. & Kitchen H. (1973) Hemoglobin function in the horse: the role of 2,3-diphosphoglycerate in modifying the oxygen affinity of maternal and fetal blood. *Blood*, **42**, 471–9.

Burd L.J., Jones M.D., Simmonds M.A., Makowski E.L., Meschia G. & Battaglia F.C. (1975) Placental production and foetal utilization of lactate and pyruvate. *Nature*, **254**, 710–11.

Campbell S., Griffin D.R., Pearce J.M. *et al.* (1983) New Doppler technique for assessing uteroplacental blood flow. *Lancet*, **i**, 675–7.

Clapp J.F. (1978) The relationship between blood flow and oxygen uptake in the uterine and umbilical circulations. *Am. J. Obstet. Gynecol.*, **132**, 410–13.

Comline R.S. and Silver M. (1970) pO_2, pCO_2 and pH levels in the umbilical and uterine blood of the mare and ewe. *J. Physiol.*, **209**, 587–608.

Comline R.S. & Silver M. (1974) A comparative study of blood gas tensions, oxygen affinity and red cell 2,3-DPG concentrations in foetal and maternal blood in the mare, cow and sow. *J. Physiol.*, **242**, 805–26.

Crawford J.S. (1965) Maternal and cord blood at delivery. *Am. J. Obstet. Gynecol.*, **93**, 37–43.

Creasy R.K., Barrett C.T., deSwiet M., Kahanpaa K.V. & Rudolph A.M. (1972) Experimental intrauterine growth retardation in the sheep. *Am. J. Obstet. Gynecol.*, **112**, 566−73.

Cummings J.N. & Kaiser I.H. (1959) The blood gases, pH, and plasma electrolytes of the sow and fetal pig at 106 days of pregnancy. *Am. J. Obstet. Gynecol.*, **77**, 10−17.

Daffos F., Cappella-Pavlovsky M. & Forestier F. (1983) Fetal blood sampling via the umbilical cord using a needle guided by ultrasound. Report of 66 cases. *Prenat. Diagn.*, **3**, 271−7.

Daffos F., Capella-Pavlovsky M. & Forestier F. (1985) Fetal blood sampling during pregnancy with use of a needle guided by ultrasound: a study of 606 consecutive cases. *Am. J. Obstet. Gynecol.*, **153**, 655−60.

deVerdier C.H. & Garby L. (1969) Low binding of 2,3-diphosphoglycerate to haemoglobin F. *Scand. J. Clin. Lab. Invest.*, **23**, 149−51.

Edelstone D.I., Caine M.E. & Fumia F.D. (1985) Relationship of fetal oxygen consumption and acid−base balance to fetal hematocrit. *Am. J. Obstet. Gynecol.*, **151**, 844−51.

Eguiluz A., Bernal L., McPherson K., Parrilla J.J. & Abad L. (1983) The use of intrapartum fetal blood lactate measurements for the early diagnosis of fetal distress. *Am. J. Obstet. Gynecol.*, **147**, 949−54.

Emmanoulides G.C., Townsend D.E. & Bauer R.A. (1968) Effects of single umbilical artery ligation in the lamb fetus. *Pediatrics*, **42**, 919−27.

Finne P.H. (1966) Erythropoietin levels in cord blood as an indicator of intrauterine hypoxia. *Acta Paediatr. Scand.*, **55**, 478−89.

Forfar J.O., Simpson H. & Russell G. (1973) Respiratory disorders. In *Textbook of Paediatrics* (Ed. by J.O. Forfar & G.C. Arneil). Churchill Livingstone, London.

Fuchs F., Spakman T. & Assali N.S. (1963) Complexity and nonhomogeneity of the intervillous space. *Am. J. Obstet. Gynecol.*, **86**, 226−33.

Fumia F.D., Edelstone D.I. & Holzman I.R. (1984) Blood flow and oxygen delivery to fetal organs as functions of fetal hematocrit. *Am. J. Obstet. Gynecol.*, **150**, 274−82.

Gahlenbeck H., Frerking H., Rathschlag-Schaefer A.M. & Bartels H. (1968) Oxygen and carbon dioxide exchange across the cow placenta during the second part of pregnancy. *Resp. Physiol.*, **4**, 119−31.

Hackett G.A., Campbell S., Gamsu H., Cohen-Overbeek T. & Pearce J.M.F. (1987) Doppler studies in the growth-retarded fetus predict neonatal necrotising enterocolitis, and haemorrhage, and neonatal morbidity. *Br. Med. J.*, **i**, 13−16.

Harington J.T., Cohen J.J. & Kassirer J.P. (1982) Introduction to the clinical acid−base disturbances. In *Acid Base* (Ed. by J.J. Cohen & J.P. Kassirer), pp. 113−20. Little, Brown, Boston.

Hochberg H.M. (1978) New instrument developments for fetal pH monitoring. In *Proceedings of the First International Workshop on Continuous Tissue pH Measurement in Obstetrics, Heidelberg. Arch. Gynaekol.*, **226**, 79−84.

Huber G.L. (1978) *Arterial Blood Gas and Acid−Base Physiology. Current concepts.* Upjohn, Kalamazoo.

Huch A., Huch R., Schneider H. & Rooth G. (1977) Continuous transcutaneous monitoring of fetal oxygen tension during labour. *Br. J. Obstet. Gynaecol.*, **84**, Suppl. 1, 1−39.

Huggett A. StG. (1927) Foetal blood-gas tensions and gas transfusion through the placenta of the goat. *J. Physiol.*, **62**, 373−84.

Illingworth R.S. (1979) Why blame the obstetrician? A review. *Br. Med. J.*, **1**, 797−801.

Itskovitz J., LaGamma E.F. & Rudolph A.M. (1983) The effect of reducing umbilical blood flow on fetal oxygenation. *Am. J. Obstet. Gynecol.*, **145**, 813−18.

Jouppila P. & Kirkinen P. (1984) Increased resistance in the descending aorta of the human fetus in hypoxia. *Br. J. Obstet. Gynaecol.*, **91**, 107−10.

Kaiser I.H. & Cummings J.N. (1957) Hydrogen ion and hemoglobin concentration, carbon dioxide and oxygen content of blood of the pregnant ewe and fetal lamb. *J. Appl. Physiol.*, **10**, 484−92.

Kaiser I.H. & Cummings J.N. (1958) pH, carbon dioxide, hemoglobin and plasma electrolytes in blood of pregnant goats and their fetuses. *Am. J. Physiol.*, **195**, 481—6.

Koresawa M., Shigemitsu S., Inaba J., Shibata J., Kubo T. & Iwasaki H. (1986) Amniotic gas analysis as an indicator of placental function. Personal communication.

Kubli F. & Berg D. (1965) The early diagnosis of foetal distress. *J. Obstet. Gynecol.*, 507—12.

Lafeber H.N. (1981) *Experimental intrauterine growth retardation in the guinea pig.* Thesis, University of Rotterdam.

Low J.A., Boston R.W. & Pancham S.R. (1972) Fetal asphyxia during the intrapartum period in intrauterine growth-retarded infants. *Am. J. Obstet. Gynecol.*, **113**, 351—7.

Low J.A., Pancham S.R., Worthington D. & Boston R.W. (1975) Clinical characteristics of pregnancies complicated by intrapartum fetal asphyxia. *Am. J. Obstet. Gynecol.*, **121**, 452—5.

Lumley J., Hammond J. & Wood C. (1969) Effects of maternal hypertension on fetal scalp blood pH, pCO_2 and pO_2. *J. Obstet. Gynaec. Br. Cwlth.*, **76**, 512—17.

Lysikeiwicz A., Vetter K., Huch R. & Huch A. (1981) Fetal transcutaneous pCO_2 during labour. Presented at the Second International Symposium on Continuous Transcutaneous Blood Gas Monitoring, Zurich, Switzerland.

Makowski E.L., Battaglia F.C., Meschia G. *et al.* (1968) Effect of maternal exposure to altitude upon fetal oxygenation. *Am J. Obstet. Gynecol.*, **100**, 852—61.

Makowski E.L., Hertz R.H. & Meschia G. (1973) Effects of acute maternal hypoxia and hyperoxia on the blood flow to the pregnant uterus. *Am. J. Obstet. Gynecol.*, **115**, 624—31.

Mann L.I. (1970) Effects in sheep of hypoxia on levels of lactate, pyruvate, and glucose in blood of mothers and fetuses. *Pediatr. Res.*, **4**, 46—54.

Maurer H.S., Behrman R.E. & Honig G.R. (1970) Dependence of the oxygen affinity of blood on the presence of foetal or adult haemoglobin. *Nature*, **227**, 388—90.

Meschia G., Prystowsky H., Hellegers A., Huckabee W., Metcalfe J. & Barron D.H. (1960) Observations on the oxygen supply to the fetal llama. *Quart. J. Exp. Physiol.*, **45**, 284—91.

Meschia G., Cotter J.R., Breathnach C.S. & Barron D.H. (1965) The haemoglobin, oxygen, carbon dioxide and hydrogen ion concentrations in the umbilical bloods of sheep and goats as sampled by indwelling catheters. *Q. J. Exp. Physiol.*, **50**, 185—95.

Meschia G., Battaglia F.C., Makowski E.L. & Droegemueller W. (1969) Effect of varying umbilical blood O_2 affinity on umbilical vein pO_2. *J. Appl. Physiol.*, **26**, 410—16.

Modanlou H., Yeh S. & Hon E.H. (1974) Fetal and neonatal acid—base balance in normal and high-risk pregnancies. *Obstet. Gynecol.*, **43**, 347—53.

Morris J.A., Hustead R.F., Robinson R.G. & Haswell G.L. (1974) Measurement of fetoplacental blood volume in the human previable fetus. *Am. J. Obstet. Gynecol.*, **118**, 927—34.

Myers R.E., de Courten-Myers G.M. & Wagner K.R. (1984) Effect of hypoxia on fetal brain. In *Fetal Physiology and Medicine* (Ed. by R. Beard & P.W. Nathanielsz). Marcel Dekker, New York.

Nelson N.M. (1973) The onset of respiration. In *Neonatology, Pathophysiology and Management of the Newborn* (Ed. by G.B. Avery). Lippincott, Philadelphia.

Nicolaides K.H., Soothill P.W., Rodeck C.H. & Campbell S. (1986a) Ultrasound-guided sampling of umbilical cord and placental blood to assess fetal wellbeing. *Lancet*, **i**, 1065—7.

Nicolaides K.H., Rodeck C.H. & Gosden C.M. (1986b) Rapid karyotyping in non-lethal malformations. *Lancet*, **i**, 283—6.

Nicolaides K.H., Soothill P.W., Rodeck C.H., Warren R.C. & Gosden C.M. (1986c) Why confine chorionic villus (placental) biopsy to the first trimester? *Lancet*, **i**, 543—4.

Nicolaides K.H., Soothill P.W., Clewell W., Rodeck C.H. & Campbell S. (1987a) Rh disease: intravascular fetal blood transfusion by cordocentesis. *Fetal Therapy*, **1**, 166—73.

Nicolaides K.H., Campbell S., Bradley R.J. Bilardo C.M, Soothill P.W. & Gibb D. (1987b) Maternal oxygen therapy for intrauterine growth retardation. *Lancet*, **i**, 942−5.

Novy M.J. & Parer J.T. (1969) Absence of high blood oxygen affinity in the fetal cat. *Resp. Physiol.*, **6**, 144−50.

O'Connor M.C., Hytten F.E. & Zanelli G.D. (1979) Is the fetus 'scalped' in labour? *Lancet*, **ii**, 947−8.

Paul R.H., Yonekura M.L., Cantrell C.J., Turkel S., Pavlova Z. & Sipos L. (1986) Fetal injury prior to labour: does it happen? *Am J. Obstet. Gynecol.*, **154**, 1187−93.

Peeters L.L.H., Sheldon R.F., Jones M.D., Mokowski E.L. & Meschia G. (1979) Blood flow to fetal organs as a function of arterial oxygen content. *Am. J. Obstet Gynecol.*, **135**, 639−46.

Pickart L.R., Creasy R.K. & Thaller M.M. (1976) Hyperfibrinogenemia and polycythemia with intrauterine growth retardation in fetal lambs. *Am. J. Obstet. Gynecol*, **124**, 268−71.

Prystowsky H., Meschia G. & Barron D.H. (1960) The oxygen tension in the placental bloods of goats. *Yale J. Biol. Med.*, **32**, 411−8.

Quilligan E.J. (1962) Amniotic fluid gas tensions. *Am. J. Obstet. Gynecol.*, **84**, 20−4.

Quilligan E.J. & Cibils L. (1964) Oxygen tension in the intervillous space. *Am. J. Obstet. Gynecol.*, **88**, 572−7.

Quilligan E.J., Vasicka A., Aznar R., Lipsitz P.J., Moore T. & Bloor B.M. (1960) Partial pressure of oxygen in the intervillous space and the umbilical vessels. *Am. J. Obstet. Gynecol.*, **79**, 1048−52.

Rivard G., Motoyama E.K., Acheson F.M., Cook C.D. & Reynolds E.O.R. (1969) The relationship between maternal and fetal oxygen tensions in sheep. *Am. J. Obstet. Gynecol.*, **97**, 925−30.

Robinson J.S., Kingston E.J., Jones C.T. & Thornburg G.D. (1979) Studies on experimental growth retardation in sheep. The effect of removal of endometrial caruncles on fetal size and metabolism. *J. Dev. Physiol.*, **1**, 379−98.

Rodeck C.H. & Campbell S. (1978) Sampling pure fetal blood by fetoscopy in the second trimester of pregnancy. *Br. Med. J.*, **ii**, 728−30.

Rodeck C.H. & Campbell S. (1979) Umbilical cord insertion as a source of pure fetal blood for prenatal diagnosis. *Lancet*, **i**, 1244−5.

Rodeck C.H., Nicolaides K.H., Warsof S.L. *et al.* (1984) The management of severe rhesus isoimmunization by fetoscopic intravascular transfusions. *Am. J. Obstet. Gynecol.*, **150**, 769−74.

Romney S.L., Kaneoka T. & Gabel P.V. (1962) Perinatal oxygen environment. *Am. J. Obstet. Gynecol.*, **84**, 25−31.

Rooth G. & Sjostedt S. (1962) The placental transfer of gases and fixed acids. *Arch. Dis. Child.*, **37**, 366−70.

Saling E. (1963) Dic Blutgasverhaeltnisse und der Saeure−Basen-Inhalt des Feten bei ungestoertem Geburtsablauf. *Z. Geburtsh Frauenheilk.*, **161**, 262−92.

Saling E. (1968) *Foetal and Neonatal Hypoxia*. Trans. F.E. Loeffler. Arnold, London.

Sheppard B.L. & Bonnar J. (1981) An ultrastructural study of the utero-placental spiral arteries in hypertensive and normotensive pregnancy and fetal growth retardation. *Br. J. Obstet. Gynaecol.*, **88**, 695−705.

Sjostedt S., Rooth G. & Caligara F. (1960) The oxygen tension of the blood in the umbilical cord and intervillous space. *Arch. Dis. Child.*, **35**, 529−33.

Sjostedt S., Rooth G. & Caligara F. (1961) The oxygen tension in amniotic fluid. *Am. J. Obstet. Gynecol.*, **81**, 1−7.

Soothill P.W., Nicolaides K.H., Rodeck C.H. & Gamsu H. (1986a) Blood gases and acid−base status of the human second trimester fetus. *Obstet. Gynecol.*, **68**, 173−6.

Soothill P.W., Nicolaides K.H., Rodeck C.H. & Campbell S. (1986b) The effect of gestational age on blood gas and acid−base values in human pregnancy. *Fetal Therapy*, **1:4**, 166−73.

Soothill P.W., Nicolaides K.H., Bilardo C., Hackett G. & Campbell S. (1986c) Utero-placental blood velocity resistance index and umbilical venous pO_2, pCO_2, pH, lactate and erythroblast count in growth retarded fetuses. *Fetal Therapy*, **1:4**, 174−8.

Soothill P.W., Nicolaides K.H., Bilardo C. & Campbell S. (1986d) The relationship of fetal hypoxia in growth retardation to the mean velocity of blood in the fetal aorta. *Lancet*, **ii**, 1118−20.

Soothill P.W., Nicolaides K.H., Rodeck C.H. & Campbell S. (1987a) Amniotic fluid and fetal tissues are not heated by obstetric ultrasound scanning. *Br. J. Obstet. Gynaecol.*, **94**, 675−7.

Soothill P.W., Nicolaides K.H., Rodeck C.H., Clewell W. & Lindridge J. (1987b) The relationship of fetal haemoglobin and oxygen content to lactate concentration in rhesus isoimmunized pregnancies. *Obstet. Gynecol.*, **69**, 268−71.

Soothill P.W., Nicolaides K.H. & Rodeck C.H. (1987c) The effect of anaemia on fetal acid−base status. *Br. J. Obstet Gynaecol.*, **94**, 880−3.

Soothill P.W., Nicolaides K.H. & Campbell S. (1987d) Prenatal asphyxia, hyperlactaemia and erythroblastosis in growth retarded fetuses. *Br. Med. J.*, **i**, 1051−3.

Soothill P.W., Lestas A.N., Nicolaides K.H., Rodeck C.H. & Bellingham A.J. (1988a) 2,3-Diphosphoglycerate in normal, anemic and transfused human pregnancies. *Clin. Sci.*, **74**, 527−30.

Soothill P.W., Nicolaides K.H., Rodeck C.H. & Bellingham A.J. (1988b) The effect of replacing fetal with adult haemoglobin on blood gas and acid−base parameters in human fetuses. *Am. J. Obstet. Gynecol.*, **158**, 66−9.

Stamm O., Latscha U., Janecek P. & Campana A. (1976) Development of a special electrode for continuous subcutaneous pH measurements in the infant scalp. *Am. J. Obstet. Gynecol.*, **124**, 193−5.

Sykes J.B. (1979) *The Concise Oxford Dictionary*, 6th edn. Oxford University Press, Oxford.

Tejani N., Mann L.I. & Bhakthavathsalan A. (1976) Correlation of fetal heart rate patterns and fetal pH with neonatal outcome. *Obstet. Gynecol.*, **48**, 460−3.

Torrance J., Jacobs P., Restrepo A., Eschback J., Lenfant C. & Finch C.A. (1970) Intra-erythrocytic adaptation to anaemia. *New Engl. J. Med.*, **283**, 165−9.

Van Geijn H.P., Kaylor W.M., Nicola K.R. & Zuspan F.P. (1980) Induction of severe intrauterine growth retardation in the Sprague−Dawley rat. *Am. J. Obstet. Gynecol.*, **137**, 43−7.

Vasicka A. (1966) Oxygen in the amniotic fluid. *Clin. Obstet. Gynecol.*, **9**, 461−71.

Vasicka A., Quilligan E.J., Aznar R., Lipsitz P.J. & Bloor B.M. (1960) Oxygen tension in maternal and fetal blood, amniotic fluid, and cerebrospinal fluid of the mother and the baby. *Am. J. Obstet. Gynecol.*, **79**, 1041−7.

Westin B. (1957) Technique and estimation of oxygenation of the human fetus *in utero* by means of hystero-photography. *Acta Paediatr.*, **46**, 117−24.

Wigglesworth J.S. (1964) Experimental growth retardation in the foetal rat. *J. Pathol. Bacteriol.*, **88**, 1−13.

Wilkening R.B. & Meschia G. (1983) Fetal oxygen uptake, oxygenation, and acid−base balance as a function of uterine blood flow. *Am. J. Physiol.*, **244**, H749−55.

Wirth F.H., Goldberg K.E. & Lubchenco L.O. (1979) Neonatal hyperviscosity: 1. incidence. *Pediatrics*, **63**, 833−6.

Yeomans E.R., Hauth J.C., Gilstrap L.C. & Strickland D.M. (1985) Umbilical cord pH, pCO_2, and bicarbonate following uncomplicated term vaginal deliveries. *Am. J. Obstet. Gynecol.*, **151**, 798−800.

Young I.M. (1952) CO_2 tension across the placental barrier and acid−base relationship between fetus and mother in the rabbit. *Am. J. Physiol.*, **170**, 434−41.

Zalar R.W. & Quilligan E.J. (1979) The influence of scalp sampling on the incidence of caesarean section performed for fetal distress. *Am. J. Obstet. Gynecol.*, **135**, 239−46.

5

Experimental Malformations and Their Correction

A.W. FLAKE & M.R. HARRISON

Introduction

> And in my mother's womb was fashioned to be flesh in the time
> of ten months, being compacted in blood, of the seed of man, and
> the pleasure that came with sleep. (Wisdom of Solomon 7.2)

Historically, our knowledge of matters within the womb has been in the realm of Solomon's wisdom. Profound and unassailable, but lacking in detail. Only in the last few decades have techniques for visualizing, monitoring, measuring and prodding the fetus begun to alter our perceptions of, and consequently our behaviour towards, the fetus. The fetus is now considered a patient, an individual whose maladies are a proper subject for medical treatment, as well as scientific observation (Harrison *et al.* 1984). The prenatal diagnosis of a fetal malformation may now allow therapeutic alternatives, such as changing the mode of delivery, or, in a few cases, treatment before birth.

The rationale for determining how the prenatal diagnosis of any given fetal defect will affect perinatal management is quite simple (Harrison *et al.* 1981a). Lesions incompatible with postnatal life may be aborted. Most surgically correctable lesions are best treated after normal term delivery, and maternal transport to a perinatal centre may improve outcome. Lesions causing dystocia require caesarean delivery. Reversible lesions causing progressive harm may require early delivery for immediate repair *ex utero*. Finally, a few lesions that cause progressive harm or prevent adequate organ development before the time of extrauterine viability may require treatment before birth.

It should be obvious that before attempting any intervention which involves risk to either the fetus or the mother, there must be a reasonable expectation that it is feasible, safe and effective. Although careful serial sonographic evaluation is beginning to elucidate the natural history of some human fetal malformations, most of the important questions about pathophysiology, efficacy of correction, and feasibility and safety of intervention cannot be answered from clinical studies. These questions must be answered experimentally in animal models. Establishing an animal model for a human malformation that may not occur spontaneously or reliably in animals has proved to be the most difficult part of the enterprise. Once the model has been established and the human defect simulated, the model may be used to explore the feasibility and efficacy of intervention. Most studies have been performed with 'easier' non-primate models, most notably the fetal lamb. Once questions of feasibility and efficacy have been dealt with, the final question of safety of intervention must be approached in the most difficult and rigorous fetal model, the non-human primate (Harrison *et al.* 1982a). The success of these experimental studies should approximate the success or failure of subsequent clinical application.

At present only three anatomical malformations theoretically amenable to prenatal treatment have been identified: (i) congenital diaphragmatic hernia; (ii) congenital hydronephrosis; and (iii) congenital hydrocephalus. In this chapter we shall briefly discuss our progress in the experimental creation and treatment of each of these malformations in the fetal lamb model.

Congenital diaphragmatic hernia

Congenital diaphragmatic hernia (CDH) is an anatomically simple defect that is easily correctable after birth by removing the herniated viscera from the chest and closing the diaphragm. However, 50% to 80% of all infants with CDH die of pulmonary insufficiency, despite optimal postnatal care, because their lungs are too hypoplastic to support extrauterine life, even at term (Harrison *et al.* 1979; Harrison & deLorimier 1981). Since the pulmonary hypoplasia appears to be a developmental consequence of compression by the herniated viscera, removal of this space-occupying lesion *in utero* should allow pulmonary development to proceed, so that pulmonary function will be adequate to support life at birth (Fig. 5.1).

We review six years of experimental work that supports the pathophysiological rationale for correction of CDH *in utero*.

The fetal lamb model

To study the pulmonary hypoplasia that accompanies CDH and the

Growth and development of the lung

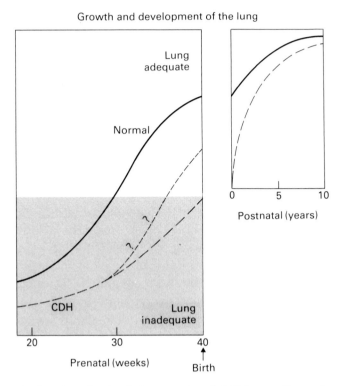

Fig. 5.1. Pathophysiological rationale for correction of CDH *in utero*. Human lung growth and development, on an arbitrary scale, are plotted against time before and after birth. The lung made hypoplastic by CDH can continue to grow and develop after neonatal correction (right inset). But most infants cannot survive the neonatal period, because the lung at birth is too small to support life. Experiments in lambs suggest that correction of CDH *in utero* will allow the lung to grow and develop enough before birth to improve survival at birth. (Reproduced, with permission, from Harrison *et al.* 1980b.)

possibility of reversing these changes by correcting the CDH *in utero*, we developed a model in which a conical, silicone-rubber balloon was progressively inflated in the left hemithorax of fetal lambs over the last trimester, to simulate compression by growing viscera (Harrison *et al.* 1980a). Lambs with inflated intrathoracic balloons, although vigorous at delivery, deteriorated rapidly, despite maximal resuscitation and ventilatory support. Deflation of the intrathoracic balloon in the neonatal period (simulating postnatal correction of the diaphragmatic hernia) did not significantly improve survival, because the lungs were already hypoplastic, with lung weight and air capacity significantly reduced ($P < 0.01$) compared with controls. Pressure–volume curves revealed decreased compliance, and barium–gelatin injections demonstrated a decreased cross-sectional area of the pulmonary vascular bed.

This model produced a clinical and pathological picture strikingly similar to that seen in infants with CDH. As in the human neonate with CDH, the neonatal clinical condition appeared to be a pathophysiological consequence of pulmonary hypoplasia. Once satisfied with the model, we could ask the crucial question: would the compressed lung grow and develop if decompressed *in utero* by deflating the balloon (Harrison *et al.* 1980b)? We found that deflation of the balloon at day 120 (simulated 'correction') allowed sufficient lung growth and development to alleviate respiratory insufficiency and to ensure survival in five of five lambs delivered by caesarean section. Lambs with simulated correction of CDH were easily resuscitated and were viable when resuscitation was discontinued after two hours. Because all lambs with simulated CDH died, it was apparent that simulated correction accounted for the improved survival. Simulated correction produced a significant ($P < 0.01$) increase in lung weight, air capacity, compliance and area of the pulmonary vascular bed (Fig. 5.2). The efficacy of *in utero* correction was confirmed by three studies of twins in which simulated CDH in one twin (uncorrected) was compared with simulated correction in the other. The twin

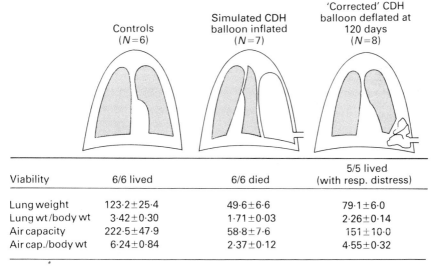

	Controls (N=6)	Simulated CDH balloon inflated (N=7)	'Corrected' CDH balloon deflated at 120 days (N=8)
Viability	6/6 lived	6/6 died	5/5 lived (with resp. distress)
Lung weight	123·2±25·4	49·6±6·6	79·1±6·0
Lung wt/body wt	3·42±0·30	1·71±0·03	2·26±0·14
Air capacity	222·5±47·9	58·8±7·6	151±10·0
Air cap./body wt	6·24±0·84	2·37±0·12	4·55±0·32

Groups are significantly different $P<0.01$ by analysis of variance or *T* test

Fig. 5.2. Summary of data in the fetal lamb model. Lambs with simulated CDH died, despite maximal resuscitation, and had severely hypoplastic lungs. Lambs 'corrected' by balloon deflation in the middle of the last trimester had sufficient lung growth and development to permit survival at birth. Lung weight and air capacity were greater than in lambs with CDH, but less than in controls. One lamb with CDH and three corrected lambs were delivered prior to planned caesarian section so viability could not be assessed. (Reproduced, with permission, from Harrison *et al.* 1980b.)

with simulated CDH died, whereas the corrected twin survived. The lungs of the corrected twin were larger and more compliant and had an increased pulmonary vascular bed. These studies demonstrated that simulated correction of CDH by deflating the thoracic balloon allowed sufficient lung growth to ensure survival at birth.

Feasibility and technique of fetal surgical correction

Although the balloon model established the pathophysiological efficacy of *in utero* repair, it could not be used to study the feasibility of correction or to develop the surgical techniques necessary for actual successful surgical repair. For this purpose we had to create, and then attempt to repair surgically, actual diaphragmatic hernias. We created diaphragmatic hernias by making a hole in the left diaphragm and demonstrated that herniated viscera produced pulmonary hypoplasia comparable to that produced by the balloon. We then tried to repair the CDH surgically at a second operation (Harrison *et al.* 1981b).

The first attempts at repair were unsuccessful. When we reduced the hernia and closed the diaphragm and abdominal wall, the first six fetuses all died in the perioperative period. To define the mechanism of fetal demise, the effects of intrathoracic and intra-abdominal pressure shifts secondary to returning the viscera from the chest to the abdomen were investigated. Acute studies showed that increased intra-abdominal pressure secondary to volume displacement severely compromised blood flow in the umbilical vein (Fig. 5.3). Intrathoracic volume displacement also affects umbilical flow, probably by shifting the mediastinum and impeding venous return. Because the fetus, unlike the neonate, is totally dependent on the umbilical circulation, it cannot tolerate the pressure shifts secondary to repair of CDH. This striking physiological difference between the fetus and the neonate must be considered in any surgical procedure on the fetal chest or abdomen.

From these experiments, it became clear that the abdominal cavity would have to be enlarged to prevent increased intra-abdominal pressure after CDH repair. Leaving a skin-covered ventral hernia proved unsatisfactory, because the fetal skin was too delicate. In addition, the fascial defect might continue to enlarge with the growth of the fetus, making subsequent abdominal wall closure difficult. Incorporating a piece of silastic into the abdominal wall and closing skin over it proved to be a satisfactory solution. The abdominal contents were accommodated without increased pressure, and the abdominal cavity and viscera grew concurrently, thus avoiding the problem of a massive abdominal wall hernia

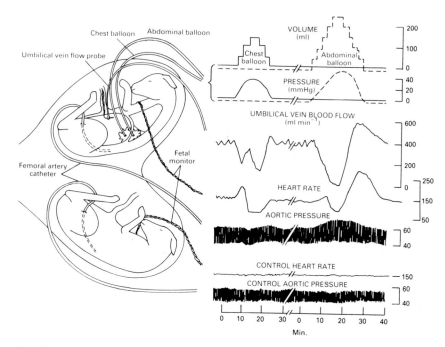

Fig. 5.3. To study the effect of increased intra-abdominal and intrathoracic pressure, silastic balloons in the fetal chest and abdomen were gradually inflated and deflated while umbilical-vein blood flow, aortic pressure and heart rate were continuously monitored. Increased pressure markedly reduced umbilical-vein flow. Bradycardia reflected fetal distress, and compensatory tachycardia occurred when pressure was released. Blood pressure changed little and was a poor monitor of fetal condition. (Reproduced, with permission, from Harrison *et al.* 1981b.)

with continued growth. To stabilize the mediastinum and minimize pressure–volume changes in the chest, the air in the partially empty left chest was replaced with warm Ringer's lactate solution before closing the diaphragm. Because this physiological solution can equilibrate and be absorbed, it provides volume replacement to offset fetal 'third-space' losses of surgery.

When we used these techniques (Fig. 5.4) for repair of the diaphragmatic hernia, six of ten lambs were viable after term delivery. In autopsied lambs, the lungs were well expanded, histologically mature, and much larger than those of the controls. These studies with surgically created CDH showed that correction of diaphragmatic hernia is technically feasible when an appropriate procedure is employed. The lamb model allowed us to develop the technique and prove its safety and feasibility.

Taken together, the studies with the intrathoracic balloon and the surgically created CDH in fetal lambs demonstrated that correction of

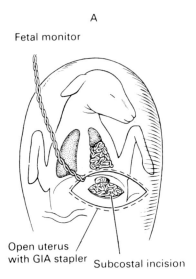

A

Fetal monitor

Open uterus
with GIA stapler   Subcostal incision

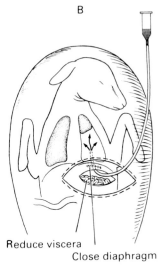

B

Reduce viscera
Close diaphragm

Fill chest with warm saline
and remove catheter

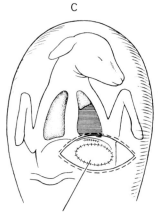

C

Silastic patch enlarges abdominal cavity
(close skin over patch)

Close hysterotomy with TA 90 stapler

Fig. 5.4. Technique for correction of CDH *in utero*. (A) Surgical exposure through a stapled hysterotomy. A screw-in fetal scalp electrode monitors fetal heart rate and variability during surgery. (B) The herniated viscera are reduced, the air in the chest replaced with warm Ringer's lactate, and the diaphragm closed with a single layer of nonabsorbable sutures. (C) The abdomen is enlarged by Silastic abdominoplasty, and the uterus closed with staples. Fetal operating time is less than 30 minutes. (Reproduced, with permission, from Harrison *et al.* 1981b.)

CDH *in utero*, with continued gestation to allow the lung to grow and develop enough to ensure survival at birth, is not only physiologically sound, but also technically feasible. However, this model differs from human CDH in several respects. Though death from human diaphragmatic hernia (CDH) has been attributed to respiratory insufficiency secondary to pulmonary hypoplasia, the major physiological abnormality is persistent fetal circulation. This correlates pathologically with an increase in muscle mass within the pulmonary arterioles. To answer these objections to our original model, we recently created CDH in fetal lambs very early in gestation, and subsequently performed morphometric analyses of the pulmonary vascular beds (Adzick *et al.* 1985).

Five fetal lambs had CDH created at 60 to 63 days' gestation (term = 140 to 145 days). The CDH was repaired in two lambs at 100 days' gestation, and left unrepaired in two others. All four lambs were delivered by caesarean section at term. The fifth CDH lamb was sacrificed at 100 days' gestation to assess morphometrics at that age. Preacinar arterioles were analysed for medial muscle thickness expressed as per cent external diameter (% ED) of the vessel (mean ± SEM). All lung specimens were compared with control lungs from age-matched, unoperated lambs.

The CDH group demonstrated smaller pulmonary arterial vessels, with a significant increase in pulmonary arteriolar medial wall thickness in the small preacinar (resistance) vessels. This effect was quite striking by 100 days' gestation, and it persisted until term. *In utero* repair of CDH at 100 days partially ameliorated this abnormal pulmonary arteriolar muscle hyperplasia and allowed impressive restoration of lung volume (Fig. 5.5) (Adzick *et al.* 1985).

From these studies, we conclude that the fetal lamb model simulates the pulmonary vascular morphological changes that correlate with fatal outcome for human neonates with CDH and persistent fetal circulation, and that fetal surgical repair of CDH ameliorates these vascular changes and permits compensatory lung growth and development.

Congenital hydronephrosis

Unrelieved urinary tract obstruction interferes with fetal development. The severity of damage at birth depends on the type, degree and duration of the obstruction (Harrison *et al.* 1981a,c, 1982b, 1983). Although children born with partial bilateral obstruction may have only mild hydronephrosis that is reversible with decompression after birth, children born at term with high-grade obstruction may already have advanced

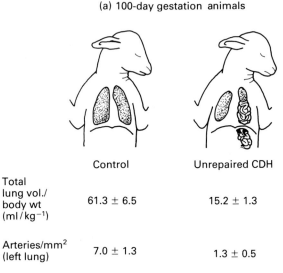

(a) 100-day gestation animals

	Control	Unrepaired CDH
Total lung vol./ body wt (ml/kg^{-1})	61.3 ± 6.5	15.2 ± 1.3
Arteries/mm^2 (left lung)	7.0 ± 1.3	1.3 ± 0.5

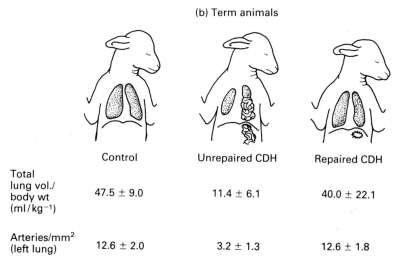

(b) Term animals

	Control	Unrepaired CDH	Repaired CDH
Total lung vol./ body wt (ml/kg^{-1})	47.5 ± 9.0	11.4 ± 6.1	40.0 ± 22.1
Arteries/mm^2 (left lung)	12.6 ± 2.0	3.2 ± 1.3	12.6 ± 1.8

Fig. 5.5. Pulmonary vascular morphometric analysis. (a) The CDH group demonstrated smaller pulmonary arterial vessels, with a significant increase in pulmonary arteriolar medial wall thickness in the small preacinar (resistance) vessels. This effect was quite striking by 100 days' gestation, and it persisted until term. (b) *In utero* repair of CDH at 100 days partially ameliorated this abnormal pulmonary arteriolar muscle hyperplasia and allowed impressive restoration of lung volume.

hydronephrosis (type 4 cystic dysplasia) that is incompatible with life. In addition, oligohydramnios secondary to decreased fetal urine output produces pulmonary hypoplasia, which is often fatal at birth.

It is possible that the life-threatening problems of respiratory and renal insufficiency may be averted or ameliorated if the obstruction is relieved early enough in gestation to allow normal development to proceed.

The fetal lamb model

In order to study the pathophysiology of fetal urethral obstruction and the efficacy and feasibility of correction *in utero*, it was necessary to develop an animal model with the following characteristics: (i) the model must simulate congenital hydronephrosis secondary to urethral obstruction in human infants (i.e. a high-grade obstruction to the flow of urine from the bladder into the amniotic fluid that produces severe bilateral hydronephrosis, hydroureter and megacystis and is associated with extrarenal manifestations such as pulmonary hypoplasia and skeletal deformities); (ii) the model must permit quantitative assessment of the effects of the obstruction on clinical condition at birth (i.e. survival) and on renal and pulmonary parenchymal development; and (iii) it must be possible to correct the obstruction *in utero* to restore urine flow into the amniotic cavity and to assess the consequences of correction on renal and pulmonary parenchymal development.

Despite our experience with the fetal lamb model for congenital diaphragmatic hernia (Harrison *et al.* 1980a,b, 1981b), we had great difficulty in developing a satisfactory model of human congenital hydronephrosis secondary to urethral obstruction in the fetal lamb (Fig. 5.6). Simple ligation of the urethra produced a urachal fistula, and ligation of both urethra and urachus produced such severe disease that the newborns did not survive. We then tried to produce a partial, graded urethral obstruction that would mimic posterior urethral valves in the human infant. Attempts to create a partial obstruction by passing the urine through a Pudenz catheter with a high opening pressure were unsuccessful. Attempts to intermittently occlude the flow of urine by compressing the urethra with a balloon constrictor or by exteriorizing the flow of urine with catheters also proved unsuccessful.

Finally, we produced the desired clinical and pathological findings by ligating the urachus and occluding the urethra with an ameroid constrictor or a ligature. Newborn lambs had respiratory distress and small lungs, but were viable with support. The bladder, ureters and renal pelves were severely dilated, mimicking the morphological disease in human neonates. The kidneys were hydronephrotic, but this relatively late obstruction did not lead to changes of cystic dysplasia.

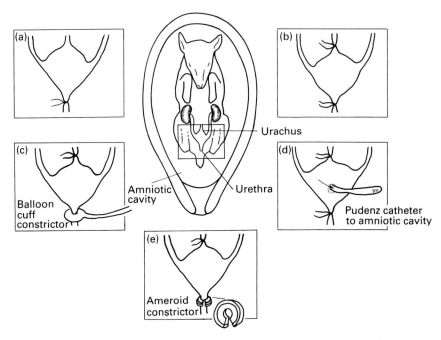

Fig. 5.6. Attempts to simulate urethral obstruction and congenital hydronephrosis in fetal lambs. (a) Ligation of the urethra. (b) Ligation of urethra and urachus. (c) Ligation of urachus and intermittent occlusion of the urethra with a balloon constrictor. (d) Ligation of urachus and pressure-limited obstruction with a Pudenz catheter (suprapubic, as shown, or transurethral). (e) Ligation of urachus and gradual occlusion of the urethra with an ameroid constrictor. (Reproduced, with permission, from Harrison *et al*. 1983.)

This model mimicked the clinical and pathological features of bilateral congenital hydronephrosis secondary to urethral obstruction in the human neonate and made it possible to study whether decompression of the obstructed urinary tract before birth would affect development of the fetal kidneys and lungs.

Feasibility and technique of fetal surgical correction

With the fetal lamb model described above, we could study the effect of obstruction and its subsequent correction on pulmonary and renal development. We obstructed the urethra of 43 fetal lambs at 95 to 105 days' gestation (Fig. 5.7). As in all fetal work, there was a frustratingly high rate of fetal loss. We then decompressed some of the obstructed fetuses by performing a suprapubic cystostomy at a second operation about three weeks later.

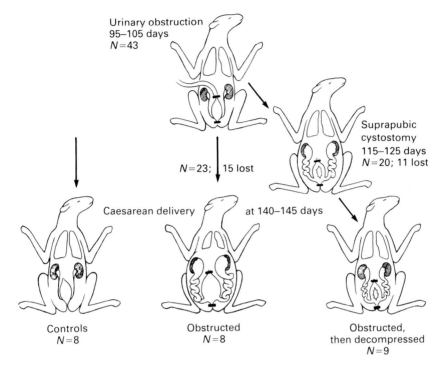

Urinary obstruction
95–105 days
N=43

Suprapubic
cystostomy
115–125 days
N=20; 11 lost

N=23; | 15 lost

Caesarean delivery　　　at 140–145 days

Controls
N=8

Obstructed
N=8

Obstructed,
then decompressed
N=9

Fig. 5.7. The fetal lamb model: summary of procedures. Pregnancy losses make these experiments difficult and expensive. (Reproduced, with permission, from Harrison *et al.* 1982b.)

We were able to compare obstructed, decompressed and control lambs after birth (Fig. 5.8). Urethral obstruction and urachal ligation produced severe hydronephrosis, hydroureter, megacystis, and urinary ascites, as well as significant pulmonary hypoplasia. The eight uncorrected lambs did poorly. At birth, all four liveborn obstructed lambs had respiratory insufficiency, and only one survived. Four others were stillborn. The lungs were significantly hypoplastic by weight and volume ($P < 0.025$). All eight had advanced megacystis, hydroureter and hydronephrosis, but no cystic dysplastic renal changes. By contrast, the corrected lambs fared much better. Seven liveborn lambs diverted *in utero* had far less respiratory difficulty, and all survived. Two others were stillborn. The lung weight was significantly increased $P < 0.05$). All lambs undergoing *in utero* decompression showed significant resolution of the severe urinary tract dilatation seen in the obstructed lambs.

These studies began to address some of the important questions about congenital hydronephrosis and the possibility of correction *in*

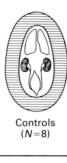

	Controls (N=8)	Obstructed (N=8)	Obstructed, decompressed (cystostomy) (N=9)
Viability	8/8	1/4 (with resp. distress)	7/7 (with resp. distress)
(Stillborn)	0	4	2
Urinary tract dilatation	none	2+ to 4+	1+ to 2+
Lung wt/body wt %±SD	3·03±0·90	1·85±0·46	2·61±0·48
Air cap./body wt %±SD	5·64±2·07	2·59±0·76	4·34±1·26

Fig. 5.8. Summary of data. Obstructed lambs had a high mortality, small lungs and grossly dilated urinary tracts. Decompression *in utero* significantly improved survival, lung size and urinary tract dilatation. Four obstructed lambs and two decompressed lambs delivered vaginally prior to planned caesarean section so viability could not be assessed. (Reprinted, with permission, from Harrison *et al.* 1982b.)

utero. What is the effect of fetal urethral obstruction and decompression on pulmonary development? It is clear that the lamb whose urinary tract is obstructed over the last trimester is born with very small lungs, which usually prevent survival, whereas the lamb whose obstruction is decompressed in the middle of the last trimester is born with lungs that are significantly larger and usually adequate to support postnatal life.

How closely does this study of pulmonary hypoplasia in fetal lambs parallel the human situation? The principal problem with all animal models of fetal malformations, such as those we have developed for urinary tract obstruction and congenital diaphragmatic hernia, is that the surgical alterations in lambs have been created relatively late in gestation, compared with the human counterpart. Although the lungs in lambs with urinary tract obstruction are small, their histology and developmental stage are not different from fully mature lungs of normal controls. Clinical evidence suggests that the developmental insult causing pulmonary hypoplasia in both congenital diaphragmatic hernia and congenital hydronephrosis occurs much earlier in gestation. In human newborns with these conditions, the hypoplastic lungs have a decreased number of airway branches from segmental bronchi, reflecting compromised development during the first half of gestation (Reid 1977; Inselman & Mellins 1981; Liggins & Kitterman 1981; Wigglesworth *et al.* 1981).

Our experiments demonstrate that the lung compressed later in gestation is capable of resuming normal growth and development if decompressed during the last trimester (when total lung growth is greatest). Although the human lung made hypoplastic by an earlier insult would not be expected to produce new airway branches, it retains the capacity to make new alveoli and new intra-acinar vessels well into the postnatal period (Reid 1977; Inselman & Mellins 1981; Liggins & Kitterman 1981; Wigglesworth *et al.* 1981; Hislop *et al.* 1979). Therefore, prenatal pulmonary decompression to allow continued growth should be clinically applicable. The lung with a reduced number of bronchial branches from an early insult, but with adequate alveolar development from later decompression, may eventually function normally, as seen in children surviving repair of congenital diaphragmatic hernia.

What is the effect of fetal urethral obstruction and its later correction on development of the urinary tract and kidneys? Urethral obstruction during the last trimester produces progressive distortion of the urinary tract: bladder dilatation and hypertrophy, massive megaureters and bilateral hydronephrosis. The fetal abdomen is distended not only from the massively dilated urinary tract, but often from urinary ascites formed from either transudation or a small (usually undetectable) direct leak (Griscom *et al.* 1977). In our fetal lambs, decompression of the obstructed urinary tract into the amniotic fluid reversed all of these ill effects to a dramatic degree.

Because the typical cystic and dysplastic changes seen in human urinary tract malformations were not produced by this relatively late obstruction, we could not ask what effect decompression had on dysplasia. Cystic dysplasia may be the consequence of urinary obstruction at an earlier stage of gestation than that used in this experiment (90 to 100 days). Unfortunately, when the fetal lamb urethra is ligated before 90 days, spontaneous urachal decompression protects the renal parenchyma from obstructive damage (Tanagho 1972a; Harrison *et al.* 1983). In order to answer the crucial question about the relationship between early fetal obstruction and the development of dysplasia, we needed a new experimental model.

The renal dysplasia model

Are renal dysplastic changes secondary to obstruction, or is dysplasia an independent process? Previous experimental studies have failed to resolve this controversy (Thomasson *et al.* 1970; Beck 1971; Tanagho 1972a, b, c; Harrison *et al.* 1982b, 1983). In most fetal models, including our own, obstruction produced late in gestation (third trimester) does not lead to renal dysplasia, possibly because the obstruction occurs too late in gestation to affect a crucial stage of kidney development. In an attempt to clarify this problem, we sought a fetal animal model with the following characteristics: (i) fetal urinary tract obstruction early enough in gestation to affect the nephrogenic phase of kidney development (i.e. early second trimester); (ii) avoidance of oligohydramnios and its life-limiting sequelae of pulmonary hypoplasia; (iii) ability to study the developmental effect of obstruction on the kidney at term; (iv) ability to study the developmental effect of decompression of the obstructed kidney.

To test whether obstruction earlier in fetal life leads to renal dysplasia, we produced unilateral obstruction in fetal lambs at 55 to 65 days' gestation (term = 140 to 145 days) (Glick *et al.* 1984a). The lambs were delivered by caesarean section near term and were resuscitated, and viability was determined prior to sacrifice. At autopsy, we found that the affected kidney was both hydronephrotic, with ureteral and calyceal dilatation proximal to the ligation, and dysplastic (Figs 5.9 and 5.10). Cut sections showed capsular scarring and numerous cortical cysts (Fig. 5.10, group 4). Microscopy of the atrophic obstructed kidney showed diffuse fibrosis, especially in the peripelvic area, which extended into the renal interstitium and around large vessels. Numerous dilated tubules and ectatic lymphatics, which form subcapsular microcysts, were present. Although foci of reactive and metaplastic tubular epithelium were identified, no heterotopic tissue was present. These changes, in particular the fibrosis, distort the cortex and medulla, producing focal parenchymal disorganization. The unobstructed contralateral kidney was unaffected. These pathological changes are strikingly similar to those seen in the kidneys of human neonates with obstructive uropathy (Potter & Craig 1975).

These experiments suggest that the renal dysplasia associated with obstructive uropathy may in fact be caused by simple obstruction to the flow of fetal urine early in gestation. This model allowed us to determine whether dysplasia secondary to obstructive uropathy is reversible by decompression before birth.

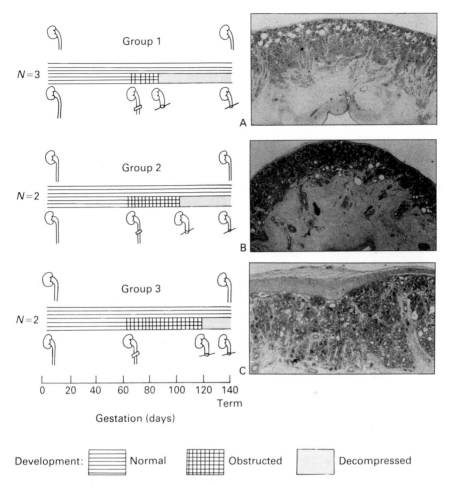

Fig. 5.9. Fetal lamb renal dysplasia model, histopathological changes. Histology of kidneys obstructed for different lengths of time prior to decompression *in utero*. (A) Kidney from group 1 lamb (obstructed 65 days, decompressed 85 days) shows minimal cortical changes and minimal interstitial fibrosis associated with small subcapsular dilated structures. There is atrophy of medullary pyramids with loose pericalyceal fibrosis (haematoxylin−eosin; magnification × 6·5). (B) Kidney from group 2 lamb (obstructed 65 days, decompressed 105 days) shows cortical features similar to group 1, but slightly increased pericalyceal fibrosis (haematoxylin−eosin; magnification × 6·5). (C) Kidney from group 3 lamb (obstructed 65 days, decompressed 125 days) shows cortical features similar to A and B, but increased pericalyceal and corticomedullary pyramid atrophy. There is a marked histological difference between this group and group 5B (see Fig. 5.10) (haematoxylin−eosin; magnification × 5·5. (Reproduced, with permission, from Glick *et al.* 1984a.)

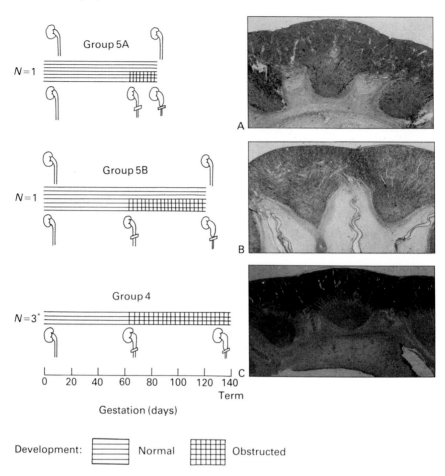

Fig. 5.10. Histology of the kidneys still obstructed at time of sacrifice. (A) Kidney from group 5A lamb (obstructed 65 days, sacrificed 85 days) shows dilatation of subcapsular structures with some dilated medullary tubules. There is increased interstitial fibrosis tissue throughout, especially in pericalyceal area (haematoxylin–eosin; magnification × 5·5). (B) Kidney from group 5B (obstructed 65 days, sacrificed 125 days) shows severe interstitial fibrosis in cortex, severe calyceal fibrosis, marked medullary pyramid atrophy and few dilated subcortical structures. Although distorted by fibrosis, the changes are insufficient for dysplasia (haematoxylin–eosin; magnification × 5·5). (C) Kidney from group 4 lamb (obstructed 65 days, sacrificed 140 days) shows parenchymal atrophy and severe fibrosis throughout. Resulting disorganization is consistent with renal dysplasia (haematoxylin–eosin; magnification × 5·5). (Reproduced, with permission, from Glick *et al.* 1984a.)

In utero decompression prevents renal dysplasia

We used the fetal lamb renal dysplasia model to attempt to answer two questions (Glick *et al.* 1984a). First, is renal dysplasia associated with congenital urinary tract obstruction preventable/reversible by *in utero* decompression? And, second, if it is, at what stage of development must this decompression be done? Following early second-trimester unilateral ureteral ligation in 25 fetal lambs, the fetuses underwent reoperation after one of three predetermined intervals (group 1, 20 days: group 2, 40 days; group 3, 60 days). At reoperation, the obstructed ureter was dissected and a percutaneous end-ureterostomy was performed. The fetus was then returned to the uterus, and was subsequently delivered at term by caesarean section. Each newborn had a ureterostomy catheter, suprapubic catheter, and umbilical vein catheter inserted, and the function of the previously obstructed kidney (obstructed) was compared to the contralateral control kidney (con). Hourly urine volume was measured separately for each kidney for four hours. To measure glomerular filtration rate (GFR), iothalamate (150 mg kg^{-1}) was given intravenously (IV) to each newborn prior to collecting hourly urines and an aliquot of each hourly urine sample was analysed for iothalamate concentration ([iothal]) by excitation electron analysis (Guesry *et al.* 1975). An iothalamate clearance ratio (ICR) was calculated for each hourly sample and the ICR results in each group were combined:

$$ICR = \frac{([iothal])_{obstructed} \times (vol)_{obstructed}}{([iothal])_{con} \times (vol)_{con}}$$

Theoretically, if each lamb's kidneys had an equivalent GFR, then the ICR would be equal to one.

The renal function and autopsy data are summarized in Table 5.1. When compared to the contralateral unobstructed kidney, there was a significant correlation between the duration of *in utero* ureteral decompression and urine output at birth. The ICR was similarly affected, except that the ICR for group 2 was better than that for group 1.

At term, the severity of histopathological changes seen in the various groups formed a continuum and was proportional to the length of time the obstruction existed; group 1 had less severe changes than group 2, where changes were less severe than in group 3. All of the decompressed kidneys were less severely affected than those of group 4 (Figs 5.9 and 5.10). Generally, the renal parenchyma on the side of the previously obstructed ureter appeared thinner than that of the contralateral control, with the medulla being the most severely affected portion of the renal parenchyma. The size of the medullary pyramids was decreased in proportion to the length of time the kidney was obstructed.

This study demonstrates that ureteral obstruction at 65 days, with

Table 5.1. Renal function and autopsy data of the fetal lamb dysplasia model (reproduced, with permission, from Glick *et al.* 1984a)

Treatment group	Days of gestation		Viability/ N*	Kidney designation	Findings at birth			
	Obstructed	Decompressed			Renal function		Autopsy data	
					Urine output (ml h⁻¹ kg⁻¹)	ICR	Weight (mg kg⁻¹)	Histopathology

	Obstructed	Decompressed	N*	designation	Urine output	ICR	Weight	Histopathology
1	65 to 85	86 to 140	3/8	Obstructed	2·8 ± 1·2 $P = 0.06$	0·39 ± 0·14	1·4 ± 0·3 $P > 0·05$	Minimal obstructive changes
2	65 to 105	106 to 140	2/5	Control	4·8 ± 2·6		3·7 ± 1·1	Normal
				Obstructed	3·8 ± 1·8 $P < 0·05$	0·47 ± 0·23	1·4 ± 0·3 $P > 0·05$	Moderate obstructive changes
3	65 to 125	126 to 140	2/6	Control	7·0 ± 4·5		3·3 ± 0·0	Normal
				Obstructed	2·9 ± 1·2 $P < 0·01$	0·22 ± 0·11 $P = 0·05$	1·9 ± 0·4 $P = 0·05$	Severe obstructive changes
4†	65 to 140	NA	3/6	Control	5·9 ± 2·2		4·8 ± 0·1	Normal
				Obstructed	NA	NA	2·6 ± 1·3 $P > 0·05$	Renal dysplasia
				Control	NA		4·2 ± 0·9	Normal

* *N* represents initially obstructed fetuses minus excluded fetuses.
† Previously reported data.
ICR = iothalamate clearance ratio.

subsequent decompression prior to term, prevents renal dysplasia and produces reversible postobstructive changes. At term, the degree of pathological changes seen in the obstructed and then decompressed kidneys was proportional to the length of time the obstruction existed. Thus, both the timing and duration of obstruction are crucial in producing dysplastic morphogenesis.

The recovery of renal function after experimental fetal urinary tract obstruction has not been previously reported. In this experiment, recovery of renal function was directly proportional to the duration of decompression and inversely proportional to the duration of obstruction. However, in every instance, the obstructed kidney had inferior renal function to its contralateral control.

Fetal hydrocephalus

Hydrocephalus can result in significant neurological impairment and a poor prognosis despite early detection and treatment after birth (Harrison *et al.* 1984). The frequent detection of fetal hydrocephalus by prenatal sonography has prompted consideration of decompression of the ventricles before birth, to ameliorate maldevelopment and functional impairment before it occurs (Birnholz & Frigoletto 1981; Michejda & Hodgen 1981; Clewell *et al.* 1982; Harrison *et al.* 1984). The rationale for prenatal treatment depends on two assumptions: first, that dilatation of the fetal ventricles, and its deleterious effect on brain development, is the result of obstruction of the cerebrospinal fluid (CSF) pathways and secondary increased intraventricular pressure; and, second, that early gestational relief of this increased pressure can avert the irreversible damage seen at term and allow normal development to proceed.

The fetal lamb and rhesus monkey models

To develop a model of congenital hydrocephalus in the fetus, we operated on time-dated pregnant ewes and rhesus monkeys (Nakayama *et al.* 1983). Fetal lambs and fetal monkeys underwent one of two procedures designed to obstruct CSF flow at the outlet foramina of the fourth ventricle.

1 Four fetal rhesus monkeys and five fetal lambs underwent percutaneous, subarachnoid injection of silicone oil through the posterior atlanto-occipital membrane. Silicone oil is a high-viscosity, non-reactive substance which has been used to obstruct CSF flow by its immiscible bulk.

2   Six fetal monkeys and twelve fetal lambs underwent subarachnoid injection of kaolin (J.T. Baker Chemical Co., Phillipsburg, NJ, USA) through the posterior atlanto-occipital membrane. Kaolin is an irritative substance which blocks CSF flow by inciting an inflammatory reaction.

The progression of ventriculomegaly was followed by sonography until delivery. Animals underwent caesarean delivery at 160−165 days' gestation.

Newborns with gross head enlargement were sacrificed 2 hours after birth and autopsies were performed. Newborns without gross head enlargement were followed closely for clinical signs of hydrocephalus, i.e. rapid head enlargement, bulging fontanelle or behavioural abnormality. If no CNS abnormalities were noted either clinically or sonographically, the animals were considered not to have hydrocephalus and were not sacrificed.

The surgical outcome is summarized in Table 5.2. Kaolin reproducibly caused hydrocephalus in our model, while silicone oil failed to occlude CSF flow. The high viscosity of silicone oil made injection unwieldy and poorly reproducible. None of these fetuses had evidence of hydrocephalus on prenatal sonography or postnatal observation.

In contrast, the watery kaolin suspension was easily injected with reproducible results. Marked ventriculomegaly was noted on prenatal sonography within 2−4 weeks after kaolin injection and the fetuses were born with enlarged heads, diastasis of cranial sutures and bulging fontanelles. The gross and histologic findings after kaolin injection were similar to those reported by other investigators who used the same technique in other species (Schurr *et al.* 1953; Wisniewski *et al.* 1969). Gross examination of cut sections of the brain after harvest and fixation revealed marked ventricular dilatation and a small degree of cortical thinning. The leptomeninges were thickened in the area of kaolin injection and microscopic examination revealed mild fibrous and inflammatory cell response in the areas of leptomeningeal thickening. This infiltrate into the subarachnoid space obstructed the foramina of Luschka and Magendie, and in some cases extended into the fourth ventricle and the aqueduct of Sylvius. Hydrocephalic brains showed marked thinning of the mantle with relative preservation of the cortex. The architecture of the grey matter was essentially normal. Neural processes were of normal complexity and density on Bodian stain sections. In contrast cerebral white matter was severely attenuated.

The histological and morphological changes seen in our model of kaolin-induced ventriculomegaly closely parallel those seen clinically

Table 5.2. Effects of silicone oil or kaolin injection in cisterna magna of fetal monkeys

	Silicone oil ($N = 4$)	Kaolin ($N = 6$)
Gestation (days)		
Injection	96–109	96–115
Delivery	106–160	119–160
Viability	2/4	1/6
Ventriculomegaly at autopsy	0/4	5/6*
Presence of injected substance in cisterna magna	2/4	5/6*

* All fetuses with kaolin properly placed in the cisterna magna developed ventriculomegaly. Early in our experience, some kaolin was misinjected.

(Weller & Shulman 1972; Weller *et al.* 1973; Eisenberg *et al.* 1974; Milhorat 1978).

Feasibility and technique of fetal surgical correction

This model allowed us to develop techniques of prenatal ventricular shunting (Fig. 5.11) and to evaluate the role of prenatal intervention in the treatment of human congenital hydrocephalus.

Eighteen time-dated fetal rhesus monkeys were injected with 2% kaolin (0·5–1·0 ml) at 96–134 days' gestation (Glick *et al.* 1984b). Fourteen to 21 days after injection, eight fetuses underwent ventriculoamniotic (V–A) shunting and were allowed to continue development until term. Nine hydrocephalic fetuses were not shunted and served as untreated controls, and one fetus was excluded from the study because of a uterine dehiscence. To follow ventricular size during development of hydrocephalus and after shunting, selected monkeys underwent *in utero* real-time ultrasound scanning and a postnatal CT scan. Outcome of the shunted fetuses versus non-shunted controls is summarized in Table 5.3.

Prenatal sonography demonstrated gradual ventricular dilatation after kaolin injection with a return to normal size immediately after shunt placement. Subsequent ventricular enlargement occurred due to shunt failure. Amorphous debris was the cause of shunt occlusion, limiting efficacy. We have noted similar problems in the fetal lamb hydrocephalus model.

Shunting did not significantly alter histopathology. The shunted newborn monkeys still had enlarged ventricles, subependymal kaolin

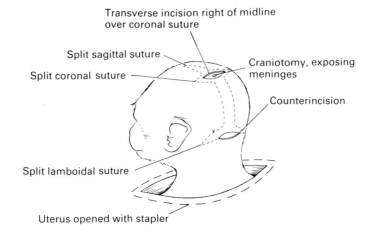

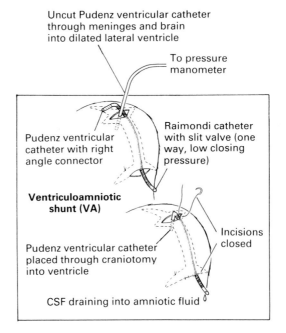

Fig. 5.11. Shunting technique in fetal monkeys performed 14−21 days after kaolin injection. (Reproduced, with permission, from Glick *et al.* 1984b.)

deposits and acute inflammatory infiltrates. The cerebral cortex appeared normal.

Using both the fetal rhesus monkey and fetal lamb hydrocephalus models, we have observed that: (i) ICP rises in a linear fashion after kaolin injection; (ii) *in utero* shunting decreases head and ventricular

Table 5.3. Fetal monkey hydrocephalus model

	VA	Unshunted controls
Group *N*	8	9
Viability*	4/8	1/9
Mean preshunt ICP (cm H$_2$O)	29·1 ± 13·6	–
Shunt patency†	1/4	–
Normal ventricular size†	0/4	0/1
Shunt infection†	0/4	0/1
Subdural haematoma†	0/4	0/1
Subdural hygroma†	0/4	0/1
Improper shunt tip placement†	1/4	–

*Viability of all shunted fetuses compared to unshunted fetuses by chi-square analysis, $P < 0.05$.
† Survivors only.

size, but fails to improve histophatological changes; and (iii) currently available shunt designs and shunting techniques are associated with a variety of complications, which makes us question their clinical efficacy (Glick *et al.* 1984b).

Our studies indicate that the CSF dynamics (i.e. gradually increasing ICP) and the histopathological changes (i.e. periventricular white matter injury with sparing of cortical grey matter) are remarkably similar to those seen in postnatal hydrocephalus in children. It was surprising that prenatal shunting did not result in improvement of the severity of histological brain injury. It is probable that reflux of kaolin into the lateral ventricles during either injection or shunting caused local tissue injury, explaining the lack of microscopic improvement in shunted fetuses. This technical problem with kaolin reflux makes it difficult to study the effects of *in utero* shunting. Preliminary results indicate that kaolin reflux and kaolin-associated changes can be prevented by injecting smaller volumes into the cisterna magna and by closely monitoring ventricular decompression.

Technical shunt problems were a major limitation to these studies. The ideal shunt for fetal hydrocephalus should: (i) re-establish normal ICP; (ii) prevent reflux of amniotic fluid and bacteria into the CSF; (iii) provide prolonged drainage without occlusion, malfunction or migration; and (iv) allow safe insertion by percutaneous, sonographically guided, techniques or limited hysterotomy. Unfortunately, the ideal shunt does not currently exist. Based on our hydrocephalus study as well as our clinical experience and research efforts in the management of fetal obstructive uropathy (Glick *et al.* 1985), we seriously question the efficacy of currently available shunting techniques and are in the process of designing a more reliable system.

We feel that the pathophysiology, the impact of prenatal shunting on neurological development and the technology of *in utero* shunting need to be more rigorously evaluated in animal models prior to clinical application.

Clinical perspective

Fetal treatment cannot prosper without fetal experimentation. Indeed, experimental fetal animal models are the key to the future. Any human intervention requires reliable information about the natural history and pathophysiology of the disease process, the efficacy of intervention in ameliorating the disease, and the feasibility and safety of the proposed intervention. These questions must be answered experimentally if possible.

Prospects for fetal experimentation remain as exciting as ever. There may be other anatomical lesions which require prenatal intervention for which suitable animal models are not currently available. Models for congenital heart disease are being developed which may yield exciting results (Slate *et al.* 1985). Enlarging mass lesions like congenital cystic adenomatoid malformation, fetal sacrococcygeal teratoma, or unilateral ureteropelvic junction obstruction with or without an associated perirenal urinoma may, under certain circumstances, require fetal intervention and should be amenable to experimental investigation (Sauer *et al.* 1987). Intrauterine pacemakers for the treatment of congenital heart block is an intriguing concept. Much remains to be done in the field of anaesthetic and tocolytic management for fetal intervention. Finally, and perhaps most exciting, is the possibility of correction of certain non-anatomical defects by fetal stem cell transplantation (Flake *et al.* 1986).

However, experience with fetal surgery in animal models may not be readily translatable to the human. The three best studied examples of animal models of correctable fetal malformations, congenital diaphragmatic hernia, congenital hydronephrosis and congenital hydrocephalus, have certain theoretical limitations. The principal problem with any animal model of fetal malformation is that the surgical alteration is created relatively late in gestation, compared with the human counterpart. Is experimentally produced renal dysplasia or pulmonary hypoplasia equivalent to that seen in human fetuses? Is the severity of malformation in our models comparable to the human disease process? Is the patho-physiology produced by complete urinary obstruction created in our lamb model equivalent to the partial obstruction frequently seen clin-ically? Are there important differences in human anatomy or human fetal tolerance of stress which might prohibit application of experimental techniques? These theoretical objections to our experimental findings can only be answered by clinical experience.

Thus far, our clinical experience has supported our findings in ani-mals. Congenital hydronephrosis is the best example of application of an experimental model of fetal malformation to the correction of human disease (Glick *et al.* 1985). Development of the lamb models allowed delineation of the pathophysiology of obstruction, and its effect on renal and pulmonary development, and led to the development of diagnostic and therapeutic techniques for relief of obstruction. Application of this work to human fetuses has generally supported our experimental findings, and many human fetuses have benefited from management strategies developed in the laboratory. In contrast, our experimental work on fetal hydrocephalus was not supportive of prenatal correction in human fetuses and, to date, efforts by others in human fetuses have been disappointing (Birnholz & Frigoletto 1981; Clewell *et al.* 1982). Finally, although we have satisfied our experimental criteria for clinical application, the repair of human CDH remains a formidable challenge which should only be attempted under ideal circumstances. Diaphrag-matic hernia remains the best studied and most compelling example of a defect requiring correction before birth and corroboration of our exper-imental findings awaits clinical application.

References

Adzick N.S., Davies P., Harrison M.R. *et al.* (1985) Correction of congenital diaphragmatic hernia *in utero*. IV. An early gestational fetal lamb model for pulmonary vascular morphometric analysis. *J. Pediatr. Surg.*, **20**, 673–80.

Beck A.D. (1971) The effect of intra-uterine urinary obstruction upon the development of the fetal kidney. *J. Urol.*, **105**, 784–9.

Birnholz J.C. & Frigoletto F.D. (1981) Antenatal treatment of hydrocephalus. *N. Engl. J. Med.*, **304**, 1021–3.

Clewell W.H., Johnson M.L., Meier P.R. *et al.* (1982) A surgical approach to the treatment of fetal hydrocephalus. *N. Engl. J. Med.*, **306**, 1320–5.

Eisenberg H.M., McLennan J.E. & Welch K. (1974) Ventricular perfusion in cats with kaolin-induced hydrocephalus. *J. Neurosurg.*, **41**, 20–7.

Flake A.W., Harrison M.R., Adzick N.S. & Zanjani E.D. (1986) Transplantation of fetal hematopoietic stem cells *in utero*: the creation of hematopoietic chimeras. *Science*, **233**, 776–8.

Glick P.L., Harrison M.R., Adzick N.S. *et al.* (1984a) Correction of congenital hydronephrosis *in utero*. IV. *In utero* decompression prevents renal dysplasia. *J. Pediatr. Surg.*, **19**, 649—57.

Glick P.L., Harrison M.R., Halks-Miller M. *et al.* (1984b) Correction of congenital hydrocephalus *in utero*. II. Efficacy of *in utero* shunting. *J. Pediatr. Surg.*, **19**, 851—9.

Glick P.L., Harrison M.R., Golbus M.S. *et al.* (1985) Management of the fetus with congenital hydronephrosis. II. Prognostic criteria and selection for treatment. *J. Pediatr. Surg.*, **20**, 376—87.

Griscom N.T., Colodny A.H., Rosenberg H.K. *et al.* (1977) Diagnostic aspects of neonatal ascites: report of 27 cases. *AJR*, **128**, 961—70.

Guesry P., Kaufman L., Orloff S. *et al.* (1975) Measurement of glomerular filtration rate by fluorescent excitation of nonradioactive meglumine iothalamate. *Clin. Nephrol.*, **3**, 134—8.

Harrison M.R. & deLorimier A.A. (1981) Congenital diaphragmatic hernia. *Surg. Clin. North. Am.*, **61**, 1023—35.

Harrison M.R., Bjordal R.I., Landmark F. *et al.* (1979) Congenital diaphragmatic hernia: the hidden mortality. *J. Pediatr. Surg.*, **13**, 227—30.

Harrison M.R., Jester J.A. & Ross N.A. (1980a) Correction of congenital diaphragmatic hernia *in utero*. I. The model: intrathoracic balloon produces fetal pulmonary hypoplasia. *Surgery*, **88**, 174—82.

Harrison M.R., Bressack M.A., Churg A.M. *et al.* (1980b) Correction of congenital diaphragmatic hernia *in utero*. II. Simulated correction permits fetal lung growth with survival at birth. *Surgery*, **88**, 260—8.

Harrison M.R., Golbus M.S. & Filly R.A. (1981a) Management of the fetus with a correctable congenital defect. *JAMA*, **246**, 774—7.

Harrison M.R., Ross N.A. & deLorimier A.A. (1981b) Correction of congenital diaphragmatic hernia *in utero*. III. Development of a successful surgical technique using abdominoplasty to avoid compromise of umbilical blood flow. *J. Pediatr. Surg.*, **16**, 934—42.

Harrison M.R., Filly R.A., Parer J.R.T. *et al.* (1981c) Management of the fetus with a urinary tract malformation. *JAMA*, **246**, 635—9.

Harrison M.R., Anderson J., Rosen M.A. *et al.* (1982a) Fetal surgery in the primate. I. Anesthetic, surgical, and tocolytic management to maximize fetal-neonatal survival. *J. Pediatr. Surg.*, **17**, 115—22.

Harrison M.R., Nakayama D.K., Noall R. *et al.* (1982b) Correction of congenital hydronephrosis *in utero*. II. Decompression reverses the effects of obstruction on the fetal lung and urinary tract. *J. Pediatr. Surg.*, **17**, 965—74.

Harrison M.R., Ross N.A., Noall R. *et al.* (1983) Correction of congenital hydronephrosis *in utero*. I. The model: fetal urethral obstruction produces hydronephrosis and pulmonary hypoplasia in fetal lambs. *J. Pediatr. Surg.*, **18**, 247—56.

Harrison M.R., Golbus M.S. & Filly R.A. (1984) *The Unborn Patient: Prenatal Diagnosis and Treatment*, pp. 1—230. Grune & Stratton, New York.

Hislop A., Hey E. & Reid L. (1979) The lungs in congenital bilateral renal agenesis and dysplasia. *Arch. Dis. Child.*, **54**, 32—8.

Inselman L.S. & Mellins R.B. (1981) Growth and development of the lung. *J. Pediatr.*, **98**, 1—15.

Liggins G.C. & Kitterman J.A. (1981) Development of the fetal lung. In *The Fetus and Independent Life (Ciba Foundation Symposium 86)* (Ed. by G.R. Dawes), pp. 308—29. Pittman, London.

Michejda A. & Hodgen G.D. (1981) *In utero* diagnosis and treatment of nonhuman primate skeletal anomalies: I. Hydrocephalus. *JAMA*, **246**, 1093—7.

Milhorat T.H. (1978) *Hydrocephalus in Pediatric Neurosurgery*, pp. 91—135. F.A. Davis, Philadelphia.

Nakayama D.K., Harrison M.R., Berger M.S., Chinn D.H., Halks-Miller M. & Edwards M.S.B. (1983) Correction of congenital hydrocephalus *in utero*. I. The model: intracisternal kaolin produces hydrocephalus in fetal lambs and rhesus monkeys. *J. Pediatr. Surg.*, **18**, 331−8.

Potter E.L. & Craig J.M. (1975) *Pathology of the Fetus and the Infant*, 3rd edn, pp. 458−9. Year Book, Chicago.

Reid L. (1977) The lung: its growth and remodeling in health and disease. *AJR*, **129**, 777−88.

Sauer L., Harrison M.R., & Flake A.W. (1987) Does an expanding fetal abdominal mass produce pulmonary hypoplasia? *J. Pediatr. Surg.*, **22**, 508−12.

Schurr P.H., McLaurin R.L., & Ingraham F.D. (1953) Experimental studies in the circulation of the cerebrospinal fluid: methods of producing communicating hydrocephalus in dogs. *J. Neurosurg.*, **10**, 515−23.

Slate R.K., Verrier E.D., Stevens M. *et al.* (1985) Intrauterine repair of pulmonic stenosis in fetal lambs. *Surg. Forum*, **36**, 246−7.

Tanagho E.A. (1972a) Surgically induced partial urinary obstruction in the fetal lamb. I. Technique. *Invest. Urol.*, **10**, 19−24.

Tanagho E.A. (1972b) Surgically induced partial urinary obstruction in the fetal lamb. II. Urethral obstruction. *Invest. Urol.*, **10**, 25−34.

Tanagho E.A. (1972c) Surgically induced partial urinary obstruction in the fetal lamb. III. Ureteral obstruction. *Invest. Urol.*, **10**, 35−52.

Thomasson B.M., Easterly J.R., & Ravitch M.M. (1970) Morphologic changes in the fetal kidney after intrauterine ureteral ligation. *Invest. Urol.*, **8**, 261−72.

Weller R.O., & Shulman K. (1972) Infantile hydrocephalus: clinical histological and ultrastructural study of brain damage. *J. Neurosurg.*, **36**, 255−65.

Weller R.O., Wisniewski H. & Shulman K. (1973) Experimental hydrocephalus in young dogs: histological and ultrastructural study of brain tissue damage. *J. Neuropath. Exp. Neurol.*, **30**, 613−27.

Wigglesworth J.S., Dejai R. & Guerrini P. (1981) Fetal lung hypoplasia: biochemical and structural variations and their possible significance. *Arch. Dis. Child.*, **56**, 606−15.

Wisniewski H., Weller R.O. & Terry R.D. (1969) Experimental hydrocephalus produced by the subarachnoid infusion of silicone oil. *J. Neurosurg.*, **31**, 10−19.

6

Invasive Fetal Therapy

L. LYNCH, K. MEHALEK &
R.L. BERKOWITZ

During the 1970s, perinatologists focused their efforts on developing techniques for diagnosing fetal disorders and congenital anomalies. With improved diagnostic acuity came the opportunity to prospectively observe the antenatal course of these diseases, and their ultimate outcome. It soon became evident that some fetal disorders might be amenable to invasive therapy *in utero*. Although fetal transfusions have been performed for more than 20 years, it was only fairly recently that *in utero* shunting procedures were used to treat conditions such as obstructive uropathy and hydrocephalus. Furthermore, the approach to intrauterine transfusions has evolved dramatically.

This chapter will review the history of, recent experience in and techniques for performing transfusions and shunting procedures *in utero*, and the current role of invasive fetal therapy will be assessed.

Intrauterine transfusions

The introduction of Rho(D) immune globulin (RhoGam) in 1968 has dramatically reduced the incidence of Rh haemolytic disease. Unfortunately, however, it has not eliminated the condition entirely. In addition, sensitization to red cell antigens other than the D antigen continues to occur.

The primary problem in erythroblastosis fetalis is haemolysis of fetal red blood cells by maternal IgG antibodies that have crossed the placenta. This results in fetal anaemia with secondary extramedullary haematopoiesis, primarily in the liver and spleen. Distortion and enlargement of the hepatic parenchyma by this process results in portal hypertension and decreased ability of the liver to synthesize albumin. These factors lead to the creation of fetal ascites and eventually anasarca, a condition referred to as 'hydrops fetalis'. Although congestive heart failure will develop terminally it does not seem to be the primary cause of hydrops.

Transfused blood that is compatible with that of the mother will not be haemolysed by her antibodies. The administration of this blood *in utero* obviates the need for immediate delivery and accomplishes two purposes. First, it corrects the fetal anaemia and consequently improves tissue oxygenation. Second, it reduces production of fetal erythropoietin and extramedullary erythropoiesis. This in turn causes a fall in portal and umbilical venous pressures and improves hepatic circulation and hepatocellular function.

In 1963, Liley successfully performed the first intraperitoneal transfusion on a severely sensitized erythroblastotic infant *in utero* and in doing so created new horizons in obstetric care. Following this successful introduction of invasive fetal therapy, Freda and Adamsons (1964) performed an 'open' intrauterine exchange transfusion. The leg of a 27-week fetus was delivered up to the groin through a hysterotomy incision. A 22-gauge polyethylene catheter was inserted into the femoral artery, and an exchange transfusion with a total of 220 ml of fresh O Rh-negative blood was performed. Although both mother and fetus tolerated the procedure well, on the second postoperative day, premature labour resulted in the delivery of an 800 gm infant who died in the neonatal period from respiratory distress. Asensio *et al.* (1966) used a similar technique and successfully performed an exchange transfusion through the saphenous vein of a 31-week fetus. The postoperative period was uneventful and the infant, who was delivered after spontaneous labour at 34 weeks, survived. However, since this type of operative therapeutic intervention is surgically complex and offers significant risks to both mother and fetus, it has never gained acceptance.

For more than 20 years the traditional method for performing transfusions *in utero* has utilized the intraperitoneal approach. This procedure has been modified from one dependent on X-ray and fluoroscopic imaging to an ultrasound-guided technique in which placement of the needle, transfusion of the blood and fetal heart activity can be continuously monitored without exposing the fetus to radiation. As expected, earlier series show poorer results after intraperitoneal transfusion than those reported later, because of improved techniques and the greater experience of operators. In a review by Bock (1976), overall survival rates from 12 series of intraperitoneal transfusions were presented. These studies were published between 1966 and 1976, and the number of patients transfused ranged from 30 to 238. Survival rates varied from a low of 24% in a series of 55 patients reported in 1968 to a high of 56% in the authors' series of 34 patients published in 1976. In 1977, Hamilton published the 13-year experience at his institution, which included 182 intrauterine transfusions on 82 patients. The overall neonatal survival rate was 67%, with 75·7% of the non-hydropic fetuses and 16·6% of those with hydrops surviving. When the five years immediately preceding publication were compared with the eight years prior to that period, the survival rate for the non-hydropic fetuses improved from 64.5% to 84·6%, but no change was noted in that of fetuses with hydrops. In 1978, Bowman published the results of the 14-year experience at his institution, which included 611 transfusions in 257 infants. The overall neonatal survival rate was 59%, with 68% of the non-hydropic fetuses and 36% of those with hydrops surviving. When the final eight years of the study were considered independently, the overall survival was 70%, with 78% of the non-hydropic fetuses and 50% of those with hydrops surviving the neonatal period. In 1983, the same group (Bowman & Manning) published impressive outcome data following the institution of real-time ultrasound surveillance during and after the transfusions. Overall survival for the interval from 1980 to 1982 was 92% (22 of 24 fetuses transfused), with 75% good outcomes in the hydropic fetuses. These are by far the best survival rates reported for fetuses treated with intraperitoneal transfusions.

Despite the success of intraperitoneal transfusions, a more direct approach to the fetal circulation has recently been advocated. Until 1981, fetoscopic blood sampling was performed only for diagnostic purposes but, in that year, Rodeck *et al.* (1981) reported on the first intravascular transfusion performed through the fetoscope. In 1982, MacKenzie *et al.* performed 37 exchange transfusions *in utero* under direct fetoscopic visualization in fetuses at 15–23 weeks before therapeutic abortion. Two years later Rodeck *et al.* (1984) described their experience with the fetoscopically guided intravascular approach in 25 severely Rh-sensitized fetuses who underwent a total of 77 intrauterine transfusions. The overall survival rate in this series was 72%. Furthermore, in fetuses who received their first transfusion before 25 weeks, the survival rate was 84%, including 11 of 13 fetuses who had antenatal evidence of hydrops.

In 1982, Bang *et al.* published a case report of a severely erythroblastotic fetus which had been successfully transfused directly into the intrahepatic portion of the umbilical vein at 29 and again at 30 weeks. In these procedures the needle was introduced percutaneously under ultrasound guidance. A recent report by Ch de Crespigny *et al.* (1985) described the use of this technique to perform a series of 16 transfusions in four Rh-sensitized pregnancies. In 1983, Daffos *et al.* published a series of 66 cases in which fetal blood was obtained for diagnostic purposes by the percutaneous introduction of a 20-gauge needle directly into the umbilical vein near the placental cord insertion site. More recently, the same group reported a series of more than 600 patients in which percutaneous umbilical blood sampling (PUBS) was performed for diagnostic purposes (Daffos *et al.* 1985). The procedure-related pregnancy loss rate in this series was less than 1%, which is four to five times lower than that generally associated with fetoscopic blood sampling. These reports led to the adaptation of the percutaneous approach for intravascular transfusions into various sites within the fetal circulation.

In 1986, Grannum *et al.* reported on nine intravascular transfusions in four patients, six of which were exchange transfusions. The outcome was successful in three of the patients. Simultaneously, our group (Berkowitz *et al.* 1986) published a series of eight patients who underwent 16 intravascular transfusions. The percutaneous intravascular technique was successful in 16 of 18 attempts (89%) and a successful outcome was achieved in six of the eight cases (75%). One of the two deaths *in utero* was probably due to the advanced nature of the disease prior to transfusion. The other death, however, may have been related to the procedure itself. In that case a technically successful intraperitoneal transfusion was administered after a failed attempt to perform the patient's third intravascular transfusion, and death *in utero* occurred eight hours later. We have since expanded our experience with this technique. Up to January 1987, 43 intravascular transfusions have been attempted, 38 (88%) of which have been technically successful. These procedures have been performed on a total of 17 patients. There have been three fetal losses before 26 weeks and none after this gestational age. Out of 14 completed pregnancies, 11 infants have survived (79%). Three additional pregnancies are continuing. The survival rate for hydropic fetuses has been two out of four (50%).

Intraperitoneal transfusion

The technique for intraperitoneal transfusions varies somewhat among institutions but typically is as follows: the mother is sedated with a combination of intravenous medications such as a narcotic and a tranquillizer. After aseptic and local anaesthetic preparation, a 16- or 18-gauge Tuohy needle is inserted into the fetal abdominal cavity under ultrasound guidance. A small incision in the maternal skin and fascia facilitates the introduction of these large-bore needles. The ideal site of entry into the fetus is below the umbilical vein but above the bladder, as this minimizes the risk of traumatizing an enlarged liver. Proper needle placement is verified by aspirating ascitic fluid in the hydropic fetus or by injecting a small amount of sterile saline solution and observing layering of fluid in the peritoneal cavity in the non-hydropic fetus. Once proper placement has been verified, one can transfuse directly through the needle or a polyvinyl catheter can be threaded into the fetal abdomen, and the needle removed. Injection is performed at an average of $5-10$ ml per minute and the infusion is periodically 'broken' by detaching the tubing from the needle to look for back flow. If the latter occurs or persistent bradycardia is observed, the transfusion should be discontinued before giving the full amount of blood calculated as necessary. The fetal heart rate should be monitored with ultrasonic visualization throughout the procedure.

The amount of blood transfused into the peritoneal cavity is estimated by the following formula: gestation in weeks minus 20×10 ml (Bowman 1975). If ultrasonography demonstrates a large amount of ascites, most of it should be removed before transfusing and the red cell volume should not be greater than the volume of ascitic fluid removed. The type of blood for transfusion is group O Rh-negative packed red cells which have been cross-matched against the mother's blood.

Once the fetus has been transfused, amniotic fluid delta OD_{450} levels cannot be relied on for diagnostic purposes because of the interference of blood breakdown products in amniotic fluid. Thus, once intraperitoneal transfusions are initiated, they should be continued on schedule until delivery.

Bowman (1978) uses the following protocol for the interval between transfusions: 9 to 12 days between first and second transfusion, 25 to 30 days between subsequent transfusions; and delivery 25 to 30 days after the last one, at or after 33 weeks' gestation, provided that fetal pulmonary maturity has been attained. Hydropic fetuses, however, are not managed according to this scheme since they have slow and erratic absorption. In these fetuses optimal transfusion intervals may be as short as 4 or 5 days depending on the ultrasound findings. Ultrasound evidence of increasing or decreasing peritoneal fluid accumulations and subcutaneous oedema determines whether transfusion intervals should be decreased or increased.

Intravascular transfusions

Why transfuse intravascularly?

There are several major advantages to the intravascular approach. One of these is the ability to document that the fetal red blood cells carry the antigen of concern. This information is of utmost importance in cases in which the father is a heterozygote for the antigen involved. If the fetus did not inherit the antigen, unnecessary further intervention is avoided.

Determination of the fetal haematocrit is a better tool in the assessment of the severity of the disease than amniotic fluid levels of bilirubin pigment, especially in the second-trimester fetus. The amount of fetal haemolysis can be estimated by spectrophotometric analysis for bilirubin pigment in amniotic fluid. This is done by measurement of optical density differences at 450 nm wavelength. In 1961, Liley developed gestational age-dependent curves relating the delta OD_{450} values to fetal haemoglobin in Rh-immunized pregnancies at 27 to 41 weeks, and proposed three zones: zone I representing an unaffected or mildly affected fetus, zone II a moderately to severely affected fetus, and zone III a severely affected fetus. This curve has subsequently been extrapolated linearly back into the second trimester. However, Nicolaides *et al.* (1986), in a study involving 59 Rh-immunized pregnancies between 18 and 25 weeks' gestation, simultaneously obtained amniotic fluid for delta OD_{450} analysis and fetal blood by fetoscopy. Thirty-one of 59 fetuses were judged to have very severe disease by cord haemoglobins of less than 6 g dl^{-1}. (Fourteen of these 31 also had ultrasonic evidence of hydrops.) Only 10 of these 31 (32%), however, had delta OD_{450} values in the extrapolated zone III; some even had values in zone I. This yielded a 68% false negative rate. In addition, one fetus with normal haemoglobin had a delta OD_{450} in zone III. These data show that the only reliable method to determine the severity of the haemolytic process during the second trimester is direct measurement of fetal haemoglobin. This is particularly true in patients with history of severe disease in prior pregnancies.

Measurement of the fetal haematocrit before the transfusion allows a more accurate estimation of the amount of blood required and the post-transfusion haematocrit verifies that an optimal amount of blood has been administered. This information together with a Kleihauer–Betke test (i.e. the proportion of adult to fetal cells determined by slide analysis following acid elution) provides a more accurate guide for timing of the next transfusion or delivery.

Blood placed into the fetal peritoneal cavity is absorbed via the subdiaphragmatic lymphatics, from which it gains access to the circulation. This process, however, may be erratic, especially in hydropic fetuses. Therefore, delivery of the blood directly into the vascular compartment is a more physiological and predictable form of therapy. Furthermore, trauma to internal organs associated with the introduction of the transfusion needle into the fetal abdomen had in some cases resulted in death *in utero*.

Although the intravascular approach offers obvious theoretical advantages, in some cases in which access to the fetal circulation is difficult or impossible for technical reasons intraperitoneal transfusions should be performed. Thus, there is still a place for intraperitoneal transfusions in the modern management of the isoimmunized fetus and this technique cannot be forgotten.

Techniques for intravascular transfusions

The fetoscopic approach described by Rodeck *et al.* (1981, 1984) employs a 1·7 mm endoscope housed in a 2·4 × 3·0 mm cannula. This is introduced transabdominally into the amniotic cavity after the patient has been sedated. Following introduction of the fetoscope and identification of the cord entry site into either the placenta or the fetus, a 21-gauge needle with a 3 mm, 26-gauge tip is introduced through the side channel of the cannula. Under direct vision, an umbilical cord vessel is punctured and a sample of blood obtained for analysis. Blood is then transfused at a rate of 1 to 3 ml per minute. Approximately two-thirds of the way through the transfusion, the fetal haematocrit is checked and the volume given is adjusted to bring the fetal haematocrit into the normal range of 35% to 45%. Fetal cardiac activity is monitored throughout the procedure.

The major problem with the fetoscopic approach to intravascular transfusion is that it is technically difficult to perform. Amniotic fluid becomes progressively more opaque as pregnancy progresses, particularly when it becomes stained with bilirubin or haemoglobin pigments. Moreover, the fetoscope needle has a 26-gauge tip, making the passage of packed cells with a haematocrit greater than 75% sometimes difficult. When using the percutaneous route a 22- or 20-gauge needle is used, making the transfusion of such concentrated blood products easier and faster. Rodeck's group has considerable experience with fetoscopic blood sampling, but it is not at all clear that other centres will be able to duplicate their excellent results with this technically demanding procedure.

At the Mount Sinai Medical Center we use the percutaneous technique. In general our approach is as follows. If the patient is considered to be a candidate for *in utero* transfusions and is seen early in pregnancy, we begin weekly ultrasound examinations looking for early evidence of erythroblastosis. In the absence of hydrops, we perform the first fetal blood sampling sometime between 20 and 26 weeks of gestation. Patients with previous severely affected fetuses or very high antibody titres are sampled at the lower end of this range.

The method used for percutaneous intravascular transfusions at our institution includes an initial ultrasound assessment of fetal lie and of placental and umbilical cord insertion-site locations. The patient is usually premedicated with a combination of a narcotic and a tranquillizer injected slowly by the intravenous route. A single dose of ritodrine (3 mg) is also administered intravenously to prevent the development of uterine contractions, and an antibiotic is administered for prophylaxis.

After aseptic preparation of the maternal abdomen, a 20- or 22-gauge spinal needle is guided with a linear-array ultrasound transducer into the umbilical cord at its insertion into the placenta. When this location cannot be accessed, the needle is directed into the umbilical vein within the fetal liver or into a cord vessel at the umbilicus. A sample of blood is then withdrawn into a heparinized syringe. Analysis of the red blood cells with an electronic cell sizer is used to confirm that the withdrawn sample is fetal in origin. At the time of the first sampling, the fetal blood type is determined. The haematocrit is measured and, if less than 30%, an immediate transfusion is performed. Washed and irradiated group O Rh-negative packed cells which have been cross-matched against the mother's blood are transfused at a rate of $2-5$ ml min^{-1} directly into the umbilical vessels. The fetal heart is visually monitored throughout the procedure. The volume of packed RBCs to be transfused is estimated, and this is titrated by checking the haematocrit after two-thirds of this amount has been administered. After completion of the transfusion a final sample is aspirated for analysis. The goal is to obtain a postprocedure haematocrit of 35 to 45%. A Kleihauer–Betke test is also performed on the final aspirate in order to determine the proportion of adult (i.e. transfused) cells in the fetal circulation. The timing of the next transfusion is individualized in each case, depending on the post-transfusion haematocrit and the Kleihauer—Betke analysis. In general the intervals range between 1 and 3 weeks. The final transfusion is done at 32 to 34 weeks depending on fetal lung maturity as shown by amniotic fluid lecithin/sphingomyelin ratio greater than or equal to 2, unless, of course, there is cardiotocographic or ultrasonic evidence of deteriorating fetal condition.

In utero exchange transfusions instead of simple transfusions have been proposed by some groups (Grannum *et al.* 1986). This, however, is controversial. The rationale for performing an exchange transfusion is the recognition that neonates can quickly become volume-overloaded if they are given excessive amounts of blood. The fetus, however, is able to accommodate relatively large increases in its intravascular volume because of its attachment to the placenta, which seems to function as a low-resistance sink. In addition, withdrawing significant volumes of fetal plasma poses at least the theoretical risk of depleting coagulation factors, which could predispose the fetus to a bleeding diathesis. In our experience non-hydropic fetuses seem to tolerate the volumes of blood being transfused very well, and exchanges have not been necessary. It may be wise, however, to utilize exchange transfusions in fetuses with severe anaemia and hydrops, in order to avoid volume overload in these cases. Clearly more research is needed in order to determine what type of transfusion is best.

Problems with intravascular transfusions

There are several issues regarding intravascular transfusions which need to be elucidated. One unanswered question is the timing of the first fetal blood sampling. Assuming that the fetus is not hydropic, sampling at a time when the fetus is not yet anaemic poses the risk of unnecessarily increasing the maternal antibody titre secondary to a fetomaternal bleed caused by the procedure. Ideally the first sample should be obtained when the fetus is already anaemic but before hydrops develops, thereby avoiding unnecessary procedures. At Mount Sinai Hospital at the present time, the first PUBS is empirically performed between 20 and 26 weeks, depending on the previous obstetrical history and antibody titres. A way of determining the optimal timing of subsequent transfusions also needs to be determined.

Another issue that must be clarified is the risk of intravascular fetal transfusions versus that of intraperitoneal transfusions. Although theoretically intravascular transfusions seem to be more physiological and less traumatic, the experience with this approach is still too limited to draw definitive conclusions.

The problem of fetal movement can be significant when one is working within the liver or with a posterior placenta. Maternal sedation is often sufficient to arrest or slow down fetal movement, but this is not always the case. Ch de Crespigny's group (1985) have administered intramuscular curare injected directly into the fetal thigh to eliminate this problem. We have utilized a short-acting neuromuscular blocker injected directly into the fetal circulation in a number of cases. Although no adverse sequelae have been detected following the administration of these agents, the experience with their use *in utero* is inadequate to be certain that they are safe.

Finally, long-term follow-up of infants transfused intravascularly *in utero* is not yet available. Follow-up studies of survivors of intraperitoneal transfusions suggest that they can be expected to develop normally if they do not suffer major hypoxic episodes during their perinatal course (Berkowitz 1980). Theoretically, the intravascular approach should not pose an increased risk of any long-term sequelae but these data are not yet available.

Intravascular transfusions of other blood products

With direct access to the fetal intravascular compartment, one is theoretically able to diagnose and treat other haematological and genetic diseases.

One such disorder is neonatal alloimmune thrombocytopenia (NAIT). NAIT is a serious condition in which central nervous system bleeding is responsible for a high rate of morbidity and mortality. In this disorder the mother produces antibodies to fetal platelet antigens, which results in thrombocytopenia *in utero*. In 1984 Daffos *et al.* reported a case in which a fetus at risk for this disorder was sampled and found to have severe thrombocytopenia. A transfusion of maternal platelets was given to the fetus before delivery by caesarean section in an attempt to minimize trauma and intracranial bleeding. Although the antenatal diagnosis of this disorder is clearly desirable in order to decide mode of delivery, whether prenatal administration of platelet transfusions to the fetus alters the outcome remains to be determined.

A new and exciting potential use of intravascular fetal therapy is *in utero* bone marrow transplantation. This approach could be potentially useful in the correction of disorders such as inherited storage diseases or defects in the immune system. Haematopoietic stem cells (HSCs) from the bone marrow of postnatal donors and from the liver of fetal donors have been used for the treatment of genetic disorders. The fetus is an ideal host for transplantation of HSC cells for two reasons: ontologically it is prepared for engraftment, and immunologically it is tolerant and should permit foreign grafts without rejections. Fetal immunotolerance obviates the need for host preparation with chemotherapy and irradiation, a disadvantage of postnatal bone marrow transplantation.

Flake *et al.* (1986) have reported the *in utero* transplantation of HSCs into the fetal sheep, with the establishment of haematopoietic chimaeras with no graft-versus-host disease. Linch *et al.* (1986) reported on a bone marrow transplant attempt in a 17-week human fetus. This was a severely Rh-immunized fetus, and the transplant, with maternal bone marrow, was done in an attempt to alter the fetus's Rh type and in this way keep the number of *in utero* transfusions to a minimum. Further fetal blood samples were obtained at subsequent transfusions at 19, 22, 27, 28 and 31 weeks' gestation. Neonatal blood was taken at the time of delivery at 33 weeks and again at 4 weeks after birth and there was no evidence of engraftment.

Despite the failure of this first attempt at *in utero* bone marrow transplantation, ongoing animal studies and the extraordinary possibilities of fetal therapy with this modality make it a remarkably promising area for further investigations.

Intrauterine shunting procedures

With intrauterine transfusion setting the foundation for successful *in utero* therapy, attention has turned to other conditions detectable *in utero* which often lead to neonatal morbidity and mortality. Improved sonographic resolution has enabled identification of structural defects which may be amenable to *in utero* therapy. The objective of such therapy is to reverse or arrest a pathological process in order to prevent damage, while allowing normal development to proceed *in utero*. Increased pressure caused by abnormal fluid collections in the fetus can cause damage to adjacent organs or tissues while prohibiting normal development. Antenatal shunting and drainage procedures have already been used to decompress hydronephrosis, hydrocephalus and fluid collections in the thorax. Other potentially correctable defects include diaphragmatic hernia and neural tube defects.

For a disorder to be amenable to *in utero* therapy, several conditions need to be satisfied. The sonographic diagnosis of the condition should be reasonably accurate. The natural history of the disease should be known, with evidence to suggest that intervention can alter outcome. Fetal surgery is only indicated for conditions which are likely to be fatal or lead to severe handicap in the absence of treatment.

In 1982, a group of perinatologists, neonatologists, paediatric surgeons, ultrasonographers and bioethicists met at a conference sponsored by the Kroc Foundation to discuss management of the fetus with a correctable congenital defect. The participants, who later established the Fetal Medicine and Surgery Society, set guidelines and selection criteria for therapy of obstructive uropathy and hydrocephalus (Harrison *et al.* 1982a). The fetus under consideration for therapy should be a singleton, so as not to jeopardize a normal twin. Coexisting anomalies which might worsen prognosis should be excluded by performing high-resolution sonography and amniocentesis for karyotype and alpha-fetoprotein determination. The fetus should be less than 32 weeks or have documented lung immaturity, as delivery with neonatal therapy is preferable to *in utero* therapy unless the neonate is unlikely to survive due to prematurity. The patient must understand the risks and benefits of the treatment and be willing to return for follow-up studies. The participants agreed that treatment should be provided by a multidisciplinary team including a perinatal obstetrician, a level II ultrasonographer, a neonatologist, and a paediatric surgeon with access to a level III high-risk obstetrical service and intensive care nursery.

Detection of a significant structural or chromosomal abnormality enables the parents to consider termination of the pregnancy (within local legal limits). Since invasive procedures on the fetus have maternal risks, fetal surgery is not indicated at any gestational age in a fetus with severe associated anomalies which may lead to problems of equal or greater magnitude for the fetus. Karyotyping is valuable even in the third-trimester fetus, as knowledge of a chromosomally abnormal fetus will influence decisions regarding shunt placement, timing of delivery, and caesarean section.

In 1982, an International Fetal Surgery Registry was established to record cases of fetal surgery for obstructive uropathy or hydrocephalus. While reporting to the registry may be biased, analysis of the cases helps to provide an evaluation of the efficacy of *in utero* therapy. In 1985, a natural history registry was added so that treated cases could be compared with those which were untreated.

Obstructive uropathy

Obstructive uropathy resulting in hydronephrosis and oligohydramnios can have a severe effect on the developing renal and pulmonary systems of the fetus. Diversion of urine from the dilated portion of the urinary tract into the amniotic fluid cavity theoretically should prevent both renal insufficiency and pulmonary hypoplasia, and allow normal development to occur.

Diagnosis

Accurate diagnosis is crucial before treatment can be considered. Routine visualization of the fetal kidneys is possible after 16 weeks. Located below the level of the stomach on either side of the spine, the kidneys are hypoechogenic and contain a central echo, the renal pelvis. Later in gestation, the capsule and collecting system are strongly echogenic, while the parenchyma remains hypoechogenic. In the presence of obstruction, the kidneys may demonstrate either hydronephrotic changes with a dilated calyceal system and thin cortex, or increased renal parenchymal echogenicity with or without pelvic and calyceal distension.

The bladder can be identified as early as 14–15 weeks. Fetal urine output increases from 2·2 ml hr^{-1} at 22 weeks to 26 ml hr^{-1} at 40 weeks (Kurjak *et al.* 1980). Micturition generally occurs at intervals of approximately 40 minutes (Kurjak *et al.* 1984). Failure to identify the bladder after one hour of scanning is highly suggestive of fetal renal failure, absent kidneys or bilateral ureteral obstruction. The presence of megacystis, a dilated bladder which fails to empty over time, suggests obstruction at or distal to the urethrovesical junction.

Obstructive uropathy is identified as being unilateral or bilateral, and can be divided according to anatomical level (Hobbins *et al.* 1984): (i) *high* — dilated renal pelvis only, seen in ureteropelvic junction (UPJ) obstruction, or ureteral atresia; (ii) *mid* — ureteral dilatation with or without a dilated renal pelvis, seen in ureterovesical junction (UVJ) obstruction, bladder atresia or transient hydroureter; (iii) *low* — dilated bladder and proximal urinary tract, seen in posterior urethral valves, or urethral atresia. Unilateral obstruction usually shows a normal-sized bladder with a dilated ureter and/or renal pelvis in association with a normal contralateral kidney and renal pelvis.

Sonographic dilatation is not diagnostic of obstruction. In Hobbins's 1984 series of obstructive uropathies, 3 of 25 cases of obstruction were misdiagnosed. All three cases involved midlevel dilatation observed *in utero*, but the neonates were found to be normal. These cases were felt to represent transient hydroureter due to vesicoureteral reflux. Avni *et al.* (1985) incorrectly diagnosed obstruction in 20 of 63 fetuses. Fourteen of these fetuses had transient dilatation; 11 involved the upper tract, and 3 involved the bladder. All neonatal radiographic examinations showed normal urinary tracts. Furthermore, in this series multicystic kidneys were misdiagnosed as ureteropelvic junction obstruction in four cases.

Once a renal anomaly is detected, a thorough search for other anomalies is indicated. According to Potter & Craig (1976), up to 50% of these fetuses may have cardiovascular, gastrointestinal, skeletal or central nervous system anomalies. Recent series of fetal obstructive uropathy have demonstrated a 23–33% incidence of associated anatomical defects (Hobbins *et al.* 1984; Quinlan *et al.* 1986; Reuss *et al.* 1988). Fetuses with low-level obstruction seem to have the highest incidence of other anomalies. Reported anomalies include: caudal regression sydrome, ranging from imperforate anus to sirenomelia, malrotation of the large or small bowel, cloacal anomalies, cardiac defects, omphalocoele, hydrocephalus, oesophageal atresia and diaphragmatic hernia.

A karyotype should be performed on fetal cells obtained from amniotic fluid, blood or urine. Rodeck & Nicolaides (1983) report a 23% incidence of chromosomal abnormalities in fetuses with obstructive uropathy where karyotyping was performed. The 1985 report from the International Fetal Surgery Registry reported 6 abnormal karyotypes in 73 shunted patients. All of these patients terminated their pregnancies once the chromosomal abnormality was known. Reported karyotypic abnormalities associated with obstructive uropathy include: trisomies 13, 18 and 21, tetraploidy, triploidy, deletions and 47, XXY (Rodeck & Nicolaides 1983; Manning *et al.* 1986; Reuss *et al.* 1988).

Natural history

Prognosis of the fetus with urinary tract obstruction depends on the level, severity and duration of obstruction. At one end of the spectrum is the fetus with severe bilateral obstruction and oligohydramnios who dies an early neonatal death from renal failure and pulmonary hypoplasia. At the other end is the fetus with mild obstruction and normal amniotic fluid who is born with normal renal and pulmonary function and who only requires neonatal urinary tract decompression.

Unilateral obstruction with a normal amount of amniotic fluid and a normal-appearing contralateral kidney carries a favourable prognosis for the fetus, and therefore does not require intrauterine therapy. Harrison *et al.* (1982b) followed eight fetuses with unilateral obstruction with expectant management. All delivered near term, and all were doing well on follow-up. Seven had UPJ obstruction, while the eighth had upper-pole hydronephrosis in a duplex left-sided system. Twenty-five per cent required nephrectomy, while 75% underwent pyeloplasty. Unilateral obstruction was also associated with a good outcome in the Yale series (Hobbins *et al.* 1984). Three patients with midlevel obstruction had transient hydroureter and normal kidneys at birth. Four patients had UVJ obstruction; one required nephrectomy for cystic dysplasia, one had surgical correction with a good result, and the other two had functional kidneys on the affected side. The eighth patient had a unilateral dysplastic kidney, but died of a cardiac anomaly.

Prognosis is more varied, and can be quite poor, with bilateral obstruction. Partial bilateral obstruction producing hydronephrosis may be reversible following decompression during the neonatal period, and renal function may be normal. Complete obstruction of long-standing duration, on the other hand, may result in cystic dysplasia with non-functioning kidneys at birth. The outcome is difficult to predict in fetuses with varying degrees of obstruction between these two extremes.

The most important non-renal sequela of obstruction is oligohydramnios, which can lead to pulmonary hypoplasia and neonatal death from respiratory insufficiency. The existence or development of oligohydramnios in a fetus with urinary tract obstruction is a poor prognostic factor. Two fetuses in Harrison's 1982 series with low-level obstruction and severe oligohydramnios diagnosed at 30 and 33 weeks died at birth. Autopsies showed small lungs, bilateral hydronephrosis, renal dysplasia and posterior urethral valves. Hobbins *et al.* (1984) expectantly followed 11 pregnancies demonstrating bilateral obstruction, with only 3 survivors. Two survivors had UVJ obstruction and oligohydramnios, while the other had bilateral transient hydroureter and normal amniotic fluid volume. All seven fetuses with low-level obstruction and oligohydramnios died.

While absence of oligohydramnios implies normal pulmonary development, it does not always correlate with normal renal function. Harrison's 1982 series included seven fetuses felt to have 'equivocal' renal function since the amniotic fluid volume was not markedly decreased. The only neonatal death was in a fetus with other anomalies.

Of the six remaining neonates, half had normal renal function, while the other half had abnormal tubular function or developed chronic renal failure.

Before prognosis can be determined, serial observations are necessary to determine if the obstruction is progressive. The San Francisco series (Harrison *et al.* 1982b) contained three cases of bilateral hydronephrosis with normal amniotic fluid. The dilatation resolved spontaneously in all cases, and the newborns were normal. In 1985, Fitzsimmons *et al.* reported spontaneous reduction of megacystis *in utero* in a fetus with prune-belly syndrome. Following reduction in bladder size, the volume of amniotic fluid increased, implying that the obstruction was relieved.

Experimental studies

Osathanondh & Potter (1964) hypothesized that urinary tract obstruction early in fetal life results in damage to developing nephrons by retrograde pressure in the collecting system. The resulting dysplastic kidney (Potter type IV) consists of disorganized epithelial structures surrounded by abundant fibrous tissue. In 1971, Beck performed ureteral ligation on the fetal lamb in order to study the morphological effect of fetal urinary tract obstruction on kidney development. He demonstrated that ureteral ligation during the first half of gestation produced contracted dysplastic kidneys containing immature glomeruli and undifferentiated mesenchymal stroma. Unilateral ligation during the last half of gestation produced hydronephrosis with preservation of renal architecture.

Harrison's group repeated Beck's study in the fetal lamb, and then carried it one step further in order to study the effect of obstruction and its subsequent reversal on renal and pulmonary development (Harrison *et al.* 1982d, 1983). They showed that uncorrected urethral obstruction produced late in gestation (100 days) resulted in pulmonary hypoplasia, hydronephrosis, hydroureter and megacystis. Lambs undergoing *in utero* correction by suprapubic cystotomy three weeks later, however, had improved survival, less respiratory distress and less urinary tract dilatation when delivered at term (140 days). The lambs undergoing correction of the obstruction had significantly higher lung weights than those lambs with uncorrected obstruction (Nakayama *et al.* 1983).

Their next series of experiments showed that unilateral ureteral ligation early in gestation produced renal dysplasia (Glick *et al.* 1983) which could be partially corrected by creating a ureterostomy three, six or nine weeks later (Glick *et al.* 1984a). The earlier the kidney was decompressed, the less severe the histological changes at birth, and the better the renal function.

These studies suggest that *in utero* decompression of urinary tract obstruction can lessen the severity of renal and pulmonary compromise. However, several questions remain unanswered. It is not known how closely the lamb urinary tract parallels that of the human. While relief of obstruction produced late in gestation partially prevents pulmonary hypoplasia, the effects of early obstruction and oligohydramnios on pulmonary hypoplasia may or may not be equally reversible.

Shunt procedure

Most intrauterine fetal shunting procedures have utilized ultrasound-guided percutaneous placement of a vesicoamniotic catheter. Early shunting procedures that attempted to pass a catheter over a guide wire were unsuccessful. Recent procedures have used a polyethylene catheter, with a memory coil at one or both ends, which is loaded on a needle. A pigtail coil placed in the bladder helps to prevent the catheter from falling out of the bladder. The amniotic end of the shunt usually has a second pigtail, or a bend, to prevent the catheter from being drawn into the fetus. Under ultrasonic visualization, the catheter-loaded needle is placed through the maternal abdomen and uterus and then directed into the site of obstruction (usually the bladder). Once the needle tip is visualized within the bladder, a separate piece of preloaded tubing which is seated on the needle above the catheter is used to push the shunt far enough off the needle so that the coil is constituted in the bladder. The needle is then withdrawn while the catheter is held in place with the pusher.

In cases of oligohydramnios, catheter placement can be facilitated by prior infusion of warmed normal saline into the amniotic cavity. This ensures an adequate pocket of fluid external to the fetal abdominal wall for placement of the distal end of the catheter. Correct placement of the catheter is verified by a decrease in size of the dilated bladder. Weekly assessment of amniotic fluid volume, urinary tract dilatation and catheter location should be made, as it is not uncommon for the catheter to stop functioning. The side holes of the catheter can become clogged or, as the fetus grows, the catheter can be pulled out of the bladder or withdrawn into either the abdominal cavity or the bladder. If the distal end is within the abdominal cavity and the proximal end remains in the bladder, urinary ascites may be seen. We have managed this problem by placing an abdominoamniotic shunt, thereby creating a two-step system in which fetal urine gains access to the amniotic cavity via the abdominal cavity.

Clinical studies

The first human shunts established the technical feasibility of *in utero* shunting, but identified the problem of patient selection. In 1982, Golbus *et al.* placed the first suprapubic catheter in a 32-week fetus with low-level obstruction, hydronephrosis and decreased amniotic fluid. Intra-uterine therapy was selected for this fetus because it was felt that early delivery would subject the coexisting twin to the morbidity of premature delivery. Delivery occurred two weeks after shunt placement, and the hydronephrotic twin underwent bilateral ureterostomies. Renal biopsy showed mild dysplasia, but the infant's serum creatinine was normal following diversion.

The outcome in subsequent procedures was less favourable. Berkowitz *et al.* (1982) placed a percutaneous bladder–amniotic fluid shunt in a fetus with marked oligohydramnios and low-level severe obstruction at 24 weeks. The shunt appeared to function optimally for three weeks and thereafter moderate hydronephrosis and a reduced quantity of amniotic fluid were noted to recur, but these remained stable. Eight weeks after shunt placement, a 2470 gm male infant was delivered which died at 12 hours of respiratory insufficiency. Autopsy showed a posterior urethral valve, severe bilateral renal dysplasia, early hyaline membrane formation and atelectasis.

A different technique was used by Harrison *et al.* (1982c) in a 21-week-old fetus with severe oligohydramnios, bilateral hydronephrosis, dilated ureters and enlarged bladder. These investigators performed bilateral ureterostomies through a hysterotomy incision. The procedure decompressed the urinary tract, but oligohydramnios persisted. The infant, delivered at 35 weeks by caesarean section, had mild facial deformities, limb contractures, bilateral undescended testes and a small chest. He expired nine hours later, despite maximum respiratory support. Autopsy showed a posterior urethral valve, hypoplastic lungs and small dysmorphic kidneys with Potter type IV cystic dysplasia.

Manning reported two similar cases, both managed with vesicoamniotic shunts for massively enlarged fetal bladders, but with very different outcomes (Manning *et al.* 1983). Both fetuses had severe oligohydramnios at the time of shunt placement at 16 weeks, and normal fluid volume subsequently. The first shunt failed at 35 weeks, and an infant with normal pulmonary and renal function was delivered. The shunt in the second fetus failed after 48 hours and another shunt was inserted. Amniotic fluid volume was reported as remaining near normal, despite partial bladder refilling. The infant delivered at 31 weeks after rupture of membranes and died of pulmonary hypoplasia.

These initial cases illustrate the problem of determining which obstructed fetuses will benefit from shunting, which would have a favourable prognosis without the risk of fetal surgery, and which have irreversible pulmonary and renal disease that will not benefit from shunting.

Diagnostic tests for evaluation of renal function

Multiple parameters have been studied to assess prognosis and evaluate residual renal function before considering shunt placement in patients with bilateral obstruction. Quantity of amniotic fluid, renal sonographic appearance, amount of urine production and the biochemical composition of the urine have provided some insight into prognosis.

Quantity of amniotic fluid is most important. In the absence of gut obstruction or neurological impairment, normal fluid usually signifies reasonable renal function and adequate pulmonary development. Decreased fluid before shunting implies urethral or bilateral upper-tract obstruction. After shunt placement, persistence of decreased fluid signifies either shunt failure or inability of the kidneys to produce urine. As previously mentioned, the sequelae of oligohydramnios will depend on the duration, degree and gestational age. Prolonged severe oligohydramnios prior to 20 weeks of gestation usually has an unfavourable prognosis (Harrison *et al.* 1982b). Diversion procedures attempted in this situation have led to perinatal deaths from respiratory failure, often with dysplastic kidneys (Berkowitz *et al.* 1982; Manning *et al.* 1983; Hobbins *et al.* 1984). On the other hand, isolated reports illustrate that prognosis is not uniformly poor (Manning *et al.* 1983). There may be a critical time in gestation before which damage to the lung and/or kidneys associated with severe obstruction and oligohydramnios is reversible. Alternatively, the cases with normal renal and pulmonary development may be those in which the oligohydramnios had been brief in duration. When oligohydramnios develops later in gestation, lung development may be normal but renal function can be permanently impaired and not correctable by drainage of the urinary tract (Harrison *et al.* 1982d; Golbus *et al.* 1982).

Between the two extremes of normal fluid and severe oligohydramnios are cases with a decreased or decreasing amount of fluid. In these cases, it is impossible to determine renal function by fluid quantity alone, especially if the fetus is seen for the first time during the late second or early third trimester of pregnancy and the duration of fluid diminution is unknown. Fetuses with bilateral obstruction and a reduced volume of amniotic fluid may benefit from *in utero* shunting, but further evaluation of the kidneys is required in order to determine residual renal function.

Measurement of urine production *in utero* has been performed to better identify non-functioning kidneys. While absence of bladder-refilling following aspiration or failure to respond to furosemide (Wladimiroff 1975) are ominous signs, the presence of 'urine production' does not guarantee good renal function. The bladder may refill following aspiration with urine from the dilated upper tracts, even in the absence of new urine formation. Prolonged drainage of the urinary tract, by an epidural or balloon-tipped catheter, into an external system has been performed in order to measure urine production and fetal creatinine clearance (McFadyen *et al.* 1983; Adzick *et al.* 1985). While these methods may provide useful data about the natural history of urinary tract obstruction *in utero*, their routine use for measurement of residual renal function is hampered by the risk of infection and the likelihood of the catheter being dislodged and causing trauma. Placement of a vesicoamniotic fluid shunt to assess fetal urine production can provide valuable information, especially in the second trimester where options include prolonged shunting, expectant management and pregnancy termination. Lack of amniotic fluid reaccumulation after shunt placement has a poor prognosis. Persistence of normal amniotic fluid is usually favourable, but does not guarantee normal renal function.

Abnormal sonographic appearance of the kidneys has a high specificity but a low sensitivity in predicting dysplasia. The cysts in Potter type IV dysplasia are usually too small to be visible on ultrasound but, if visible, the presence of cortical cysts implies dysplasia. More often, renal dysplasia is identified by increased echogenicity of the renal parenchyma. Mahoney *et al.* (1984) compared sonographic findings with renal pathology and found that visible cortical cysts had a sensitivity of 44% and a specificity of 100% in predicting dysplasia. Increased echogenicity of the renal parenchyma had a sensitivity of 57% and a specificity of 89%. Least predictive was the severity of hydronephrosis, with a sensitivity of 35% and a specificity of 78%. Unfortunately, normal appearance of the kidneys on ultrasound does not exclude dysplasia. Among 34 kidneys with histological documentation of dysplasia, 15 had cortical cysts on sonography, 20 had only increased echogenicity and 9 were normal in appearance.

Normal fetal urine production involves selective tubular absorption of sodium and chloride from an ultrafiltrate of fetal serum. Golbus *et al.* (1985) found measurements of urine electrolytes and osmolality to be useful in predicting prognosis. In their retrospective study of 18 fetuses with obstructive uropathy, hypotonic urine predicted good function, while isotonic urine with high sodium and chloride concentrations was found in fetuses with poor renal function. Values predictive of good function were: osmolality less than 210 mosm, sodium less than 100 meq dl^{-1}, and chloride less than 90 meq dl^{-1}. Nicolaides & Rodeck (1985) reported similar results in 16 patients with obstructive uropathy. Twelve patients with dysplastic kidneys on autopsy where the pregnancies were terminated because of suspected poor renal function had fetal urinary sodium greater than 95 mmol l^{-1} with no increase in amniotic fluid volume after vesicoamniotic shunting. Four infants delivered with good renal function had fetal urinary sodium of less than 60 mmol l^{-1} at the time of *in utero* catheterization.

Our experience at Mount Sinai with fetal urinary electrolytes is somewhat different (Wilkins *et al.* 1987). In a series of nine fetuses with sonographic evidence of obstruction, none of the four fetuses with elevated urinary electrolytes survived. Two of these pregnancies were electively terminated, and the fetal kidneys demonstrated renal dysplasia on autopsy. The other two neonates died shortly after birth of pulmonary hypoplasia, but only one had renal dysplasia on autopsy. Urine electrolytes predicted good function in the other five fetuses, but only one is alive with normal renal function. Three of the others were born alive; two died of renal failure at six weeks of life, while the third is alive with chronic renal failure. The fifth pregnancy was electively terminated despite the normal electrolytes, and autopsy showed renal dysplasia. In our series, therefore, abnormally high fetal urinary electrolytes were predictive of poor outcome, but normal electrolytes did not accurately predict normal renal function during the neonatal period.

International Fetal Surgery Registry

From 1982 to 1986, 79 cases of catheter shunts for obstructive uropathy were reported to the International Fetal Surgery Registry, held at the University of Manitoba (Manning 1986; F.A. Manning, personal communication, 1987). Eleven of the 79 fetuses were electively terminated subsequent to catheter placement, six for abnormal karyotype, five others for suspected severe renal disease. Of the 68 cases where the pregnancy was continued, the survival rate was 50%. Survival was 100% for prune-belly syndrome; all three cases showed no anatomical evidence of urethral obstruction. Lowest survival was seen with urethral atresia; all three fetuses died.

The most common diagnosis was posterior urethral valve, which had a survival of 74%. The mortality of untreated posterior urethral valve syndrome detected at birth is about 45% (Nakayama *et al.* 1986). While the number of patients in both series is small, this suggests that *in utero* therapy for posterior urethral valves may be of benefit.

Sixty-three of the fetuses with ongoing pregnancies were male, while only five were female. This is not surprising, as posterior urethral valves, the most common diagnosis in the treated series, are almost exclusively a male disease (Grupe 1984). Overall survival for males was 50·9%, while only 20% of females survived. Three female fetuses had isolated urethral atresia, and two had urethral atresia with persistent cloacal syndrome. One of the latter survived.

Procedure-related mortality in ongoing pregnancies was 4·8%. Two deaths occurred at the time of shunt placement and were presumed to be due to trauma. The other procedure-related loss occurred in a premature neonate born as a result of premature labour 48 hours after shunt placement. Pulmonary hypoplasia was the major cause of death in the remaining fetuses. Twenty-seven neonates died from respiratory insufficiency while only one died of chronic renal failure. Quality of life in the survivors was good, as only two of the 34 survivors have chronic illness.

The registry data illustrate the feasibility and possible utility of *in utero* shunting for obstructive uropathy, but also highlight the problem of our inability to diagnose pulmonary hypoplasia in the fetus. Harrison's group has shown that, in animals, pulmonary hypoplasia can be improved, or partially prevented, by decompression of the urinary tract *in utero* (Nakayama *et al.* 1983). The critical periods and duration of obstruction resulting in renal dysplasia also require elucidation, as normal pulmonary function at birth does not guarantee normal renal function.

Management of fetal obstructive uropathy

Patients with a suspected fetal urinary tract obstruction should undergo high resolution sonography at a centre experienced in the diagnosis and management of this disorder. Serial examinations may be required to determine the level, degree and progression of obstruction. Special attention should be given to the appearance of the fetal kidneys, amount of amniotic fluid and presence of non-renal anomalies. Chromosomal analysis is mandatory. Aspiration of urine from the dilated portion of the tract may provide additional prognostic information (e.g. urine electrolytes, reaccumulation of urine documenting ongoing production).

Expectant management should be selected for fetuses with a normal amount of amniotic fluid, regardless of whether the obstruction is unilateral or bilateral. These fetuses are expected to have a good prognosis, but require serial follow-up ultrasound examinations to look for worsening upper tract dilatation and decrease in amniotic fluid volume. If the fluid volume decreases in a premature fetus who has no other anomalies, shunt placement is recommended.

Fetuses with severe bilateral obstruction (bilateral hydronephrosis and/or megacystis) associated with marked oligohydramnios are suspected to have a poor prognosis. Additional prognostic information may be gained from aspiration of urine in order to observe urine production and to measure electrolytes. *In utero* shunting is unlikely to improve outcome in this group of fetuses unless rapid urine reaccumulation is demonstrated, urine electrolytes are normal and the kidneys lack cortical cysts and increased echogenicity on sonography. Even then, pulmonary hypoplasia may already be present and may be irreversible. Bladder—amniotic shunts can be placed in gestations less than 24 weeks to achieve decompression and assess renal function. If amniotic fluid does not reaccumulate, the prognosis for normal renal function and adequate lung development is poor. In those cases, pregnancy termination should be considered.

Treatment may improve the prognosis in those fetuses with bilateral obstruction, no associated abnormalities, and progressive decrease in amniotic fluid quantity. If evaluation of renal function suggests good prognosis, then intrauterine therapy should be considered for fetuses who are immature.

Improved success with shunting for obstructive uropathy will require better selection of fetuses as well as improvements in shunt technique. Accurate antenatal assessment of adequate pulmonary and renal function would improve selection. Ability to maintain shunt patency would decrease morbidity by requiring fewer procedures. Further study is required to determine if open surgical techniques yield results which are sufficiently superior to percutaneous shunt placement to justify the added maternal risks involved.

Hydrocephalus

Most children born with severe congenital obstructive hydrocephalus die or are left severely retarded. Milder cases treated with early neonatal shunting can have a favourable prognosis. It therefore became logical to question whether *in utero* shunting of mild, yet progressive, hydrocephalus could prevent ongoing damage and allow normal brain development to proceed. The results of intrauterine shunting procedures have not yet met these expectations, primarily due to a failure to identify those fetuses who would benefit from decompression. The diverse aetiologies of hydrocephalus, the lack of information on their natural histories and the inability to accurately exclude other major anomalies have contributed to suboptimal selection.

Diagnosis

By the 12th week of gestation, the lateral ventricles of the fetus can be recognized filling the cranial vault, while the ventricles are filled in turn with the highly echogenic choroid plexuses. At 15 to 17 weeks, the lateral wall of the ventricles can clearly be distinguished from the calvarium, and the intervening mantle identified. As gestation advances, the ventricles appear to shrink as rapid proliferation and growth of the cerebral hemispheres occur. The diagnosis of early hydrocephalus is made by an elevated lateral ventricular width to hemispheric width ratio (LVW/HW) according to the nomograms of Johnson *et al.* (1980) and Jeanty *et al.* (1981). At 15 weeks' gestation, the LVW/HW averages 56% but ranges from 40 to 71%, while at term it should not be greater than 35%, and usually averages 28% (Johnson *et al.* 1980). As a general rule, the lateral ventricle extends about two-thirds the distance from the midline to the inner edge of the skull at 15 weeks, then decreases to one-half, one-third and one quarter the distance by 18, 22 and 40 weeks, respectively.

The diagnosis of early hydrocephalus should be confirmed by evidence of progressive ventricular enlargement. As pointed out by Chervenak *et al.* (1983), approximately 2·5% of the normal population will have an abnormally elevated LVW/HW as defined by the nomograms of Johnson or Jeanty. Persistent elevation of LVW/HW ratio has been shown to be a reliable predictor of ventriculomegaly (Chervenak *et al.* 1983, 1984a). Enlargement of the skull seen in late hydrocephaly usually does not occur until after 28 weeks. In severe cases, cortical echoes are replaced by those from the fluid-filled ventricles extending laterally to the skull.

Aetiology

Hydrocephalus is a morphological finding which can result from a variety of causes. Once hydrocephalus is identified, an attempt to determine aetiology should be made, as the clinical course and the prognosis will differ depending on aetiology. The two mechanisms responsible for ventricular enlargement are (i) elevation of intracranial pressure (ICP) due to obstruction of fluid flow or to increased rate of fluid production, and (ii) decrease in brain substance. Ventriculoamniotic shunts are only useful in cases resulting from the first mechanism where a high ventricular/amniotic fluid pressure gradient will result in passive flow out of the ventricles. Most cases of prenatally diagnosed ventriculomegaly are due to elevation in ICP, either from blockage within the ventricular system (obstructive) or from lack of reabsorption due to blockade in the subarachnoid pathways (communicating). Choroid plexus papilloma, a tumour which secretes cerebrospinal fluid and causes elevated ICP, has not yet been reported in a fetus (Clewell *et al.* 1986).

Environmental and genetic causes of hydrocephalus have been identified in some cases, while other cases are only identified by their structural abnormalities. Intrauterine infections can cause inflammation or haemorrhage resulting in scarring and obstruction at the aqueduct of Sylvius or at the subarachnoid granulations. Toxoplasmosis, cytomegalovirus, syphilis and rubella may cause ventriculomegaly by either obstruction or degeneration of brain substance. Sonographic identification of cerebral calcifications may be suggestive of an infectious aetiology.

Genetic causes of hydrocephalus range from those with multifactorial inheritance with a low recurrence risk, to autosomal recessive syndromes with a 25% recurrence risk. X-linked aqueductal stenosis accounts for 2% of all cases of isolated hydrocephalus, but may be responsible for up to 25% of aqueductal stenosis in males (Burton 1979). Dandy–Walker syndrome, congenital atresia of the foramina of the ventricle, may be of autosomal recessive inheritance in some cases (Burton 1979). Ultrasound findings include a large cystic structure in the posterior fossa continuous with the fourth ventricle. Cerebellar agenesis, which may show an X-linked inheritance, has a poor prognosis and should be distinguished from Dandy–Walker syndrome (Ricardi & Marcus 1978). Chromosomal anomalies, such as trisomy 18 or 13, may cause brain malformation with obstruction at the cerebral aqueduct or fourth ventricle.

The presence or absence of associated anomalies may aid in determining the aetiology and prognosis of the ventriculomegaly. Recent series have shown major malformations occurring in 70–83% of fetuses with hydrocephalus, with only a small percentage of these attributable to chromosomal aberrations (Glick *et al.* 1984c; Chervenak *et al.* 1985; Pretorius *et al.* 1985). Spina bifida is the most common associated abnormality, present in 25–30% of the cases of fetal hydrocephalus. The Arnold–Chiari malformation, obstruction at the foramen magnum or fourth ventricle caused by downward displacement of the medulla oblongata and of the cerebellum, causes hydrocephalus in approximately 80% of cases of spina bifida. While prognosis for intelligence depends on the site of the lesion, almost all of these children are physically handicapped. Thirty-seven per cent of the hydrocephalic fetuses in Chervenak's 1985 series had intracranial anomalies, including microcephaly, agenesis of the corpus callosum, encephalocoele, arteriovenous malformation, arachnoid cyst and cebocephaly.

Anomalies have also been reported in the cardiovascular, renal, gastrointestinal, skeletal, respiratory and reproductive systems. Severe anomalies are important to diagnose, as their poor prognosis would preclude intervention for hydrocephalus. The identification of minor anomalies is also important as they may identify syndromes. Microcephaly, encephalocoele, polycystic kidneys or polycystic liver in combination with hydrocephalus would suggest Meckel syndrome. Hypotelorism in addition to hydrocephaly might suggest holoprosencephaly (Chervenak *et al.* 1983).

Of concern is the failure to detect these malformations before birth. In the combined experience of three recent series of fetal hydrocephalus, failure to diagnose a severe associated anomaly before birth occurred in 26 of the 95 (27%) cases (Glick *et al.* 1984c; Chervenak *et al.* 1985; Clewell *et al.* 1985). Major malformations not identified before delivery included: spina bifida, cardiac malformations, oesophageal atresia, tracheo-oesophageal fistula, eventration of the diaphragm, sirenomelia, agenesis of the corpus callosum, alobar holoprosencephaly, AV malformation of the thalamus, cerebellar cyst, porencephalic cyst, polymicrogyria and congenital toxoplasmosis.

Ultrasound can accurately diagnose fetal ventriculomegaly, even in the early second trimester, but the reported accuracy in diagnosing associated anomalies is suboptimal. Accuracy is likely to improve with experience, improving resolution of sonography and adjuvant use of other modalities such as echocardiography, computerized tomography and magnetic resonance imaging in selected cases.

Natural history of fetal hydrocephalus

The natural history of ventriculomegaly in the fetus, particularly if found in the second trimester, is unclear. It is therefore difficult to determine prognosis for the fetus with isolated hydrocephalus, and difficult to determine the effect of *in utero* treatment.

Glick *et al.* (1984c) reported outcomes in 11 fetuses thought to have isolated ventriculomegaly. Nine fetuses had stable ventricular size on serial sonography, one had progressive dilatation, and one had resolution of the ventriculomegaly. After birth, only six of the neonates had isolated hydrocephalus. Five neonates had associated anomalies: two with agenesis of the corpus callosum, one each with myelomeningocoele, septo-optic dysplasia and porencephalic cyst. Only one of the neonates with an associated anomaly had normal motor and mental development. On the other hand, only one of the five neonates with isolated hydrocephalus at birth demonstrated any developmental delay after an average follow-up of 10 months. Two of the three infants with neonatal shunts had normal development, as did the other three with no evidence of raised ICP.

Clewell's 1985 series included 13 patients who were candidates for, but declined, *in utero* shunt placement. Of the eight fetuses who had isolated hydrocephalus at birth, only three survived. Two of the survivors had normal mental and motor development. In Chervenak's 1984b series of 48 patients with fetal hydrocephalus managed expectantly, only eight patients had isolated ventriculomegaly. Four of these were born alive, two were electively terminated and two with severe ventriculomegaly had intrapartum deaths. One of the four liveborns was alive at seven months, and this infant, while shunt-dependent, had normal mental and motor development. The other three liveborns died in the early neonatal period. Vintzileos *et al.* (1987) reported the outcome of 20 fetuses with ventriculomegaly; five with isolated hydrocephalus were all born alive. After an average follow-up of 12 months, all were shunt-dependent, three had normal development and two had mild retardation.

These series report a total of 26 fetuses with isolated ventriculomegaly at birth who were managed expectantly *in utero*. Sixteen (61·5%) neonates survived and 13 (81%) of the survivors were normal at follow-up. Since this is a small series which only includes infants found to have no associated anomalies at birth, the true incidence of normal outcome for fetuses thought to have isolated ventriculomegaly requires larger series with longer follow-up.

Natural history of neonatal hydrocephalus

Much of the support for *in utero* shunting comes from the fact that neonatal shunts have improved the prognosis for infants with hydrocephalus. Laurence & Coates (1962) reported a series of 182 hydrocephalic infants managed expectantly between 1938 and 1957: 46% had spontaneous arrest of hydrocephalus, 49% died and 5% had progressive hydrocephalus. By 1974, only 5 of 200 consecutively shunted infants in one series had died (Raimondi & Soare 1974). Early shunting and absence of congenital malformations were the best prognostic factors in this series. Infants with macrocephaly or reduced cortical mantle thickness may have good outcomes if shunted in the early neonatal period. McCullough & Barbzer-Martin's 1982 study of 37 infants with macrocephaly demonstrated an 86% survival rate. Of the survivors, 53% had normal IQs and 19% had borderline IQs. Lorber & Bassi's 1965 series of neonates with a cortical mantle thickness of less than 10 mm demonstrated an overall survival rate of 78·5%, with 82% of the survivors having IQs over 80. While these studies suffer from selection bias, it is clear that early neonatal shunting offers the best prognosis for survival and intellectual development in newborns with congenital hydrocephalus.

It is not clear whether the improved prognosis with neonatal shunting can be expected with *in utero* shunting. The spectrum of diseases seen in the fetus may differ from those seen in the neonate. In addition, the diagnosis of associated anomalies is more clearly made in the newborn than in the fetus. In Lorber's 1968 neonatal series of congenital hydrocephalus, 81% had an associated meningomyelocoele, while 29·8% of the cases without a neural tube defect had a different associated anomaly. Recent series of fetal hydrocephalus, on the other hand, show a 30% incidence of meningomyelocoele, while 40−80% of the fetuses without a neural tube defect have another anomaly (Chervenak *et al.* 1983; Glick *et al.* 1984c; Pretorius *et al.* 1985). It is not known whether this difference in associated anomalies is geographic or truly represents a difference in neonatal compared with fetal hydrocephalus.

Experimental studies

Animal studies have demonstrated the feasibility and efficacy of intra-uterine shunting procedures. Michejda & Hodgen (1981) induced hydrocephalus in rhesus monkeys by maternal injection of a corticosteroid, triamcinolone acetonide. When this teratogen is administered early in gestation, days 18−22 (term, 164±5 days), the fetuses showed extensive occipital bone hypoplasia resulting in large cranium bifidum, encephalocoele and hydrocephalus. Treatment later in gestation, days 21−25, resulted in hydrocephalus associated with less severe or no cranial malformations. Thirty of their 60 affected fetuses underwent *in utero* placement of a valved ventriculoamniotic shunt, placed through a maternal hysterotomy incision, between days 115 and 125. Their results showed a clear benefit of *in utero* shunting, in both the early and the late treatment groups. Only 23 of 30 animals with induced hydrocephalus not shunted *in utero* survived to birth, and 6 died in the neonatal period. Of the 17 survivors, 5 underwent cranioplasty and had delayed motor development and blindness, 10 had seizures and muscle weakness, and 2 had slow neurobehavioural development. In the shunted group, 28 of the 30 treated animals survived and had normal development, while 2 animals died as a result of the surgical procedure. Examination of the CNS with both computerized tomography and microscopic sections demonstrated that fetal monkey brain resumes its ability to grow rapidly and to reorganize its cytoarchitecture when hydrocephalus is effectively shunted *in utero* (Michejda *et al.* 1986).

Glick *et al.* (1984b) induced hydrocephalus in fetal lambs and monkeys by a different method. While their series demonstrated improvement in gross ventriculomegaly and overall survival with shunting, *in utero* treatment was associated with significant complications and did not improve histopathological brain damage. They injected kaolin into the cisterna magna, causing inflammation and obstruction of the foramina of Luschka and Magendie. Eight of 18 rhesus monkeys treated with kaolin at 96−134 days' gestation underwent shunting 14−21 days later. Valveless shunts were placed through a small hysterotomy incision, and the monkeys were delivered at 160 days' gestation. Thirty-five fetal lambs were injected with kaolin at 100 days' gestation, 20 were shunted at 120−125 days, and all were delivered at 140 days' gestation. Eighteen of the 28 shunted animals survived, while only 2 of the 16 unshunted controls lived. Complications of shunting seen in the survivors included: shunt blockage, improper shunt tip placement, shunt infection, subdural haematoma and subdural hygroma.

Histological examination of the brains of the unshunted fetal animals showed ependymal and periventricular white matter injury with relative sparing of the cortical grey matter. The changes are similar to those found in neonates and children with hydrocephalus (Weller & Shulman 1972). The shunted lambs, however, also showed white matter damage thought to be directly related to the kaolin. The authors hypothesized that kaolin refluxed into the lateral ventricles, causing a severe inflammatory ventriculitis and local tissue injury. It is not clear, therefore, if increased ICP, kaolin or shunting with reflux of amniotic fluid was responsible for the white matter damage in the shunted animals. Nevertheless, their series demonstrated improved survival with shunting.

Shunt procedure

Most of the shunts placed in human fetuses to date have been similar to the shunt used by the Denver group (Clewell *et al.* 1982), with or without the valve. The Denver shunt is made of silicone rubber tubing and contains a valve to avoid sudden decompression of the ventricle and to prevent back flow of amniotic fluid into the ventricle. The amniotic end of the shunt has a thickened collar to prevent the shunt from being pushed into the fetal head. Modification of the original shunt has included placement of two rubber flanges that fold flat along the shunt during placement and then expand to keep the shunt anchored in the fetal skull.

Following maternal sedation and/or local anaesthesia, a 13-gauge needle with a sharp stylet is inserted through the maternal abdomen and uterus into the fetal lateral ventricle. Entry through the fetal calvarium is usually through the posterior parietal region above the level of the trigone. As a ventriculoamniotic shunt will be of benefit only in cases of elevated intracranial pressure, measurements of pressure within the amniotic fluid and the fetal ventricle are taken during placement of the needle. Once the needle is in place within the ventricle, the shunt is pushed through the needle and held in position with a blunt stylet as the needle is withdrawn.

Proper shunt placement can be determined by sonographically locating the catheter ends, and confirmed by the gradual decrease in the LVW/HW ratio. Malfunction due to obstruction or migration from proper location is diagnosed by a rapid increase in the LVH/HW ratio.

Clinical studies

The first attempt at intrauterine treatment of fetal hydrocephalus was performed by Birnholz & Frigoletto (1981). They performed six serial sonographically guided cephalocenteses on a fetus from 25 to 32 weeks' gestation. The fetus had moderate, asymmetrical dilatation of the ventricles, and later in gestation was noted to have a posterior midline cyst. The first two taps did not reveal any evidence of increased ICP. Following delivery by caesarean section at 34 weeks, the neonate had a ventriculoposterior midline intracranial cyst, absent corpus callosum, developmental delay and hypotonia. A diagnosis of Becker's muscular dystrophy was made. It is not clear whether or not antenatal treatment affected the outcome.

Clewell *et al.* (1982), realizing that serial aspirations may be traumatic and can only offer temporary relief of elevated ICP, developed an indwelling ventriculoamniotic shunt with a one-way valve. The first shunt was placed percutaneously in a hydrocephalic fetus with a family history of X-linked aqueductal stenosis. The fetus had progressively elevated LVW/HW ratios at 21 and 23 weeks. Following shunt placement at 24 weeks, a decrease in LVW/HW ratio, an increase in cortical mantle thickness and a normal BPD were observed. Delivery by caesarean section occurred at 34 weeks, after sudden ventricular dilatation and increase in BPD suggested shunt occlusion. The neonate underwent ventriculoperitoneal shunting, and on follow-up at 10 months had dysmorphic ears, flexion contractures of the hands and fingers, and delayed neurological development (Hect & Grix 1982).

As the natural history of ventriculomegaly in a given fetus is difficult to predict, the benefit of *in utero* shunting for a given fetus is hard to evaluate.

International Fetal Surgery Registry

From 1982 to 1985, the International Fetal Surgery Registry contained 39 reported cases of fetal hydrocephalus treated by *in utero* decompression (Manning *et al.* 1986). Thirty-seven of the the 39 cases were treated with indwelling shunts for a mean duration of $2\cdot1\pm1\cdot3$ weeks (range less than 1 to 7 weeks). The average gestational age at diagnosis was $25\pm2\cdot7$ weeks, while the mean age at treatment was $27\pm2\cdot6$ weeks. Survival rate was $82\cdot1\%$, with a procedure-related death rate of $10\cdot25\%$. One fetus died at the time of shunt placement from brain trauma, while three others died from premature delivery related to the surgical procedure. Three deaths occurred that were not procedure-related: two with severe associated anomalies, one was unexplained.

Neonatal diagnoses were: aqueductal stenosis (32 cases) and one case each of Dandy—Walker syndrome, holoprosencephaly, Arnold—Chiari syndrome and porencephalic cyst. In three cases, the cause of hydrocyphalus was unknown. Associated anomalies in other organ systems were found in 15·4% of the fetuses: diaphragmatic hernia, arthrogryposis multiplex congenita, myelomeningocoele, trisomy 21, massive facial cleft, pulmonary hypoplasia and multiple anomalies.

Follow-up of the survivors for a mean of 8·2±6 months showed the majority to be abnormal (65·6%). Eighteen of 39 treated fetuses (56·25%) have severe handicap, and all tested exhibited developmental quotients of less than 50. Five of these infants have cortical blindness, two have severe seizure disorders and two have spastic dysplegia. The only neurologically normal fetuses in the series were those with aqueductal stenosis. Of the 32 cases with this diagnosis, 34% are normal, 50% have a severe handicap and 12·5% died of procedure-related complications.

It is difficult to compare outcomes in groups of untreated and treated fetuses with hydrocephalus, as both groups suffer from selection bias. However, a prospective randomized controlled trial does not exist. Preliminary analysis of treated fetuses with isolated hydrocephalus compared with historical controls indicates that *in utero* treatment may increase survival by allowing severely handicapped fetuses to survive. Manning *et al.* (1986) compared the above registry statistics for aqueductal stenosis with published reports of the outcome of fetal aqueductal stenosis managed expectantly. Only 40% of the 20 reported cases which were not shunted *in utero* survived (two elective terminations, three intrapartum cephalocenteses), but six of the eight survivors (75%) were normal at follow-up. In the registry's treated group, 87·5% survived but only 37·5% of these were normal.

At the present time, *in utero* shunting for hydrocephalus offers no clear benefit to the fetus. While intrauterine therapy may improve outcome for a small group of fetuses, accurate antenatal selection of that group has not yet been demonstrated. Improvements are needed in our ability to diagnose aetiology, to document increased intracranial pressure and to rule out irreversible brain damage. More information on the natural history and long-term outcome of fetal hydrocephalus is essential before the role of *in utero* treatment can be properly evaluated. At the same time, experimental studies should be continued in order to develop a model which more closely parallels isolated human hydrocephalus. Experimental models can also help in refining shunt procedures in order to lower the morbidity of shunt placement and decrease the need for repeated procedures.

References

Adzick N.S., Harrison M.R., Glick P.L. *et al.* (1985) Fetal urinary tract obstruction: experimental pathophysiology. *Sem. Perinatol.,* **9**(2), 79–90.

Asensio S.H., Figueroa-Longo J.G. & Pelegrina I.A. (1966) Intrauterine exchange transfusion. *Am. J. Obstet. Gynecol.,* **95**, 1129–33.

Avni E.F., Rodesch F. & Schulman C.C. (1985) Fetal uropathies: diagnostic pitfalls and, management. *J. Urol.,* **134**, 921–5.

Bang J., Bock J.E. & Trolle D. (1982) Ultrasound-guided fetal intravenous transfusion for severe rhesus haemolytic disease. *Br. Med. J.,* **284**, 373–4.

Beck A.D. (1971) The effects of intrauterine urinary obstruction upon the development of the fetal kidneys. *J. Urol.,* **105**, 784–9.

Berkowitz R.L. (1980) Intrauterine transfusion 1980. An update. *Clin. Perinatol.,* **7**, 285–97.

Berkowitz R.L., Glickman M.G., Smith G.J.W. *et al.* (1982) Fetal urinary tract obstruction: what is the role of surgical intervention *in utero? Am J. Obstet. Gynecol.,* **144**(4), 367–75.

Berkowitz R.L., Chitkara U., Goldberg J.D., Wilkins I., Chervenak F.A. & Lynch L. (1986) Intrauterine intravascular transfusions for severe red blood cell isoimmunization: ultrasound-guided percutaneous approach. *Am. J. Obstet. Gynecol.,* **155**, 574–81.

Birnholz J.C. & Frigoletto F.D. (1981) Antenatal treatment of hydrocephalus. *N. Engl. J. Med.,* **303**(17), 1021–3.

Bock J.E. (1976) Intrauterine transfusion in the management of pregnant women with severe rhesus isoimmunization. II Results and discussion. *Acta Obstet. Gynecol. Scand. (Suppl.),* **53**, 29–36.

Bowman J.M. (1975) Rh erythroblastosis 1975. *Sem. Hematol.,* **12**, 189–207.

Bowman J.M. (1978) The management of Rh-isoimmunization. *Obstet. Gynecol.,* **52**, 1–16.

Bowman J.M. & Manning F.A. (1983) Intrauterine Fetal Transfusions: Winnipeg 1982. *Obstet. Gynecol.,* **61**, 203–9.

Burton B.K. (1979) Recurrence risk for congenital hydrocephalus. *Clin. Genet.,* **16**, 47–53.

Ch de Crespigny L., Robinson H.P., Quinn M., Doyle L., Ross A. & Cauchi M. (1985) Ultrasound-guided fetal blood transfusion for severe rhesus isoimmunization. *Obstet. Gynecol.,* **66**, 529–32.

Chervenak F.A., Berkowitz R.L., Romero R. *et al.* (1983) The diagnosis of fetal hydrocephalus. *Am. J. Obstet. Gynecol.,* **147**, 703–16.

Chervenak F.A., Berkowitz R.L., Tortora M. *et al.* (1984a) Diagnosis of ventriculomegaly before fetal viability. *Obstet. Gynecol.,* **64**, 652–6.

Chervenak F.A., Duncan C., Ment L.R. *et al.* (1984b) Outcome of fetal ventriculomegaly. *Lancet,* **ii**, 179–81.

Chervenak F.A., Berkowitz R.L., Tortora M. *et al.* (1985) The management of fetal hydrocephalus. *Am. J. Obstet. Gynecol.,* **151**, 933–42.

Clewell W.H., Johnson M.L., Meier P.R. *et al.* (1982) A surgical approach to the treatment of fetal hydrocephalus. *N. Engl. J. Med.,* **306**(22), 1320–5.

Clewell W.H., Meier P.R., Manchester D.K. *et al.* (1985). Ventriculomegaly: evaluation and management. *Sem. Perinatol.,* **9**(2), 98–102.

Clewell W.H., Manco-Johnson M.L., Manchester D.K. *et al.* (1986) Diagnosis and management of fetal hydrocephalus. *Clin. Obstet. Gynecol.,* **29**(3), 514–22.

Daffos F., Capella-Pavlosky M. & Forestier F. (1983) Fetal blood sampling via the umbilical cord using a needle guided by ultrasound. *Prenat. Diagn.,* **3**, 271–7.

Daffos F., Forestier F., Muller J.Y. *et al.* (1984) Prenatal treatment of alloimmune thrombocytopenia. *Lancet,* **ii**, 63–2.

Daffos F., Capella-Pavlosky M. & Forestier F. (1985) Fetal blood sampling during pregnancy with use of a needle guided by ultrasound: a study of 606 consecutive cases. *Obstet. Gynecol.,* **153**, 655–60.

Fitzsimmons R.B., Keohane C. & Galvin J. (1985) Prune belly syndrome with ultrasound demonstration of reduction of megacystis *in utero*. *Br. J. Radiol.*, **58**, 374−6.

Flake A.W., Harrison M.R., Adzick N.S. & Zanjani E.D. (1986) Transplantation of fetal haematopoietic stem cells *in utero*: the creation of haematopoietic chimeras. *Science*, **233**, 776−8.

Freda V.F. & Adamsons K.J. (1964) Exchange transfusion *in utero*. *Am. J. Obstet. Gynecol.*, **89**, 817−21.

Glick P.L., Harrison M.R., Noall R.A. *et al.* (1983) Correction of congenital hydronephrosis *in utero*. III. Early midtrimester ureteral obstruction produces renal dysplasia. *J. Pediatr. Surg.*, **18**, 681−7.

Glick P.L., Harrison R.M., Adzick N.S. *et al.* (1984a) Correction of congenital hydronephrosis *in utero*. IV. *In utero* decompression prevents renal dysplasia. *J. Pediatr. Surg.*, **19**, 649−57.

Glick P.L., Harrison R.M., Halks-Miller M. *et al.* (1984b) Correction of congenital hydrocephalus *in utero*. II. Efficacy of *in utero* shunting. *J. Pediatr. Surg.*, **19**(6), 870−81.

Glick P.L, Harrizon R.M., Nakayama D.K. *et al.* (1984c) Management of ventriculomegaly in the fetus. *J. Pediatr*, **105**, 97−105.

Golbus M.S., Harrison M.R., Filly R.A. *et al.* (1982) *In utero* treatment of urinary tract obstruction. *Am. J. Obstet. Gynecol.*, **142**, 383−8.

Golbus M.S., Filly R.A., Callen P. *et al.* (1985) Fetal urinary tract obstruction: management and selection for treatment. *Sem. Perinatol.*, **9**(2), 91−7.

Grannum P.A., Copel J.A., Plaxe S.C., Scioscia A.L. & Hobbins J.C. (1986) *In utero* exchange transfusion by direct intravascular injection in severe erythroblastosis fetalis. *N. Engl. J. Med.*, **314**, 1431−4.

Grupe W.E. (1984) Hydronephrosis. In *Schaffer's Diseases of the Newborn* (Ed. by M.E. Avery & H.W. Taeusch), pp. 427−36. W.B. Saunders, Philadelphia.

Hamilton E.G. (1977) Intrauterine transfusion — safeguard or peril? *Obstet. Gynecol.*, **50**, 255−60.

Harrison M.R., Filly R.A., Golbus M.S. *et al.* (1982a) Fetal treatment 1982. *N. Engl. J. Med.*, **306**(26), 1651−2.

Harrison M.R., Golbus M.S., Filly R.A. *et al.* (1982b) Management of the fetus with congenital hydronephrosis. *J. Pediatr. Surg.*, **17**(6), 728−42.

Harrison M.R., Golbus M.S., Filly R.A. *et al.* (1982c) Fetal surgery for congenital hydronephrosis. *N. Engl. J. Med.*, **306**(10), 591−3.

Harrison M.R., Nakayama D.K, Noall R. *et al.* (1982d) Correction of congenital hydronephrosis *in utero*. II. Decompression reverses the effects of obstruction on the fetal lung and urinary tract. *J. Pediatr. Surg.*, **17**, 965−74.

Harrison M.R., Ross N., Noall R. *et al.* (1983) Correction of congenital hydronephrosis *in utero*. I. The model: fetal urethral obstruction produces hydronephrosis and pulmonary hypoplasia in fetal lambs. *J. Pediatr. Surg.*, **18**, 247−56.

Hect F. & Grix A. (1982) Treatment of fetal hydrocephalus (letter). *N. Engl. J. Med.*, **307**(19), 1211.

Hobbins J.C., Romero R., Grannum P. *et al.* (1984) Antenatal diagnosis of renal anomalies with ultrasound. I. Obstructive uropathy. *Am. J. Obstet. Gynecol.*, **148**, 868−77.

Jeanty P., Dramaix-Wilmet M. & Delbeke D. (1981) Ultrasonic evaluation of fetal ventricular growth. *Neuroradiology*, **21**, 127−31.

Johnson M.L., Dunne M.G., Mack L.A. *et al.* (1980) Evaluation of fetal intracranial anatomy by static and realtime ultrasound. *J.C.U.*, **8**, 311−18.

Kurjak A., Kirkinen P., Latin V. *et al.* (1980) Diagnosis and assessment of fetal malformations and abnormalities by ultrasound. *J. Perinat. Med.*, **8**, 219−35.

Kurjak A., Latin V., Mandruzzato B. *et al.* (1984) Ultrasound diagnosis and perinatal management of fetal genitourinary abnormalities. *J. Perinat. Med.*, **12**, 291−312.

Laurence K.M. & Coates S. (1962) The natural history of hydrocephalus. *Arch. Dis. Child.*, **37**, 345−62.

Liley A.W. (1961) Liquor amnii analysis in the management of the pregnancy complicated by rhesus sensitization. *Am. J. Obstet. Gynecol.*, **82**, 1359−70.

Liley A.W. (1963) Intrauterine transfusion of foetus in haemolytic disease. *Br. Med. J.*, **2**, 1107−9.

Linch D.C., Rodeck C.H., Nicolaides K., Jones H.M. & Brent L. (1986) Attempted bone-marrow transplantation in a 17-week fetus. *Lancet*, **ii**, 1453.

Lorber J. (1968) The results of early treatment of extreme hydrocephalus. *Dev. Med. Child Neurol.*, **16** (suppl.), 21−9.

Lorber J. & Bassi V. (1965) The etiology of neonatal hydrocephalus (excluding cases of spina bifida). *Dev. Med. Child Neurol.*, **7**, 289−94.

McCullough D.C. & Barlzer-Martin L.A. (1982) Current prognosis in overt neonatal hydrocephalus. *J. Neurosurg.*, **57**, 378−83.

McFayden I.R., Wigglesworth J.S. & Dillon M.J. (1983) Fetal urinary tract obstruction: is active intervention before delivery indicated? *Br. J. Obstet. Gynaecol.*, **90**, 342−9.

MacKenzie F.Z., MacLeass D.A., Fryu A. & Evans S.L. (1982) Midtrimester intrauterine exchange transfusion of the fetus. *Am. J. Obstet. Gynecol.*, **143**, 555−9.

Mahoney B.S., Filly R.A., Callen P.W. *et al.* (1984) Sonographic evaluation of renal dysplasia. *Radiology*, **152**, 143−6.

Manning F.A. (1986) International Fetal Surgery Registry: 1985 update. *Clin. Obstet. Gynecol.*, **29**(3), 551−7.

Manning F.A., Harmon C.R., Lange I.R. *et al.* (1983) Antepartum chronic fetal vesico-amniotic shunts for obstructive uropathy: a report of two cases. *Am. J. Obstet. Gynecol.*, **145**, 819−22.

Manning F.A., Harrison M.R., Rodeck C. *et al.* (1986) Catheter shunts for fetal hydronephrosis and hydrocephalus. Report of the International Fetal Surgery Registry. *N. Engl. J. Med.*, **315**(5), 336−40.

Michejda M. & Hodgen G.D. (1981) *In utero* diagnosis and treatment of nonhuman primate fetal skeletal anomalies. I. Hydrocephalus. *JAMA*, **246**, 1093−7.

Michejda M., Queenan J.T. & McCullough D. (1986) Present status of intrauterine treatment of hydrocephalus and its future. *Am. J. Obstet. Gynecol.*, **155**, 873−82.

Nakayama D.K., Glick P.L., Villa R.L. *et al.* (1983) Experimental pulmonary hyperplasia due to oligohydramnios and its reversal by relieving thoracic compression. *J. Pediatr. Surg.*, **18**, 347−53.

Nakayama D.K., Harrison M.R. & deLorimer A.A. (1986) Prognosis of posterior urethral valves presenting at birth. *J. Pediatr. Surg.*, **21**, 43−5.

Nicolaides K.H. & Rodeck C.H. (1985) Fetal therapy. In *Progress in Obstetrics and Gynecology*, Vol. 5 (Ed. by J. Studd), pp. 40−57. Churchill Livingstone, Edinburgh.

Nicolaides K.H., Rodeck C.H., Mibashan R.S. & Kemp J.R. (1986) Have Liley charts outlived their usefulness? *Am. J. Obstet. Gynecol.*, **155**, 90−4.

Osathanondh V. & Potter E.L. (1964) Pathogenesis of polycystic kidneys. Type I due to hyperplasia of interstitial portion of collecting tubules. *Arch. Pathol.*, **77**, 510−14.

Potter E.L. & Craig J.M. (1976) *Pathology of the Fetus and Infant*, pp. 447−60. Year Book, Chicago.

Pretorius D.H., Davis K., Manco-Johnson M.L. *et al.* (1985) Clinical course of fetal hydrocephalus: 40 cases. *Am. J. Radiol.*, **144**, 827−31.

Quinlan R.W., Cruz A.C. & Huddleston J.F. (1986) Sonographic detection of fetal urinary tract anomalies. *Obstet. Gynecol.*, **67**, 558−65.

Raimondi A.J. & Soare P. (1974) Intellectual development in shunted hydrocephalic children. *Am. J. Dis. Child.*, **127**, 664−71.

Reuss A., Wladimiroff J.W., Scholtmeijer R.J. *et al.* (1988) Antenatal evaluation and outcome of fetal obstructive uropathies. *Prenat. Diagn.*, **8**, 93−102.

Riccardi V.M. & Marcus E.S. (1978) Congenital hydrocephalus and cerebellar agenesis. *Clin. Genet.*, **13**, 443−7.

Rodeck C.H. & Nicolaides K.H. (1983) Ultrasound guided invasive procedures in obstetrics. *Clin. Obstet. Gynecol.*, **10**(3), 515−39.

Rodeck C.H., Holman C.A., Karnicki J., Kemp J.R., Whitmore D.N. & Austin M.A. (1981) Direct intravascular fetal blood transfusion by fetoscopy in severe rhesus isoimmunization. *Lancet*, **i**, 625−8.

Rodeck C.H., Nicolaides K.H., Warsof L.S., Fysh W.J., Gamsu H.R., & Kemp J.R. (1984) The management of severe rhesus isoimmunization by fetoscopic intravascular transfusions. *Am. J. Obstet. Gynecol.*, **150**, 769−74.

Vintzileos A.M., Campbell W.A., Weinbaum P.J. *et al.* (1987) Perinatal management and outcome of fetal ventriculomegaly. *Obstet. Gynecol.*, **69**, 5−11.

Weller R.D. & Shulman K. (1972) Infantile hydrocephalus: clinical, histological, and ultrastructural study of brain damage. *J. Neurosurg.*, **36**, 225−65.

Wilkins I.A., Chitkara U., Lynch L. *et al.* (1987) The nonpredictive value of fetal urinary electrolytes: preliminary report of outcomes and correlations with pathologic diagnosis. *Am. J. Obstet. Gynecol.*, **157**, 694−8.

Wladimiroff J.W. (1975) Effect of furosemide on fetal urine production. *Br. J. Obstet. Gynaecol.*, **82**, 221−4.

7

Medical Treatment of the Fetus

J.W. WLADIMIROFF, P.A. STEWART & A. REUSS

Fetal treatment has become of major interest following the introduction of high-resolution ultrasound in the antenatal detection of structural defects. Increasingly, reports appear on the technical, ethical and legal aspects of fetal surgical procedures. Scarce information is available on fetal medical treatment. In a surgical procedure, there is direct structural intervention with fetal development. Medical treatment has up until now been directed at both transplacental drug administration, with the aim of creating pharmacological alterations in the fetus, and fetal blood transfusion, either via the intraperitoneal route or via the intravascular route in the treatment of immune hydrops fetalis. The disadvantages of transplacental treatment are twofold: (i) placental transfer will depend on the degree of maternal absorption and excretion of a particular drug and its metabolites as well as the quality of the placenta itself; (ii) direct monitoring of fetal drug levels is not feasible.

Fetal medical treatment is not new, a familiar example being the administration of corticosteroids for the prevention of respiratory distress syndrome in fetuses which are threatened with premature delivery. Medical treatment in relation to the developing fetus can be preventive or symptomatic. Preventive treatment has been mainly preconceptual and may vary from dietary measures in the presence of metabolic disorders such as phenylketonuria (Murphy *et al.* 1985) and galactosaemia (Chen *et al.* 1981) to vitamin supplementation as an unproven remedy in the prevention of neural tube defects (Rhoads & Mills 1986). Of a more symptomatic nature are therapies which have been applied in the presence of fetuses with vitamin B_{12} deficiency resulting in methylmalonic acidaemia (Ampola *et al.* 1975) and with metabolic disorders such as multiple carboxylase deficiency (Roth *et al.* 1982). In the first instance, maternal administration of cyanocobalamin 10 mg day^{-1} was started at 32 weeks' gestation in a pregnancy in which cultured amniotic fluid cells at 19 weeks demonstrated a deficient synthesis of 5^1-deoxy-adenosylcobalamin. An affected infant will usually die from severe acidosis and dehydration. Postnatally, the diagnosis of methylmalonic acidaemia was confirmed. Apart from protein restriction, no continuous cyanocobalamin was required. In the second instance, a fetus with suspected multiple carboxylase deficiency (two previous infants had died from the disease) was treated by maternal oral administration of biotin 10 mg day^{-1} as from 34 weeks of gestation. Affected infants present with severe metabolic acidosis and dermatitis but in this case the neonatal course was unremarkable, despite virtually complete deficiency of pyruvate carboxylase, propionyl-coenzyme A-carboxylase and B-methylcrotonoyl-coenzyme A carboxylase. Further studies are needed to substantiate these incidental data.

Fetal medical treatment has been well defined in three areas: the conversion of fetal tachyarrhythmias; the prevention of external genital masculinization in female fetuses affected by 21-hydroxylase-deficient congenital adrenal hyperplasia; and immune fetal hydrops. In this chapter attention will be focused on treatment of congenital adrenal hyperplasia, non-immune fetal hydrops and tachyarrhythmias.

Congenital adrenal hyperplasia

Evans and colleagues first demonstrated in 1985 that, in women with 21-hydroxylase deficiency, pharmacological suppression of the fetal adrenal gland can be achieved by maternal administration of dexamethasone (for review, see Evans & Schulman 1986). They described a woman with mild 21-hydroxylase deficiency whose previous female infant had classic congenital adrenal hyperplasia with masculinization. Although there was no firm evidence of congenital adrenal hyperplasia in the present pregnancy, the mother agreed to take dexamethasone 25 mg by mouth four times a day, starting at the 10th week of gestation. Amniocentesis at 17 weeks revealed a female karyotype. At 39 weeks spontaneous delivery of a female infant with normal external genitalia took place. ACTH challenge test demonstrated that she did not have the classic disease; further studies suggested carrier status. Forrest & David (1984), using the same protocol, demonstrated that fetuses who were clinically affected with the severe form of 21-hydroxylase deficiency were prevented from having congenital masculinization of the external genitalia.

Non-immune hydrops fetalis

Hydrops fetalis can be defined as pathologically increased fluid accumulation in fetal serous body cavities and/or oedema of soft tissues. It is considered non-immune if there is no sign of a fetomaternal blood group incompatibility. Lately, attention is increasingly being focused on non-immune hydrops fetalis for several reasons:

1 Parallel to the reduction in both incidence and severity of immunological hydrops, the ratio of non-immune to immune cases of hydrops fetalis is rising.

2 There is a marked heterogeneity of underlying causes.

3 A considerable percentage (30—60%) of cases of non-immune hydrops fetalis still has to be recorded as idiopathic.

4 Intrauterine treatment of non-immune hydrops fetalis has so far been disappointing.

The most common causes of non-immune hydrops fetalis are cardiac anomalies, other structural defects, chromosomal disorders and the twin—twin transfusion syndrome. Less frequent findings are infections and haematological disorders, in particular alpha-thalassaemia. For more detailed information on the aetiology on non-immune hydrops fetalis, the reader is referred to a recent review by Holzgreve *et al.* (1985).

Diagnostic work-up

As soon as fetal hydrops is recognized, almost always by ultrasonography, the following three procedures should be carried out:

1 Maternal blood sampling for:
   (a) maternal antibody screening to exclude some kind of isoimmunization;
   (b) Kleihauer—Betke test to exclude fetomaternal transfusion;
   (c) serum glucose determination to exclude diabetes;
   (d) infection screening (TORCH);
   (e) blood count and red blood cell indices to exclude alpha-thalassaemia trait (paternal blood also);
   (f) specific enzyme deficiency screening in erythrocytes, e.g. glucose 6-phosphate dehydrogenase, pyruvatekinase.

2 Detailed ultrasound scan for:
   (a) the presence of single or multiple pregnancy;
   (b) cardiac and non-cardiac structural anomalies;

(c) the degree of fetal hydrops, the degree of cardiac compromise (pulsed Doppler);

(d) cardiac rate and/or rhythm disturbances.

3 Amniocentesis or fetal blood sampling for karyotyping. If fetal blood has been obtained, chromosome analysis is possible after 2−4 days' culture of fetal lymphocytes as opposed to 2−3 weeks for culturing cells in amniotic fluid. Fetal blood can also be examined for specific IgMs for suspected intrauterine infection.

Perinatal complications

The fetus may be threatened by intrauterine death due to the severity of structural defects or the presence of markedly altered water and electrolyte homeostasis and haemodynamic disturbances. The newborn may suffer respiratory embarrassment secondary to lung hypoplasia and impaired diaphragmatic movement.

Obstetric management

Obstetric management will be determined by the gestational age at diagnosis, the nature and severity of the underlying cause, the severity of the hydrops and the options available for intrauterine treatment. Medical treatment has been both causal and symptomatic. The recognition of fetal cardiac arrhythmias in the absence of severe cardiac defects offers the opportunity for transplacental administration of antiarrhythmic drugs. In the presence of moderate to marked hydrops, the results are poor. Frusemide has been given in combination with antiarrhythmics, but its usefulness in mobilizing excessive fluid in the fetus has not been clearly established. Hypoproteinaemia and hypoalbuminaemia were a consistent finding in pure fetal blood samples obtained fetoscopically in 18 cases of unexplained fetal hydrops (Nicolaides *et al.* 1985) These authors have attempted correction through fetal intravascular albumin infusions but this appears to be of only limited benefit. Thoracocentesis and/or paracentesis only results in short-term fluid reduction. Indwelling catheters for long-term fluid drainage have been suggested as a next step (Watson & Campbell 1986). It should be realized, however, that this would be a purely symptomatic form of treatment without approaching the, often unknown, underlying cause. With these very limited options for effective treatment, it is not surprising to find perinatal losses in non-immune hydrops fetalis to be as high as 75−90% (Nicolaides *et al.* 1985; Watson & Campbell 1986).

Fetal tachyarrhythmias

Fetal tachyarrhythmias are usually first suspected on the basis of auscultatory findings during routine examination in pregnancy. With improved ultrasonic equipment, a more accurate diagnosis of the type of tachyarrhythmia can be made, associated problems such as structural cardiac defects and cardiac compromise can be recognized, and the effects of intrauterine treatment schedules can be closely monitored. In general, the decision to embark on intrauterine treatment of fetal tachyarrhythmia depends on:

1 Accurate assessment of the type of tachyarrhythmia.
2 The nature and seriousness of associated cardiac defects and the presence or absence of an abnormal karyotype.
3 The presence or absence of congestive heart failure or fetal hydrops.
4 The gestational age.
5 The presence or absence of fetal distress and/or labour.
6 The availability of appropriate neonatal and paediatric cardiac facilities.

Incidence

The estimated incidence of tachyarrhythmias is 0·4−0·6% of all pregnancies (Southall *et al.* 1980).

Diagnosis

Tachyarrthymias are almost exclusively of supraventricular origin. They may be due to:

1 Sinus tachycardia, which is characterized by a heart rate of more than 180 beats per minute (bpm) and normal conduction.
2 Paroxysmal supraventricular tachycardia (PSVT) with heart rates above 180, often above 200−220 bpm, and usually of abrupt onset and termination; this is the most frequent type of tachyarrhythmia.
3 Atrial flutter and atrial fibrillation with rates of 300−480 bpm with a variable degree of A−V conduction resulting in a ventricular rate of 60−240 bpm.

Structural heart disease is present in 5−10% of fetuses and congestive heart failure occurs in about 70%, resulting in fetal hydrops. Two-dimensional real-time directed M-mode recording of atrial and ventricular activity permits accurate diagnosis of the tachyarrhythmia (Fig. 7.1) (Stewart *et al.* 1983). Pulsed Doppler ultrasound recording of the flow velocity waveform in the fetal descending aorta has shown that, at heart rates beyond 230−250 bpm, flow velocity drops as a result of cardiac failure and is followed by the appearance of pericardial effusion within the next 24 hours (Tonge *et al.* 1984).

Aetiology

Supraventricular tachyarrhythmias may be associated with functional instability of the atrial muscle, congenital heart disease, cardiac tumour

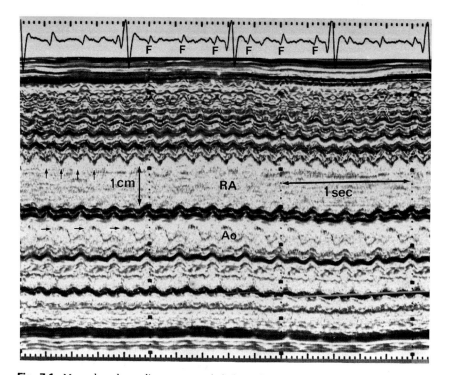

Fig. 7.1. M-mode echocardiogram recorded through fetal right atrium (RA) and aortic root (Ao) from a patient with atrial flutter with 2:1 atrioventricular conduction. F = fetal QRS complex. Vertical arrows indicate rapid, regular atrial contractions. Horizontal arrows indicate opening of aortic valve.

and cardiomyopathy (Wedemeyer & Breitfeld 1975; Pearl 1977). Increasing attention has been focused on intrauterine infections such as cytomegalovirus and Coxsackie B virus as possible causes. Amniocentesis for virus culture is therefore indicated. A common association in the presence of atrial fibrillation is the Wolff–Parkinson–White syndrome (Belhassen *et al.* 1982). Conduction system defects have been established in a number of infants with intrauterine arrhythmias (Siew Yen Ho *et al.* 1985). Sinus tachycardia is mostly secondary to causes such as maternal fever, congenital infections or drug administration.

Intrauterine treatment

This can be defined as transplacental administration of antiarrhythmic agents to the fetus with the object of normalizing fetal heart rate and rhythm and abolishing associated cardiac compromise. The rationale is that tachyarrhythmias are often not well tolerated by the fetus, resulting in cardiac compromise (Hedvall 1973; Schreiner *et al.* 1978; Valerius & Jacobson 1978). Tables 7.1 and 7.2 represent data from various reports on transplacental therapy in the management of supraventricular tachyarrhythmias, using digoxin alone (Table 7.1) or a combination of antiarrhythmic agents (Table 7.2). Data from our own unit are presented in Tables 7.3 and 7.4. We treated seven fetuses without non-immune hydrops (Table 7.3, patients 1–7) and four fetuses which had already developed hydrops at the time of cardiac rhythm analysis (Table 7.4, patients 8–11).

Age of detection and type of tachyarrhythmia

Almost all tachyarrhythmias are first diagnosed during the late second and the third trimester of pregnancy. In earlier publications, tachyarrhythmias were nearly always classified as supraventricular tachycardia (SVT) on the basis of fetal ECG recordings. Later, following the introduction of high quality two-dimensional real-time directed M-mode recordings, other tachyarrhythmias were recognized, such as atrial flutter with variable AV conduction, in which atrial rates may vary from 300 to 480 bpm. About 70% of tachyarrhythmias subjected to intrauterine therapy initially presented with signs of various degrees of cardiac compromise, from mild pericardial effusion to fully developed non-immune fetal hydrops.

Dose and mode of treatment

Digoxin

Digoxin is generally considered the drug of choice in the treatment of fetal tachyarrhythmias. Maternal digoxin levels in patients on stable dosages are 40–50% lower during the last trimester of pregnancy compared with those who are not pregnant. Explanations for this phenomenon include increased maternal intravascular volume, increased glomerular filtration rate, delayed gastric emptying, and raised fetal metabolism of digoxin (Rogers *et al.* 1972). It seems that the affinity of digoxin for the infant myocardium is higher than that for the adult (Wetzell 1976). Cord blood digoxin levels at birth have been reported to be similar to maternal levels (Rogers *et al.* 1972; Kerenyi *et al.* 1980; Lingman *et al.* 1980), indicating passive transfer of digoxin across the placenta.

Valerius & Jacobson (1978) were the first to report successful treatment of fetal SVT by maternal digitalization. No treatment schedules, however, were given. Tables 7.1–7.4 show that digoxin treatment varied both in mode (oral or intravenous) and dosage (0·5–2·0 mg daily), making comparisons as to the effect of digoxin on tachyarrhythmias very difficult. It was often not known whether therapeutic levels were reached, since maternal serum digoxin levels were not always measured. Whereas others were generally fairly successful in converting the fetal heart rate to normal, we only observed normalization of the heart rate in four non-hydropic fetuses which were treated with digoxin alone and in two hydropic fetuses which were treated with digoxin and other antiarrhythmic drugs. In patient no. 6 conversion to normal heart rate may have been coincidental, since maternal serum digoxin level was only 0·4 ng ml^{-1} (therapeutic range 0·5–1·5 ng ml^{-1}). The poor outcome in our patients was probably related to the advanced stage of fetal hydrops at the time of intrauterine treatment, which resulted in fetal or neonatal death in cases 8–11. In fetuses 9 and 10 conversion to normal heart rate did not lead to resolution of hydrops due to the marked cardiac failure as shown by aortic Doppler flow measurements. Intracardiac Doppler flow measurement at the level of the mitral and tricuspid valves, ascending aorta and pulmonary artery as described by Reed *et al.* (1986) may provide us with more detailed information on cardiac performance during various treatment regimes. It is of interest that, in the successful cases (Tables 7.3 and 7.4), there is no relationship between the therapeutic dose and termination of tachyarrhythmia, which suggests

Table 7.1. Transplacental treatment of fetal tachyarrhythmias with digoxin

Reference	Age at detection of tachyarrhythmia (weeks)	Dose and mode of therapy	Termination of tachyarrhythmia	Gestational age at delivery (weeks)	Mode of delivery	Fetal outcome
Lingman *et al.* (1980)	29	0·5 mg IV, then 0·25 mg PO daily (maternal serum level 0·9–1·6 ng ml^{-1})	yes, after 24 h	38	vaginal	NSR
Kerenyi *et al.* (1980)	29	0·25 mg PO qid, then 0·25 mg bid	yes, after 38 h	31–33	caesarean section	WPW
Harrigan *et al.* (1981)	26	1·5 mg PO over 14 h, then 0·25 mg day^{-1} (maternal serum level 0·7–0·8 ng ml^{-1})	yes, after 15 h	38	vaginal	NSR
Wiggins *et al.* (1982)	24	1 mg over 24 h, then 0·375 mg PO daily	yes, after 6 days	Term	vaginal	NSR
Belhassen *et al.* (1982)	32	IV 0·5–0·75 mg daily (maternal serum level 1·9 ng ml^{-1})	no	34	caesarean	digoxin restored NSR
Gembruch *et al.* (1982)	33	0·3 mg IV daily (maternal serum level 0·6 ng ml^{-1})	yes, after 10 days	41	vaginal	NSR
King *et al.* (1984)	20	0·125 mg PO daily	yes, after 60 h	36	caesarean	NSR
Allan *et al.* (1984)	30–38 (4 cases)	0·75 mg PO daily (maternal serum level 1·5–2·2 ng ml^{-1})	yes, after ? days	Term	vaginal	NSR

Kleinman *et al.* (1985)	24–38 (6 cases)	0·5–2·0 mg IV, then 0·25–0·75 mg PO daily	yes, after ? weeks	?	vaginal	NSR
Wiggins *et al.* (1986)	24–30 (6 cases)	0·75–1·0 mg daily (PO or IV) (maternal serum level 0·5–2·0 ng ml^{-1})	yes, after 0·6–35 days	25–36	4 vaginal 2 caesarean	4 NSR 2 WPW
Truccone & Mariona (1985)	31	digoxin 1 mg PO daily (maternal serum level 1·3 ng ml^{-1}) digoxin 0·5–0·75 PO daily verapamil 160–480 mg PO daily	no — yes, within 72 h	31+		NSR, digoxin 0·03 mg PO

SVT = supraventricular tachycardia.
NSR = normal sinus rhythm.
WPW = Wolff–Parkinson–White syndrome.
PO = *per os* (L) by mouth.
qid = *quater in die* (L) four times a day.
bid = *bis in die* (L) twice a day.

Table 7.2. Transplacental treatment of tachyarrhythmias with antiarrhythmic drugs other than digoxin

Reference	Age at detection of tachyarrhythmia (weeks)	Dose and mode of therapy	Termination of tachyarrhythmia	Gestational age at delivery (weeks)	Mode of delivery	Fetal outcome
Teuscher et al. (1978)	34	propranolol 160 mg PO daily	yes, within 12 h	37	caesarean section	SVT on day 3, digoxin + propranolol restored NSR
Wolff et al. (1980)	33	digoxin 0.5 mg IV daily + verapamil 240 mg PO daily	yes, after 5 days	34	vaginal	NSR
Dumesic et al. (1982)	29	digoxin 0.5 mg IV daily for 6 days (maternal serum level 1.3 ng ml^{-1})	no			
		propranolol 0.2 mg kg^{-1} IV at a rate of 1 mg min^{-1} to a total dose of 1 mg	no			
		digoxin 0.25 mg PO daily + procainamide 340 mg bolus IV at a rate of 50 mg min^{-1}, then 4 g daily	yes, after 60 min, for 4 weeks	33	caesarean section	SVT, digoxin + propranolol restored NSR
Given et al. (1984)	24	digoxin 1.25 mg IV over 16 h, then 0.75 mg daily (maternal serum level 2.7 ng ml^{-1})	no			
		propranolol 1.0 mg IV every 3–5 min, total dose 0.4 mg kg^{-1}	no			
		procainamide 100 mg IV every 5 min to a total dose of 1.5 g, then 2 mg min^{-1}	yes, after less than 1 h, for 9 h			
		Procainamide 750 mg bolus IV, then 4 mg min^{-1}	yes, after less than 1 h, for 6 h	27	caesarean section	SVT on 25th day, digoxin restored NSR

Allan et al. (1984)	34	digoxin 0·75 mg PO daily + verapamil 240 mg PO daily	yes, after ? days	39	vaginal	NSR
Spinnato et al. (1984)	29	Digoxin 1·5 mg IV over 36 h, then 0·5 mg daily (maternal serum level 1·2 ng ml^{-1}) Digoxin 0·5 mg IV daily + quinidine 800–1200 mg PO daily	no yes, after 24h	34	vaginal	NSR
Vintzileos et al. (1985)	32 (atrial flutter, 2:1 AV block)	digoxin 1·5 mg PO over 12 h, then 0·5 mg PO daily propranolol 100 mg PO daily verapamil 5 mg IV over 5 min, then 20 mg PO daily	no no no	38	caesarean section	worsening congestive cardiac failure; atrial flutter 2:1 + AV block; cardioversion restored NSR on day 2
Kleinman et al. (1985)	24–38 (6 cases)	digoxin 0·5–2·0 mg IV, then 0·25–0·75 mg PO daily + verapamil 5·0–10·0 mg, then 80–120 mg PO tid or qid	Yes, after ? h	?	vaginal	NSR
	(1 case)	digoxin 0·5–2·0 mg IV then 0·25–0·75 mg PO daily + propranolol 0·5 mg IV every 5 min, then 20–160 mg PO tid or qid		?	vaginal	NSR

tid = *ter in die* (L) three times a day.
qid = *quater in die* (L) four times a day.

that other factors are involved. A digoxin-like immunoreactive substance has been established in neonates and infants (Valdes *et al.* 1983) and in amniotic fluid (Graves *et al.* 1984). Experiments in which known amounts of digoxin were added to digoxin-free neonatal plasma and amniotic fluid samples have demonstrated that quantitative digoxin recoveries were obtained only if compensation was made for the measured base-line presence of the endogenous substance (Valdes *et al.* 1983). Since each fetus may have its own base-line level of endogenous digoxin-like substance, these levels should be established before initiating transplacental treatment. This can only be done through fetal blood sampling. It is particularly for this unknown endogenous factor that we raised the therapeutic digitalis level to $2-3$ ng ml^{-1}. Finally we believe that in a number of tachyarrhythmias the heart rate may have returned to normal independent of intrauterine treatment. Long-term, i.e. 24-hour, recordings of fetal tachyarrhythmias are needed to obtain a better insight into the paroxysmal nature of these arrhythmias (Southall *et al.* 1980).

Other antiarrhythmic drugs

In cases of failure of digoxin, other antiarrhythmic drugs, such as propranolol, procainamide, verapamil and amiodarone, have been used in an attempt to normalize the fetal heart rate (Tables 7.2 and 7.4). In some instances, combined treatment with digoxin and another drug was attempted (Wolff *et al.* 1980; Dumesic *et al.* 1982; Allan *et al.* 1984; Spinnato *et al.* 1984; Vintzileos *et al.* 1985).

1   *Propranolol.* Propranolol, a beta adrenergic blocking agent, has been used as a second choice in a number of cases of tachyarrhythmia (Dumesic *et al.* 1982; Given *et al.* 1984; Vintzileos *et al.* 1985) and even as a first choice by Teuscher *et al.* (1978). Propranolol crosses the placenta and appears in the fetal serum soon after administration to the mother (Langer *et al.* 1974). Fetal serum levels of propranolol are about 20% of those in the mother. Therapeutic maternal serum concentrations vary between 20 and 100 ng ml^{-1}. Because of its beta blocking effects, propranolol has been used for a variety of maternal problems such as hyperthyroidism, essential hypertension and maternal tachycardia (Gladstone *et al.* 1975; Cottrill *et al.* 1977). Since early reports indicated that the drug had no demonstrable side-effects on the fetus (Langer *et al.* 1974), it was also used to correct fetal tachycardia (Teuscher *et al.* 1978; Klein *et al.* 1979). However, several reports suggest that propranolol

Table 7.3. Transplacental treatment of fetal tachyarrhythmia in our Unit: non-hydropic cases

Case no.	Gestational age 1st visit	Dose + mode of therapy	Termination arrhythmia	Mode of delivery	Fetal outcome
1	21 SVEs → PSVT	therapeutic digoxin level 0·5–1·5 ng ml^{-1} oral digoxin 0·5 mg day^{-1} (maternal serum 1·2 ng ml^{-1})	yes	vaginal term ♂ 3970 g	NSR, digoxin *post partum*, cord + amniotic digoxin levels unsuccessful
2	23 SVEs atrial flutter → PSVT	oral digoxin 0·5 mg day^{-1} (maternal serum 0·6–1·3 ng ml^{-1})	yes	vaginal term ♀ 3270 g	SVEs → NSR, digoxin *post partum*, cord digoxin 0·8 ng ml^{-1}
3	26 SVEs → PSVT	oral digoxin 0·75 mg day^{-1} (maternal serum 1·1–1·9 ng ml^{-1})	yes	vaginal term ♀ 3550 g	NSR, digoxin *post partum*, cord digoxin 1·2 ng ml^{-1} amniotic digoxin 2·4 ng ml^{-1}
4	31 SVT	oral digoxin 0·5 mg day^{-1} (maternal serum 1·0–1·6 ng ml^{-1})	no, ↑ Rt ht size	caesarean 38 wks ♀ 2945 g	NSR, digoxin *post partum*, cord digoxin < 0·5 ng ml^{-1}
5	34 atrial flutter, variable A–V conduction	IV digoxin 0·75 mg day^{-1} (maternal serum 0·5–1·2 ng ml^{-1})	no, ↑ Rt ht size, pericardial effusion period NSR, serum level 0·5 ng ml^{-1}	caesarean 35+ wks ♂ 3250 g	NSR, digoxin *post partum*, cord digoxin < 1 ng ml^{-1}, amniotic digoxin 1·2 ng ml^{-1}
6	38 atrial flutter, 2:1 A–V conduction	IV digoxin 1·75 mg (maternal serum 0·4 ng ml^{-1})	yes, < 48 h (prob. spontaneous)	vaginal 38 wks ♂ 4150 g	NSR, digoxin *post partum*, cord digoxin 0·2 ng ml^{-1}
7	36 SVT → short bursts of atrial flutter	therapeutic digoxin level > 2 ng ml^{-1} loading: IV digoxin 2 mg day^{-1} maintenance: 3 × 0·25 mg day^{-1} (maternal serum > 2 ng ml^{-1})	no, intermittent NSR; ↑ Rt ht size, pericardial effusion	caesarean 37 wks ♀ 3535 g	NSR, one period of SVT *post partum*, cord digoxin 2·3 ng ml^{-1}, neonatal digoxin 1·2 ng ml^{-1}

Table 7.4. Transplacental treatment of fetal tachyarrhythmias in our Unit: hydropic cases

Case no.	Gestational age 1st visit	Dose + mode of therapy	Termination arrhythmia	Mode of delivery	Fetal outcome
		therapeutic levels — digitalis 0·5–1·5 ng ml⁻¹ procainamide 4–10 mg l⁻¹ NAPA 10–30 mg l⁻¹			
8	25 atrial flutter 2:1 A–V conduction severe hydrops polyhydramnios	oral digoxin 0·75 mg daily (maternal serum 0·9 ng ml⁻¹)	no	IUD 26 wks vaginal	IUD
		IV procainamide 2 × 500 mg loading 4g 24⁻¹ h maintenance (maternal serum 2·4 mg l⁻¹ NAPA 1·4 mg l⁻¹)	no ↑ hydrops pericardial effusion		block dissection SA node — no abnormalities
		IV verapamil 3 × 5 mg	no		
9		IV + oral digoxin 0·75 mg (maternal serum 2·6 ng ml⁻¹)	heart rate varied between 125 and 220 bpm	increasing hydrops + abnormal CTG	severely hydropic died 48 h *post partum*
		IV + oral verapamil		caesarean 31 wks ♂ 3·5–4 kg	block dissection SA node — no abnormalities
	SVT (240–260 bpm) severe hydrops	IV procainamide IV propranolol IV + oral amiodarone + frusemide triamterine, MgSO₄ + intra-abdominal to fetus—digoxin + frusemide			

10	26 SVEs PSVT atrial flutter chaotic atrial rhythms ascites	IV + oral digoxin (maternal serum 1·60–2·80 ng ml^{-1}) IV propranolol oral quinidine oral verapamil + frusemide Therapeutic level 0·5–1·5 ng ml^{-1}	↑ hydrops return to normal sinus rhythm at 32 weeks after addition verapamil	Severe hydrops unchanged IUD at 33 vaginal	IUD cord digoxin 1·14 ng/ml grossly abnormal posterior MV leaflet + mild hypoplasia of LV block dissection SA node — not yet known
11	27 atrial flutter, 2:1 A–V conduction severe hydrops	IV digoxin 1·25 mg loading oral digoxin 4 × 0·25 mg maintenance (maternal serum 4·5 ng ml^{-1}) IV verapamil 4 × 5 mg	yes NSR 150 bpm	despite NSR ↑ hydrops + ↓ blood flow velocity CTG—fetal hypoxia caesarean 29 wks ♀ 1200 g	severely hydropic died 24 h *post partum* block dissection SA node — no abnormalities

SVE = supraventricular extrasystoles.
PSVT = paroxysmal supraventricular tachycardia.
SVT = supraventricular tachycardia.
NSR = normal sinus rhythm.
NAPA = metabolite of procainamide.
MV = mitral valve.
LV = left ventricle.
SA = sino-atrial.

places the neonate at risk for depressed Apgar scores, hypoglycaemia and bradycardia (Gladstone *et al.* 1975; Cottrill *et al.* 1977). It therefore seems prudent to avoid the use of propranolol in initial attempts to correct fetal tachyarrhythmias. According to Table 7.2, results with propranolol have been largely disappointing.

2   *Procainamide.* Procainamide is a small compound with low protein binding, which favours placental transfer although no data are available on either the mechanism or the rate of transfer. As it is a weak base, membrane diffusion could be limited. The fetal blood pH, which is slightly more acidic than the maternal, would be expected to trap procainamide and limit back-diffusion. The efficacy of this drug in the management of fetal tachyarrhythmias has been pointed out in two reports (Dumesic *et al.* 1982; Given *et al.* 1984). If procainamide is successful, it acts quite rapidly, although both loading and maintenance dosages vary widely. The risk of maternal hypotension, leading to uteroplacental insufficiency and ventricular arrhythmias in previously digitalized patients, must be considered when choosing procainamide in any therapeutic regimen (Zapato-Dias *et al.* 1952). Therapeutic maternal serum concentrations vary between 4 and 14 µg ml^{-1}.

3   *Digoxin plus quinidine.* Successful conversion of atrial flutter into normal heart rate was achieved by Spinnato *et al.* (1984) using a combination of digoxin and quinidine (the therapeutic range of quinidine is 2·5−5·0 ng ml^{-1}). Maternal and fetal quinidine levels have been reported to approach a one-to-one relationship (Doering 1979). Quinidine is reported to have oxytocic activity (Meyer *et al.* 1930) and to be associated with rare neonatal thrombocytopenia (Domula *et al.* 1977). In doses much larger than those achieved by clinical therapy, fetal eighth nerve damage has been observed (Mendelson 1956). In spite of these concerns, the potential for benefit seems to outweigh the risks (Spinnato *et al.* 1984). Several recent reports have been published on the interaction between quinidine and digoxin (Spinnato *et al.* 1984). Most patients on a stable dose of digoxin experience a twofold to threefold rise in the serum digoxin level when quinidine is added, apparently due to a decrease in the volume of distribution and renal clearance of digoxin. This has been shown to occur in as many as 90% of patients (Bussey 1982). It suggests that the effect of quinidine might be indirect, i.e. it may act by increasing digoxin levels.

4   *Verapamil and amiodarone*: There is only limited experience with the use of verapamil and the relatively new drug, amiodarone, in fetal tachyarrhythmias. Verapamil is a calcium antagonist, and it crosses the placenta. Fetal serum levels have been reported to be about 50% of maternal levels (Strigl *et al.* 1980). Successful conversion of SVT and atrial flutter has been obtained using a combination of digoxin and verapamil (Wolff *et al.* 1980; Allan *et al.* 1984; Kleinman *et al.* 1985). The therapeutic range in maternal serum is $50-100$ ng ml^{-1}. A combination of verapamil and propranolol should be avoided because both are negative inotropic agents and poor myocardial contractility and therefore function may result.

Verapamil was used by us in two patients with fetal atrial flutter and advanced fetal hydrops. In one case (no. 11 in Table 7.4), cardioversion was achieved, but Doppler flow measurements in the fetal descending aorta revealed poor myocardial contraction force; a flat fetal heart rate tracing indicated fetal hypoxia. A caesarean section was performed at 29 weeks. Despite resuscitative measures the infant died on day 2. In case no. 9 in Table 7.4 a total of five antiarrhythmic drugs were subsequently given. Only following amiodarone treatment was a normal heart rate obtained. However, hydropic features became more prominent and Doppler flow measurement in the descending aorta clearly showed poor myocardial contraction force. A caesarean section was performed at 31 weeks. Despite cardioversion, the infant died on day 2 due to extreme cardiac compromise.

Amiodarone is a benzofuran derivative that has been shown to be extremely effective as treatment in infants and children with tachyarrhythmias resistant to conventional treatment. Its use during pregnancy has been limited by insufficient knowledge of maternal–fetal transfer and the documented adverse effects of excessive iodine (Ginsburg 1971): amiodarone 200 mg contains approximately 75 mg of iodine within its structure. The precise fate of this large amount of iodine is uncertain (Broekhuysen *et al.* 1969). Iodine is known to be:

1 Transferred rapidly across the placenta even against a concentration gradient.
2 Concentrated in the fetal thyroid gland from as early as 14 weeks.
3 Associated with neonatal goitre after as little as 12 mg is ingested (Burrow 1978).
The risk of such complications for the individual patient is unpredictable and a genetic predisposition has been suggested (Croors 1975).

Umbilical cord compression

An interesting report appeared in which correction of fetal SVT was obtained by compression of the umbilical cord (Martin *et al.* 1984). Cord compression produces a rise in fetal blood pressure and thereby stimulates the baroreceptors, inducing a vagal response. In this respect cord compression mimics the mechanism by which carotid sinus pressure or the Valsalva manoeuvre interrupts SVT. The authors would not recommend umbilical cord compression as a method of correcting SVT when fetal hypoxia or significant congestive heart failure is present, or when the mother has received digoxin or beta adrenergic blockers.

Obstetric management

When a fetal tachyarrhythmia has been discovered, obstetric management, including intrauterine treatment, depends on fetal maturity (age) and the presence or absence of an abnormal karyotype. Careful two-dimensional real-time analysis of fetal cardiac anatomy is carried out. In the presence of a structural defect, amniocentesis for karyotyping is performed, since an abnormal karyotype has been found in about 45% of structural cardiac defects (Wladimiroff *et al.* 1985). In cases of an inoperable cardiac defect and/or an abnormal karyotype, surgical intervention is avoided. When a cardiac structural defect in the presence of tachyarrhythmia has been ruled out, the initiation of intrauterine treatment mainly depends on fetal lung maturity.

Adequate lung maturity

If there is adequate lung maturity, assessed by amniotic fluid phospholipids, intrauterine treatment is not indicated and the infant is delivered. The mode of delivery depends on obstetric conditions such as cervical maturity, fetal lie, etc. The fetal heart rate and acid–base status are monitored.

Insufficient lung maturity

If there is insufficient lung maturity, maternal administration of steroids may be considered and intrauterine treatment is started. If intrauterine therapy is successful, obstetric management is no different from that in uncomplicated pregnancies. Regular two-dimensional real-time ultrasonic monitoring of the fetus for imminent signs of cardiac compromise is carried out. Vaginal delivery at term is the goal, the monitoring of fetal heart rate and acid–base status is then advisable because of the stress of

labour. When intrauterine treatment fails, one should differentiate between fetal tachyarrhythmia without and with cardiac compromise. In
the absence of cardiac compromise, delivery takes place as soon as fetal
lung maturity has been established. The mode of delivery again depends
on obstetric factors such as cervical maturity, fetal lie, etc. In case of
vaginal delivery, monitoring of the fetal heart rate and acid−base status
is mandatory. In the mean time, regular two-dimensional real-time
ultrasonic monitoring of the fetus for imminent signs of cardiac compromise is performed. In the presence of cardiac compromise, it may be
prudent to deliver the patient by caesarean section as soon as fetal lung
maturity has been established, in order to avoid the superimposed stress
of labour on an already compromised fetus. In some instances, despite
intrauterine therapy, progression to congestive heart failure may require
surgical intervention at an earlier stage. All infants should be delivered
in the vicinity of a neonatal intensive care unit under supervision of a
neonatologist together with a paediatric cardiologist, since even those
who do well during labour may develop cardiac failure in the neonatal
period.

Prognosis

The prognosis mainly depends on the type and aetiology of the tachyarrhythmia, the severity of associated cardiac structural defects, the
absence or presence of an abnormal karyotype, and the efficacy of
intrauterine and postnatal treatment. Atrial fibrillation is a common
complication of the Wolff−Parkinson−White syndrome in adult patients.
This syndrome can also occur in the fetus and newborn. Therefore, if the
Wolff−Parkinson−White syndrome is suspected on the grounds of atrial
fibrillation, the use of digoxin may result in a further increase in ventricular rate (Belhassen *et al.* 1982). Whereas viral myocarditis may have
a reasonable prognosis, fibroelastosis and conduction system defects are
associated with a high neonatal mortality.

Conclusion

Fetal tachyarrhythmia is often life-threatening. Aggressive treatment is
necessary in the presence of developing cardiac compromise and lung
immaturity. Transplacental therapy with digoxin is still considered the
approach of first choice. If this fails, a combination of digoxin and
verapamil may be contemplated. Digoxin combined with propranolol,

procainamide or quinidine may be given as a next step, whereas amiodarone is a last resort until more information about its possible effects on the fetal thyroid has been obtained. A combination of verapamil and propranolol should be avoided because both are negative inotropic agents. More information should be collected on the natural incidence and progression of tachyarrhythmias to gain more insight into the potential of adequate treatment programmes. Fetal blood sampling should be carried out to establish more exactly the transplacental passage of various antiarrhythmics under hydropic and non-hydropic circumstances as well as the endogenous production of digoxin-like immunoreactive substance.

References

Allan L.D., Crawford D.C., Anderson R.H. & Tynan M. (1984) Evaluation and treatment of fetal arrhythmias. *Clin. Cardiol.*, **7**, 467−73.

Ampola M.S., Mahoney M.J. & Nakamura E. (1975) Prenatal therapy of a patient with vitamin B responsive methylmalonic acidemia. *N. Engl. J. Med.*, **293**, 313−17.

Belhassen B., Pauzner D., Blieden L. *et al.* (1982) Intrauterine and postnatal atrial fibrillation in the Wolff−Parkinson−White syndrome. *Circulation*, **66**, 1124−7.

Broekhuysen J., Laruel R. & Sion R. (1969) Recherches dans la série des benzolyrannes. XXXVII Étude comparée du transit et du métabolisme de l'amiodarone chez diverses espèces animales et chez l'homme. *Arch. Int. Pharmacodyn. Ther.*, **177**, 340−59.

Burrow G.N. (1978) Maternal fetal consideration in hyperthyroidism. In *Clinics in Endocrinology and Metabolism* (Ed. by R. Volpe), pp. 115−25. W.B. Saunders, London.

Bussey H.L. (1982) The influence of quinidine and other agents on digitalis glycosides. *Am. Heart J.*, **104**, 289−94.

Chen Y.T., Mattison D.R. & Feigenbaum L. (1981) Reduction in oocyte number following prenatal exposure to a high galactose diet. *Science*, **214**, 1145−8.

Cottrill C.M., McAllister R.G., Gettes L. & Noonan J.A. (1977) Propranolol therapy during pregnancy, labor, and delivery: evidence for transplacental drug transfer and impaired neonatal drug disposition. *J. Pediatr.*, **91**, 812−14.

Croors J. (1975) Thyroid and antithyroid drugs. In *Meyler's Side-effects of Drugs 1972−1975* (Ed. by M.N.S. Dukes), pp. 889−98. Excerpta Medica, Amsterdam.

Doering W. (1979) Quinidine−digoxin interaction. *N. Engl. J. Med.*, **301**, 400−5.

Domula V.M., Weissach G. & Lente H. (1977) Über die Auswirkung medikamentöser Behandlung in der Schwangerschaft und das Gezennungspotential der Neugeborene. *Zentralbl. Gynaekol.*, **99**, 473−8.

Dumesic D.A., Silverman N.H., Toblas S. & Golbus M.S. (1982) Transplacental cardioversion of fetal supraventricular tachycardia with procainamide. *N. Engl. J. Med.*, **307**, 1128−31.

Evans M.I. & Schulman J.D. (1986) Biochemical fetal therapy. *Clin. Obstet. Gynecol.*, **29**, 523−32.

Forrest M. & David M. (1984) Prenatal treatment of congenital adrenal hyperplasia due to 21-hydroxylase deficiency. Quebec, Canada: *7th Intl. Cong. Endocr.*, No. 911.

Gembruch U., Venn H.J., Redel D.A. & Hansmann M. (1982) Wolff−Parkinson−White syndrom mit paroxysmalen supraventrikularen Tachykardien des Feten und des Neugeborenen: Fallbeschreibung. *Klin. Pädiat.*, **194**, 320−3.

Ginsburg J. (1971) Placental drug transfer. *Am. Rev. Pharmacol. Toxicol.,* **1**(11), 387−408.

Given B.D., Philippe M., Saunders S.P. & Dzan V.J. (1984) Procainamide cardioversion of fetal supraventricular tachyarrhythmia. *Am. J. Cardiol.,* **53**, 1460−1.

Gladstone G.R., Hordorf A. & Gersony W.M. (1975) Propranolol administration during pregnancy: effect on fetus. *J. Pediatr.,* **86**, 962−4.

Graves S.W., Valdes Jr.R., Brown B.A., Knight A.B. & Craig R.H. (1984) Endogenous digoxin—immunoreactive substance in human pregnancies. *J. Clin. Endocrinol. Metab.,* **58**, 748−51.

Harrigan J.T., Kangos J.J., Sikka A. *et al.* (1981) Successful treatment of fetal congestive heart failure secondary to tachycardia. *N. Engl. J. Med.,* **304**, 1527−9.

Hedvall G. (1973) Congenital paroxysmal tachycardia. A report of three cases. *Acta Paediatr. Scand.,* **62**, 550−4.

Holzgreve W., Holzgreve B. & Curry C.J.R. (1985) Non-immune hydrops fetalis: diagnosis and management. *Semin. Perinatol.,* **9**, 52−67.

Kerenyi Th.D., Gleicher N., Meller, J. *et al.* (1980) Transplacental cardioversion of intra-uterine supraventricular tachycardia with digitalis. *Lancet,* **ii**, 393−4.

King Ch.R., Mattioli L., Goertz K.K. & Snodgrass W. (1984) Successful treatment of fetal supraventricular tachycardia with maternal digoxin therapy. *Chest,* **85**, 573−5.

Klein A.M., Holzman I.R. & Austin E.M. (1979) Fetal tachycardia prior to development of hydrops: attempted pharmacologic cardioversion. Case report. *Am. J. Obstet. Gynecol.,* **134**, 347−8.

Kleinman Ch.S., Copel J.A., Weinstein E.M., Santulli Th.V. & Hobbins J.C. (1985) Treatment of fetal supraventricular tachyarrhythmias. *J. Clin. Ultrasound,* **13**, 265−73.

Langer A., Hung G.T., McNulty J.A., Harrigan J.Y.T. & Washington E. (1974) Adrenergic blockade. A new approach to hyperthyroidism during pregnancy. *Obstet. Gynecol.,* **44**, 181−4.

Lingman G., Ohrlander S. & Ohlin P. (1980) Intrauterine digoxin treatment of fetal paroxysmal tachycardia. Case report. *Br. J. Obstet. Gynaecol.,* **87**, 340−2.

Martin C.B., Nijhuis J.G. & Weijer A.A. (1984) Correction of fetal supraventricular tachy-cardia by compression of the umbilical cord: report of a case. *Am. J. Obstet. Gynecol.,* **150**, 324−6.

Mendelson C.L. (1956) Disorders of heart beat during pregnancy. *Am. J. Obstet. Gynecol..,* **72**, 1268−71.

Meyer J., Lackner J.E. & Schochet S.S. (1930) Paroxysmal tachycardia in pregnancy. *JAMA,* **94**, 1901−6.

Murphy D., Saul I. & Kirby M. (1985) Maternal phenylketonuria and phenylalanine restricted diet: studies of 7 pregnancies and of offspring produced. *Ir. J. Med. Sci.,* **154**, 66−72.

Nicolaides K.H., Rodeck C.H., Lange I. *et al.* (1985) Fetoscopy in the assessment of unexplained fetal hydrops. *Br. J. Obstet. Gynaecol.,* **92**, 671−8.

Pearl W. (1977) Cardiac malformations presenting as congenital atrial flutter. *South. Med. J.,* **70**, 662−5.

Reed K., Sahn D.J., Scagullti S., Anderson C.F. & Shenker L. (1986) Doppler echocardio-graphic studies of diastolic function in the human fetal heart: changes during gestation. *J. Am. Coll. Cardiol.,* **8**, 391−5.

Rhoads G.G. & Mills J.L. (1986) Can vitamin supplements prevent neural tube defects? Current evidence and ongoing investigation. *Clin. Obstet. Gynecol.,* **29**, 569−79.

Rogers M.C., Willerson J.T., Goldblatt A. & Smith T.W. (1972) Serum digoxin concentration in the human fetus, neonate and infant. *N. Engl. J. Med.,* **287**, 1010−12.

Roth K.S., Yang W. & Allen L. (1982) Prenatal administration of biotin: biotin-responsive multiple carboxylase deficiency. *Pediatr. Res.,* **16**, 126−30.

Schreiner R.L., Hurwits R.A. & Muller W. (1978) Atrial tachyarrhythmias associated with massive edema in the newborn. *J. Perinat. Med.,* **6**, 274−8.

Siew Yen Ho, Mortimer G., Anderson R.H., Pomerance A. & Keeling J.W. (1985) Conduction system defects in three perinatal patients with arrhythmia. *Br. Heart J.,* **53**, 158−63.

Southall D.P., Richard J., Hardwick R.A. *et al.* (1980) Prospective study of fetal heart rate and rhythm patterns. *Arch. Dis. Child.*, **55**, 506–11.

Spinnato J., Shaver D.C., Flinn G.S., Sibai B.M., Watson D.L. & Marin-Garcia J. (1984) Fetal supraventricular tachycardia: *in utero* therapy with digoxin and quinidine. *Obstet. Gynecol.*, **64**, 730–5.

Stewart P.A., Tonge H.M. & Wladimiroff J.W. (1983) Arrhythmia and structural abnormalities of the fetal heart. *Br. Heart J.*, **50**, 550–4.

Strigl R., Erhardt W., Hege H.G. & Bümel G. (1980) Untersuchungen zur Plazenta Passage von Verapamil beim Meerschweinchen. *Z. Geburtsh. Perinat.*, **183**, 109–12.

Teuscher A., Bossi E., Imhof P., Erb E., Stocker F.P. & Weber J.W. (1978) Effect of propranolol on fetal tachycardia in diabetic pregnancy. *Am. J. Cardiol.*, **42**, 304–7.

Tonge H.M., Stewart P.A. & Wladimiroff J.W. (1984) Fetal blood flow measurements during fetal cardiac arrhythmia. *Early Hum. Dev.*, **10**, 23–4.

Truccone N. & Mariona F. (1985) Intrauterine conversion of fetal supraventricular tachycardia with combination of digoxin and verapamil. *Pediatr. Pharmacol.*, **5**, 149–53.

Valdes R., Graves S.W., Brown B.A. & Landt M. (1983) Endogenous substance in newborn infants causing false positive digoxin measurements. *J. Pediatr.*, **102**, 947–51.

Valerius N.H. & Jacobson J.R. (1978) Intrauterine supraventricular tachycardia. *Acta Obstet. Gynecol. Scand.*, **57**, 407–10.

Vintzileos A.M., Campbell W.A., Soberman S.M. & Nochinison D.J. (1985) Fetal atrial flutter and X-linked dominant vitamin D-resistant rickets. *Obstet. Gynecol.*, **65**, 395–445.

Watson J. & Campbell S. (1986) Antenatal evaluation and management of fetal hydrops. *Obstet. Gynecol.*, **67**, 589–93.

Wedemeyer A.L. & Breitfeld V. (1975) Cardiac neoplasm, tachyarrhythmia and anasarca in an infant. *Am. J. Dis. Child.*, **129**, 738–41.

Wetzell G. (1976) Digoxin therapy in infants. *Acta Paediatr. Scand. (Suppl.)*, 257.

Wiggins W., Clewell W., Bowes W., Johnson M., Appareti K. & Wolfe R.R. (1982) Successful diagnosis and therapy of arrhythmias, congestive heart failure in the fetus with digoxin (abstract). *Pediatr. Cardiol.*, **2**, 175.

Wiggins J.W., Bowes W., Clewell W. *et al.* (1986) Echocardiographic diagnosis and intravenous digoxin management of fetal tachyarrhythmias and congestive heart failure. *Am. J. Dis. Child.*, **140**, 202–4.

Wladimiroff J.W., Stewart P.A., Sachs E.S. & Niermeijer M.F. (1985) Prenatal diagnosis and management of congenital heart defect: significance of associated fetal anomalies and prenatal chromosome studies. *Am. J. Med. Genet.*, **21**, 285–90.

Wolff F., Brenker K.H., Schlensker K.H. & Bolte A. (1980) Prenatal diagnosis and therapy of fetal heart rate anomalies with a contribution on the placental transfer of verapamil. *J. Perinat. Med.*, **8**, 203–8.

Zapato-Dias J., Cabrera E.C. & Mendez R. (1952) An experimental and clinical study on the effects of procainamide (Pronestyl) on the heart. *Am. Heart J.*, **43**, 854–70.

8

The Effects of Maternal Diabetes on the Fetus

M.B. LANDON & S.G. GABBE

Introduction

That diabetes mellitus complicating pregnancy alters fetal growth and development perhaps more than any other maternal disorder should not be surprising. Diabetes mellitus may have profound effects on glucose, a major fetal fuel, and insulin, a significant fetal growth hormone. Fetal hyperglycaemia and hyperinsulinaemia may alter fetal growth and maturation and impair the transition from the fetal to the neonatal state. Recent investigations have demonstrated that even subtle aberrations in glucose and insulin may be associated with significant derangements in fetal development. Abnormalities in the intrauterine environment caused by maternal diabetes mellitus may also contribute to a process which Freinkel (1980) has labelled 'fuel-mediated teratogenesis', producing major malformations which may result in death or marked impairment of function. This chapter will review those pathophysiological processes associated with maternal diabetes mellitus which may alter fetal growth and development.

Congenital malformations

With the reduction in intrauterine deaths and a marked decrease in neonatal mortality related to hyaline membrane disease and traumatic delivery, congenital malformations have emerged as the most important cause of perinatal loss in pregnancies complicated by insulin-dependent diabetes mellitus (IDDM) (Gabbe 1977). In the past, these anomalies were responsible for approximately 10% of all perinatal deaths. At present, however, malformations account for 30−50% of perinatal mortality (Gabbe 1985). Neonatal deaths now exceed stillbirths in pregnancies complicated by IDDM, and fatal congenital malformations account for this changing pattern.

177

Historical perspective and population studies

Most studies have documented a two- to fourfold increase in major malformations in infants of insulin-dependent diabetic mothers. While one group has suggested that the incidence of major malformations has been rising in the past decade (Ballard *et al.* 1984), little evidence is available to support this conclusion. In a prospective study at the Boston Hospital for Women, Holmes (Kitzmiller & Cloherty 1978) noted a major malformation rate of 2% in the general population as compared with 9% in offspring of insulin-dependent diabetic patients. In a recently published prospective analysis, Simpson (Simpson *et al.* 1983) observed an 8·5% incidence of major anomalies in the insulin-dependent diabetic population, while the malformation rate in a small group of concurrently gathered control subjects was 2·4%. Similar figures were obtained in the recently completed Diabetes in Early Pregnancy Study in the United States (Mills 1987). The incidence of major anomalies was 2·1% in 389 control patients and 9·0% in 279 insulin-dependent diabetic women. In general, the incidence of major malformations in worldwide studies of offspring of insulin-dependent diabetic mothers has ranged from 5 to 10%. If approximately 3600 women with IDDM are delivered each year in the United States, 180−360 malformed infants will result (Mills & Witham 1986).

The profile of a patient most likely to produce an infant with a congenital anomaly would include a woman with poor diabetic control at and around the time of conception, with onset of diabetes early in life, especially before the age of 20, and a duration of diabetes of at least five years, and with the presence of vasculopathy including benign retinopathy, proliferative retinopathy and nephropathy (Chung & Myrianthopoulos 1975; Gabbe 1977). The significance of a family history of malformations, including cardiac and neural tube defects, is not clear. Although Mills has suggested that certain maternal HLA types may more often be associated with anomalies (Koppe *et al.* 1983), data recently presented by Simpson did not reveal a specific HLA type that conferred a greater risk for such anomalies (Simpson *et al.* 1983). Furthermore, chromosomal abnormalities were not increased in frequency in malformed infants. A higher malformation rate has *not* been demonstrated in women who develop gestational diabetes or in infants of diabetic fathers, thus emphasizing the importance of the intrauterine environment as a contributing factor (Mills 1982).

The insult which causes malformations in infants of diabetic mothers has an impact on most organ systems. These abnormalities must result before the seventh week of gestation (Mills *et al.* 1979). The defect thought to be most characteristic of diabetic embryopathy is sacral agenesis or caudal dysplasia, an anomaly found 200–400 times more often in offspring of diabetic women (Kucera 1971) (Fig. 8.1). Central nervous system malformations, particularly anencephaly, open spina bifida and possibly holoprosencephaly, are increased tenfold (Reece & Hobbins 1986). Cardiac anomalies, especially ventricular septal defects, and complex lesions such as transposition of the great vessels are increased fivefold.

Aetiology of diabetic embryopathy

It appears that a derangement in maternal metabolism, possibly in association with a greater genetic susceptibility, contributes to abnormal embryogenesis. Maternal hyperglycaemia has been proposed by most investigators as the primary factor, but hyperketonaemia and hypoglycaemia have also been suggested.

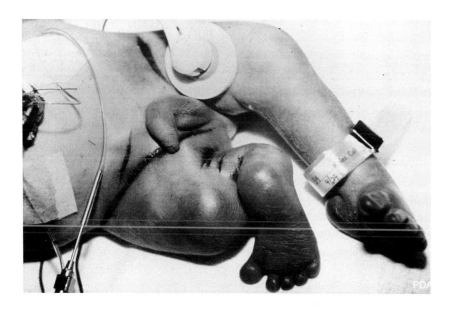

Fig. 8.1. Infant of a diabetic mother with caudal regression syndrome and hypoplastic lower extremities. Reprinted with permission from Samuels P. & Landon M.B. (1986) Medical complications. In *Obstetrics: Normal and Problem Pregnancies* (Ed. by S.G. Gabbe, J.R. Niebyl & J.L. Simpson). Churchill-Livingstone, New York.

A considerable amount of experimental animal data has linked maternal diabetes mellitus with fetal malformations. In 1963, Watanabe & Ingalls (1963) found that alloxan-induced diabetes produced anomalies in 30−45% of mouse offspring if the diabetic state were present on days 9−11 of embryogenesis. If the diabetic state were produced after day 14, malformations were not seen. Horii (Horii *et al.* 1966) confirmed the high incidence of anomalies produced in the mouse model with alloxan-induced diabetes. Furthermore, he demonstrated that insulin treatment of the diabetic mothers reduced the malformation rate to 0·2%. These early studies documented that a critical period of embryogenesis existed during which the teratogenic effects produced by maternal diabetes mellitus were likely to occur and that these effects could be offset by treatment with insulin.

Recent investigations have confirmed and expanded upon these findings. Baker (Baker *et al.* 1981) demonstrated two types of lumbar and/or sacral malformations, a fusion defect and an ossification defect, anomalies analogous to those occurring in infants of diabetic human mothers, when streptozotocin was used to induce diabetes in pregnant rats on day 6 of gestation, a critical period for fusion of the neural tube in the lumbosacral area. When diabetes was induced after day 6, the incidence of lumbosacral malformations was not increased. Furthermore, Baker was able to reduce significantly the number of lumbosacral defects when insulin therapy was used to produce normal maternal serum glucose concentrations. Baker confirmed that the quality of maternal diabetes control was critical because mothers who were treated with insulin but who were allowed to maintain moderately hyperglycaemic glucose levels delivered fetuses with an incidence of lumbosacral defects no different from those diabetic mothers who were treated with saline.

Whole-embryo culture techniques have substantiated the teratogenic effects of elevated glucose concentrations and contributed new insights about other potential teratogens. Cockroft *et al.* (1977) found that rat embryos cultured in high concentrations of D-glucose ($12−15$ mg ml^{-1}) exhibited neural tube defects. In contrast, Sadler & Horton (1986) found that insulin had no teratogenic potential in mouse embryos exposed to insulin concentrations 500 times normal. Whole-embryo cultures have also revealed the possible synergistic effect of ketones in producing diabetic embryopathy. In mouse embryos, beta-hydroxybutyrate will delay neural tube closure and retard fetal growth (Horton & Sadler 1983). Lewis (Lewis *et al.* 1983) has demonstrated that glucose and beta-hydroxybutyrate can act synergistically to produce a marked increase in neural tube, brain and cardiac defects. A third teratogenic factor has been identified in whole-embryo culture studies. Somatomedin inhibitors, which are found in increased concentrations in serum from diabetic animals, can produce malformations and growth reduction in rat embryos when added to the culture medium of rat embryos (Cockroft *et al.* 1981).

While interest in the teratogenic agents associated with diabetes mellitus has focused on the effects of hyperglycaemia, several investigators have recently demonstrated that hypoglycaemia may impair embryonic growth and induce neural tube defects in whole-embryo culture studies (Akazawas *et al.* 1986; Buchanan *et al.* 1986).

How could the teratogenic factors cited above produce the wide spectrum of malformations identified in infants of diabetic mothers? Some have suggested that non-enzymatic glycosylation of embryonic proteins may play an important role. However, Sadler was unable to show a significant increase in the glycosylated proteins of embryos cultured in a hyperglycaemic medium (Sadler & Horton 1986). Ely proposed that hyperglycaemia may inhibit mitosis by lowering intra-cellular ascorbic acid levels while increasing plasma dehydroascorbic acid concentrations (Ely 1981). Fetal malformation might arise from inhibition of glycolysis, the key energy-producing process during embryogenesis. Freinkel found that D-mannose added to the culture medium of rat embryos inhibited glycolysis and produced growth re-tardation and derangements of neural tube closure (Freinkel *et al.* 1984). The effects of mannose could be offset by adding more glucose to the medium to increase glycolytic activity, or by increasing atmospheric oxygen to enhance oxidative metabolism. Freinkel stressed the sensitivity of normal embryogenesis to alterations in these key energy-producing pathways. Goldman and Baker have suggested that the mechanism responsible for the increased incidence of neural tube defects in embryos cultured in hyperglycaemic medium may involve a functional deficiency of arachidonic acid, since supplementation with arachidonic acid or myoinositol will reduce the frequency of neural tube defects in this experimental model (Goldman *et al.* 1985). Indomethacin reversed the protection provided by myoinositol. Pinter and Reece have confirmed these studies and demonstrated that the hyperglycaemia-induced altera-tions in neural tube closure include disordered cells, decreased mitoses and increased differentiation and cell processes, changes indicative of premature maturation (Pinter & Reece 1986; Pinter *et al.* 1986).

Reece has suggested that the target site of action for these teratogenic factors may be the yolk sac. The yolk sac is a vital structure during the early stage of postimplantation development and organogenesis. Insults to the yolk sac which limit the development of vitelline vessels could impair the development of embryonic vessels and blood cells, leading to asphyxia of the embryo and anomalous fetal development. The yolk sac of rat embryos cultured in a hyperglycaemic medium demonstrated a marked reduction in vitelline vessel formation and fewer and shorter microvilli, as well as a reduction in quantity of mitochondria, endoplasmic reticulum and ribosomes (Pinter & Reece 1986; Pinter *et al.* 1986).

Early growth delay and spontaneous abortion

Pedersen and his colleagues have observed that an early growth delay may be recognized in fetuses of insulin-dependent patients on ultrasound scanning in the first trimester (Pedersen & Molsted-Pedersen 1979b). Those patients who fail to maintain good diabetic control between pregnancies are more likely to demonstrate a fetus too small for gestational age at 7–14 weeks of gestation. Furthermore, at delivery, these infants have a significantly higher incidence of congenital malformations. These data support the hypothesis of Spiers (1982) that growth retardation predisposes the fetus to a variety of malformations. Tchobroutsky has found that early growth delay may occur in pregnancies which are not complicated by diabetes mellitus (Tchobroutsky *et al.* 1985). The incidence of fetal malformations is increased in this setting as well. However, some workers believe that early growth delay is an artefact caused by a failure to detect precisely the time of ovulation (Steel *et al.* 1984).

Pedersen also suggests that early growth delay may be associated with spontaneous abortion. However, review of the literature reveals several reports, including a carefully performed prospective study (Mills 1984), in which the observed rates of spontaneous abortion for women with diabetes were consistent with the accepted incidence of spontaneous abortion for the general population. A recent study by Miodovnik did demonstrate an increased rate of spontaneous abortion in pregnancies complicated by class D diabetes (Miodovnik *et al.* 1985). In another report, Miodovnik noted that the mean glycosylated haemoglobin concentrations of diabetic women experiencing spontaneous abortions were significantly greater than those who did not abort, suggesting a contributory role for poor control of diabetes during early embryogenesis (Miodovnik *et al.* 1986).

An elevated glycosylated haemoglobin level during the first trimester

has also been associated with an increased incidence of congenital malformations. Early studies by Leslie and Ylinen demonstrated elevated
glycosylated haemoglobin levels in a small number of patients who
subsequently delivered infants with major anomalies (Leslie *et al.* 1978;
Ylinen *et al.* 1981). In 116 insulin-dependent diabetic women who had
haemoglobin A_{1c} levels measured before 14 weeks' gestation, Miller
observed a significantly higher incidence of anomalies when the
glycosylated haemoglobin values were elevated (Miller *et al.* 1981). In
58 women with normal first-trimester haemoglobin A_{1c} levels, only two
infants (3%) with major congenital anomalies were delivered. However,
in 58 patients with elevated glycosylated haemoglobin levels, 13 malformed infants (22%) were noted. In an expanded series, Ylinen found
both major and minor anomalies to be increased when glycosylated
haemoglobin values were elevated during the first trimester (Ylinen *et
al.* 1984). Overall, the risk of a major fetal anomaly may be as high as 1
in 4 or 1 in 5 when the glycosylated haemoglobin level is several per
cent above control values.

Prevention of diabetic embryopathy

Several investigators have stressed that meticulous regulation of maternal diabetes before conception and during the period of early
embryogenesis can decrease the incidence of major malformations in the
offspring of insulin-dependent diabetic women. This conclusion has been
supported by several clinical trials. In 1970, Navarette observed that
women treated with oral hypoglycaemic agents to normalize a previously
abnormal oral glucose tolerance test were subsequently delivered of
infants without congenital malformations (Navarette *et al.* 1970). Prior
to this treatment, such pregnancies had been associated with a 17·5%
incidence of malformations. Pedersen & Molsted-Pedersen (1979a) noted
a reduction in the rate of major malformations from 19·4% to 8·5% in
class D and F patients who attended a diabetic clinic to maintain
glycaemic control prior to conception. Most recently, Fuhrmann found
that intensive treatment begun before conception in 307 diabetic women
was associated with only three malformations, an incidence of 1%.
Almost 90% of the patients in this group had mean daily glucose levels
of less than 110 mg dl^{-1}. However, in 593 diabetic women who sought
care after 8 weeks of gestation, the incidence of major anomalies was
8·0% (47/593) (Fuhrmann *et al.* 1986). Only 20% of these patients had
mean daily glucose levels of less than 110 mg dl^{-1}. The incidence of

cardiac anomalies was 0·3% in the general population, 1% in diabetic women who were seen prior to pregnancy, and 3% in diabetic women who registered after 8 weeks for prenatal care. The threefold increase in cardiac lesions observed in women who were well controlled at the time of conception is worrying. The Diabetes in Early Pregnancy study has recently reported that women with diabetes who registered early and were under excellent control at conception had offspring with a lower rate of major anomalies than did diabetic women who were late registrants (4·9% vs. 9·0%) (Mills 1987). However, the incidence of 4·9% is significantly higher than that of the control population (4·9% vs. 2·0%, $P = 0.027$). Does some increase in anomalies persist even with normalization of maternal glucose levels?

Intrauterine fetal death

In the past, sudden and unexplained intrauterine fetal deaths occurred in 10–30% of pregnancies complicated by insulin-dependent diabetes (Gabbe 1980). Although relatively uncommon today, such losses still plague the pregnancies of patients who do not receive optimal care. Stillbirths have been most often observed after the 36th week of pregnancy, in patients with vascular disease, poor glycaemic control, hydramnios, fetal macrosomia or pre-eclampsia. In an effort to prevent intrauterine deaths, a strategy of scheduled preterm deliveries was established. While this empirical approach reduced the number of stillbirths, errors in estimation of fetal size and gestational age, as well as the functional immaturity characteristic of the infant of the diabetic mother (IDM), contributed to many neonatal deaths from hyaline membrane disease.

Pathophysiology of intrauterine deaths

The precise cause of the excessive stillbirth rate in pregnancies complicated by diabetes mellitus remains unknown. Yet, it has become clear that, when maternal glucose levels are maintained within physiological limits, sudden intrauterine deaths rarely occur. A considerable number of experimental data have linked derangements in maternal and fetal carbohydrate metabolism and fetal death.

Because extramedullary haematopoiesis is frequently observed in stillborn IDMs, chronic intrauterine hypoxia has been cited as a likely cause of these intrauterine fetal deaths. Madsen has provided an excellent review of those factors which may limit fetal oxygenation in pregnancies complicated by diabetes mellitus (Madsen 1986) (Table 8.1). Significant maternal factors include alterations in red blood cell oxygen release and placental blood flow. While there is little evidence that red blood cell oxygen release is impaired in well regulated pregnant diabetic women, in poorly controlled patients a shift to the left may occur in the oxyhaemoglobin dissociation curve. This change, which may be most marked in patients recovering from diabetic ketoacidosis, results in increasing haemoglobin oxygen affinity and, therefore, reduced red cell oxygen delivery at the tissue level.

Reduced uterine blood flow is thought to continue to contribute to the increased incidence of intrauterine growth retardation observed in pregnancies complicated by diabetic vasculopathy. Investigations using radioactive tracers have also suggested a relationship between poor maternal control and reduced uteroplacental blood flow (Nyland *et al.* 1982). Most recently, the antenatal assessment of uteroplacental and fetal placental blood flow using Doppler ultrasound has been applied in pregnancies complicated by diabetes mellitus (Bracero *et al.* 1986). An increase in the systolic (S) to diastolic (D) ratio of umbilical artery velocity wave forms, suggesting increased placental vascular resistance, may be observed more often in patients with poor metabolic control. Elevated S/D ratios have also been associated with an increased number

Table 8.1. Factors which reduce fetal oxygenation in pregnancies complicated by diabetes mellitus*

Maternal:
  1 Alterations in oxyhaemoglobin dissociation curve
  2 Ketoacidosis

Placental:
  1 Reduced uteroplacental blood flow
        (a) Hyperglycaemia
        (b) Ketoacidosis
        (c) Pre-eclampsia
  2 Reduced oxygen transfer
        (a) Increased diffusion distance

Fetal:
  1 Hyperglycaemia
  2 Hyperinsulinaemia
  3 Ketonaemia

* Adapted from Madsen (1986).

of stillbirths and neonatal morbidity. Ketoacidosis and pre-eclampsia, two factors known to be associated with an increased incidence of intrauterine deaths, may further decrease uterine blood flow. In diabetic ketoacidosis, hypovolaemia and hypotension due to dehydration may reduce flow through the intervillous space, while in pre-eclampsia narrowing and vasospasm of spiral arterioles may result.

Placental pathology may also impair fetal oxygenation. A decrease in the surface area of fetal capillaries available for exchange could result from obliterative lesions and thromboses in villous arteries. The diffusion distance across villous capillaries may be increased by thickening of the basement membrane of placental villi, increased proliferation of cytotrophoblastic cells and enlargement of endothelial cells. In addition, villous oedema may not only increase the diffusion distance from the intervillous space to the fetal capillaries, but also reduce the volume of the intervillous space.

How might alterations in fetal carbohydrate metabolism contribute to intrauterine asphyxia? In normally oxygenated fetal lambs, hyperglycaemia produces a small increase in plasma lactate but little change in pH (Shelley *et al.* 1975). However, when hyperglycaemia is produced in slightly hypoxic lambs, a marked rise in plasma lactate results, with a rapid fall in pH. Kitzmiller and his co-workers (1981) have made similar observations in a rhesus monkey model. Phillips described a fall in fetal arterial oxygen content when chronic hyperglycaemia is produced in the fetal lamb model (Phillips *et al.* 1982). Although plasma insulin increased, no association between fetal plasma insulin concentration and reduced fetal oxygen content was evident. Widness has recently demonstrated a relationship between maternal glycosylated haemoglobin levels during the third trimester of human pregnancies and fetal erythropoietin levels at delivery (Widness *et al.* 1987). Umbilical vein levels of glucose appeared to be a more important contributor to elevations in plasma erythropoietin than did cord insulin levels. Miodovnik and his co-workers (1982) have shown that an increase in fetal beta-hydroxybutyrate may also reduce oxygenation in the ovine fetus. When beta-hydroxybutyrate was infused into the uterine arteries, fetal lactate levels rose significantly while fetal pH fell.

There is considerable evidence linking hyperinsulinaemia and fetal hypoxia (Table 8.2). Hyperinsulinaemia induced in fetal lambs by an infusion of exogenous insulin produces an increase in oxygen consumption and a decrease in arterial oxygen content (Carson *et al.* 1980; Quissell & Bonds 1981). An elevation in fetal heart rate was noted

Table 8.2. Factors responsible for perinatal morbidity and mortality in pregnancies complicated by diabetes mellitus

	Hyperglycaemia	Hyperinsulinaemia	Ketonaemia	Hypoglycaemia
Malformations	+	−	+	+
Impaired growth	+	−	+	+
Hypoxia	+	+	+	−
Macrosomia	−	+	−	−
Delayed pulmonary maturation	+	+		
Hypoglycaemia		+		
Polycythaemia		+		
Septal hypertrophy		+		

concomitant with the fall in arterial oxygen content. Milley has observed an increase in cardiac output but a fall in fetal arterial oxygen content in association with chronic insulin infusion in the near-term ovine fetus (Milley *et al.* 1984). Blood flow increased to the brain, adrenals and carcass but placental blood flow did not change and actually fell when expressed as a percentage of cardiac output. The hypoxaemia observed during the insulin infusion occurred as a result of increased oxygen extraction by fetal tissues without a corresponding increase in oxygen delivery. Thus, hyperinsulinaemia in the fetus of the diabetic mother may increase fetal metabolic rate and oxygen requirements in the face of several factors such as hyperglycaemia, ketoacidosis, pre-eclampsia and maternal vasculopathy, which can reduce placental blood flow and fetal oxygenation.

Macrosomia

Excessive growth resulting in macrosomia can be considered the hallmark effect of maternal diabetes on fetal development. Macrosomia may pre-dispose the fetus of the diabetic mother to shoulder dystocia, traumatic birth injury and asphyxia (Resnik 1980). Newborn adiposity may also be associated with a significant risk for obesity in later life (Pettit *et al.* 1983). For these reasons, the pathogenesis, diagnosis and prevention of macrosomia in the IDM have become areas of great interest in perinatal medicine.

While some have defined macrosomia as a birthweight in excess of 4000−5000 g, others prefer categorizing infants as large for gestational age (LGA: a birthweight above the 90th percentile), using population-specific growth curves. According to these definitions, macrosomia has been observed in as many as 50% of pregnancies complicated by gestational diabetes mellitus (Sepe *et al.* 1985) and 40% of insulin-dependent pregnancies (Lavin *et al.* 1983). Since approximately 8–10% of normal pregnancies will result in infants with birthweights greater than 4000 g, the risk for delivery of a macrosomic infant may be increased as much as fivefold in women with diabetes. Delivery of an infant weighing more than 4500 g occurs *ten times* more often in diabetic women when compared with a non-diabetic control population (Spellacy *et al.* 1985).

Fetal macrosomia in the IDM is reflected by increased adiposity and muscle mass and organomegaly. Because brain growth is not increased, the head circumference usually remains in the normal range (Naeye 1965). This disproportionate increase in the size of the trunk and shoulders when compared with the head may contribute to the likelihood of a difficult vaginal delivery (Modanlou *et al.* 1982). The most eloquent descriptions of the characteristic appearance of the macrosomic IDM have been given by Farquhar (1959). In noting that these infants closely resemble each other, he stated that 'fat confers anonymity and a brotherhood of identicality in IDMs' (Fig. 8.2). An increase in total body fat in the IDM has been supported by direct measurements as well as by assessment of subcutaneous stores using skin-fold thickness measurements. Brans and colleagues (1983a) performed anthropometric measurements in a large series of IDMs and noted that 67% had increased skin-fold thickness when compared with non-diabetic controls. Skin-fold thickness can also be correlated with birthweight (Modanlou *et al.* 1982; Brans *et al.* 1983b). Enzi and co-workers (1980) found that skin-fold thickness, body-fat mass, and fat-cell weight in full-term newborns of gestational diabetic (GDM) women and insulin-dependent diabetic women were greater than in infants of non-diabetic mothers. These authors analysed gluteal fat biopsies in 8 infants of IDDM women and 17 of GDM women as well as 17 controls. Fat-cell number was similar in the diabetic and control groups, but fat-cell hypertrophy was observed in the IDM, probably secondary to an increase in triglyceride content of the adipocytes. The amount of subcutaneous fat present in the IDM may be an indication of the quality of diabetic control achieved during gestation. In Enzi's study, maternal blood glucose levels as well as neonatal immunoreactive insulin levels measured in cord blood were significantly correlated with fat-cell weight.

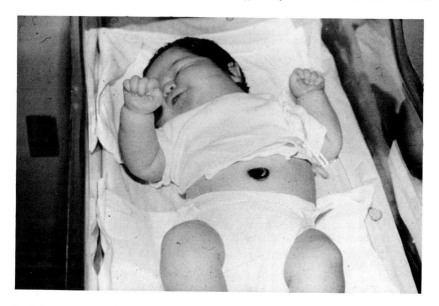

Fig. 8.2. Macrosomic infant of a diabetic mother.

Farquhar also suggested that the plethoric appearance of these new-borns was not a result of oedema, but actually reflected excess adipose tissue. Several investigations have confirmed that total body water is actually decreased in the IDM when compared to controls of similar birthweights (Osler & Pedersen 1960; Brans *et al.* 1983b). The reduction in total body water is even more pronounced in LGA IDMs, since less intracellular water may be found in cells which have increased fat content (Brans *et al.* 1983b).

The concept that maternal hyperglycaemia leading to fetal hyperglycaemia and hyperinsulinaemia (Table 8.2) results in excessive fetal growth and adipose deposition was first advanced by the Danish internist Pedersen (1954). Several autopsy studies have confirmed the existence of pancreatic islet hyperplasia in the IDM (Driscoll *et al.* 1960; Naeye 1965). Milner and colleagues (1981), using cytochemical techniques, have recently demonstrated a specific increase in beta cell mass in the pancreatic islets of IDMs when compared with control infants. This finding was observed in approximately 40% of IDMs. Increased beta cell mass may be identified as early as the second trimester (Reiher *et al.* 1983).

Using a rhesus monkey model, Susa and co-workers (1979) have confirmed the central role of excess insulin in disordered fetal growth and development. Subcutaneous minipumps were implanted in the monkeys to provide a constant insulin infusion for two weeks during the third trimester. In order to observe the independent effect of fetal hyperinsulinaemia, maternal and fetal glucose level were kept within the normal range. The findings of increased body-weight, as well as organomegaly of the liver, placenta and heart, in the infused rhesus fetuses mimic the features characteristic of the human macrosomic IDM.

Further evidence supporting the Pedersen hypothesis has come from studies of amniotic fluid (AF) and cord-blood insulin and C-peptide levels. Both are increased in the AF of insulin-treated diabetic women at term (Falluca *et al.* 1985). Elevated AF insulin levels are observed in LGA infants of insulin-dependent diabetic mothers, as well as those of women with GDM (Weiss *et al.* 1984; Falluca *et al.* 1985). Lin *et al.* (1981) found that C-peptide levels in AF could be correlated with both maternal glucose control and birthweight. These authors noted that 78% of macrosomic infants had elevated AF C-peptide levels compared with a 48% rate overall in 33 diabetic subjects. Persson and colleagues (1986) have also confirmed a positive relationship between maternal blood glucose and AF C-peptide in pregnancies complicated by IDDM and GDM.

Cord-blood levels of C-peptide are also increased in the IDM (Sosenko *et al.* 1979). IDMs exhibit a more brisk insulin response to a glucose load than infants of non-diabetic women. This response appears to be greatest in the macrosomic IDM (Phelps *et al.* 1978). Interestingly, Sosenko's study revealed that only macrosomic infants who developed hypoglycaemia had elevated C-peptide levels at birth. These data suggest that fetal hyperinsulinism cannot completely explain the high incidence of macrosomia found in the IDM.

In addition to glucose, other substrates can modify the fetal insulin secretory response (Freinkel 1980). Of the major maternal nutrients, it is likely that amino acids are important regulators of fetal insulin secretion (Milner *et al.* 1979). Milner & Hill (1984) suggested that branched-chain amino acids may act as insulin secretagogues earlier in gestation than glucose. Disturbances leading to amino acid excess in the fetus may prove to be important determinants of macrosomia. Metzger *et al.* (1980) has reported a significant elevation in plasma levels of branched-chain amino acids in gestational diabetes marked by significant carbohydrate intolerance. Insulin and C-peptide concentrations in AF increase re-markably following an arginine challenge in diabetic women when compared with controls (Falluca *et al.* 1985). Persson and colleagues (1986) have demonstrated a significant correlation between C-peptide in AF and branched-chain amino acids in maternal plasma in women with IDDM. These authors emphasize that further studies will be necessary to clarify at what stage during development and to what extent alterations in the mixture of amino acids reaching the fetus determine maturation and responsiveness of the fetal pancreas.

Over the past two decades, well-organized plans of care emphasizing control of blood glucose within physiological ranges have eliminated much of the morbidity and mortality suffered by the IDM. The results of several clinical series have validated the Pedersen hypothesis inasmuch as good maternal glycaemic control has been associated with a decline in the incidence of macrosomia. In a series of 260 insulin-dependent women achieving fasting plasma glucose levels between 109 and 140 mg dl^{-1}, Gabbe *et al.* (1977b) observed 58 (22%) macrosomic infants. Kitzmiller & Cloherty (1978) reported that 11% of 134 women achieving fasting levels between 105 and 121 mg dl^{-1} were delivered of an infant with a birthweight in excess of 4000 g. Several reports have demonstrated a reduction in the rate of macrosomia when more physiological control is achieved. Roversi *et al.* (1979) instituted a programme of 'maximally tolerated' insulin administration and observed macrosomia in only 6% of cases while Jovanovic and co-workers (1981) eliminated macrosomia in 52 women who achieved a mean glucose level of 80–87 mg dl^{-1} throughout gestation. On the other hand, it has been reported that the incidence of macrosomia in pregnancies complicated by diabetes mellitus does not increase significantly until mean glucose values approach 130 mg dl^{-1} (Willman *et al.* 1986). Differences in methodology employed in the assessment of glycaemic control may in part explain some of the disparate findings cited above. In a recent study using daily capillary glucose values obtained during the second and third trimesters in insulin-dependent patients, only 9% of infants of women with mean capillary glucose values less than 110 mg dl^{-1} were found to be LGA compared with 34% of infants of women with less optimal control (Landon *et al.* 1987). Thus, it appears that the frequency of excessive fetal growth may be reduced by maintaining excellent glucose control in women with IDDM.

Gestational diabetes is frequently complicated by fetal macrosomia. We have reviewed 13 series of women with GDM, and noted the frequency of macrosomia to be 22% (range 5–29%). When it is considered that these studies include women who have been identified and treated, it is clear that universal screening for GDM must precede any management protocol aimed at reducing morbidity, including macrosomia. Prophylactic insulin has been advocated in women with GDM who would usually be treated by diet alone (Coustan *et al.* 1984). It has been suggested that insulin may reduce minimal degrees of postprandial hyperglycaemia, which could promote excessive fetal growth. Maternal insulin therapy may also decrease other insulin secretagogues, such as branched-chain amino acids. A retrospective study demonstrated a reduction in the incidence of macrosomia from 18% in 184 gestational diabetics treated with diet alone to 7% in 155 patients receiving prophylactic insulin (Coustan *et al.* 1984). Operative delivery and birth trauma were also reduced. In contrast, Persson *et al.* (1985) failed to demonstrate a reduction in fetal macrosomia in a prospective trial of prophylactic insulin therapy in women with GDM.

The antenatal detection of fetal macrosomia could provide essential information for planning the optimal timing and safest route for delivery. To date, ultrasonography has proved to be of limited value in the prediction of macrosomia (Deter & Hadlock 1985). Because estimation of fetal weight using various formulae has been associated with far too much error, indices and ratios of differential body growth have been employed to detect macrosomia. Wladimiroff and colleagues (1978) were among the first to describe ultrasonographically derived growth characteristics in LGA infants and IDMs. These authors noted head-to-chest ratios fell below the fifth percentile in 53% of the LGA group, compared with 2% of normal-weight infants. Abdominal measurements, reflecting the size of the insulin-sensitive liver, have proved to be the most reliable sonographic parameter for the detection of macrosomia *in utero*. Eliott *et al.* (1982) analysed biparietal diameter and chest measurements in 70 diabetic women undergoing ultrasound examination within three weeks of delivery. A macrosomia index was derived for each fetus by subtracting the biparietal diameter from the chest diameter. These authors found that 20 of 23 (87%) infants weighing in excess of 4000 g exhibited a macrosomia index of 1·4 cm or greater. While this approach appears sensitive, it is associated with many false positive results. Only 61% of infants with a positive screen were found to be macrosomic at birth.

Ogata and colleagues (1980) performed serial ultrasonographic studies in 23 diabetic women during the third trimester. In 10 fetuses who proved to be macrosomic, accelerated abdominal growth was detectable by 28–32 weeks' gestation. In a series of 79 insulin-dependent women, Landon *et al.* (1988) also noted that abdominal circumference growth was accelerated at 32 weeks' gestation in LGA fetuses. These authors concluded that abdominal circumference growth >1.2 cm week^{-1} after 32 weeks' gestation could detect excessive fetal growth with an 84% sensitivity and 85% specificity.

Hypoglycaemia

Neonatal hypoglycaemia, a blood glucose below 40 mg dl^{-1} during the first 12 hours of life, results from a rapid fall in plasma glucose concentration following clamping of the umbilical cord. The degree of hypoglycaemia may be influenced by at least two factors: (i) maternal glucose control during the latter half of pregnancy; and (ii) maternal glycaemic control during labour and delivery. Maternal glucose levels greater than 90 mg dl^{-1} during delivery have been found to increase significantly the frequency of neonatal hypoglycaemia (Soler *et al.* 1978). Presumably, prior poor maternal glucose control can result in fetal β-cell hyperplasia, leading to exaggerated insulin release following delivery (Table 8.2). IDMs exhibiting hypoglycaemia have elevated cord C-peptide and free insulin levels at birth (Sosenko *et al.* 1979; Kuhl *et al.* 1982). Sosenko noted that C-peptide levels were nearly twice as high in IDMs that became hypoglycaemic. An exaggerated pancreatic response to glucose loading has also been demonstrated in the IDM (Phelps *et al.* 1978). This response is usually diminished by 7–10 days of age. Together, these studies support the concept that hypoglycaemia in the newborn IDM can be largely attributed to fetal and neonatal hyperinsulinaemia.

Other mechanisms for neonatal hypoglycaemia in the IDM have been proposed. Fetal hyperinsulinaemia is associated with suppression of plasma free fatty acid levels and diminished glycogenolysis. Limited data also suggest that the IDM may have diminished counter-regulatory responses of both glucagon and catecholamines (Bloom & Johnston 1972).

Neonatal hypoglycaemia is commonly observed in the IDM. In recently reported series, the frequency of this complication has ranged from 18 to 49% (Kitzmiller & Cloherty 1978; Coustan *et al.* 1980). Gabbe (1977) observed that 99 of 257 IDMs (39%) became hypoglycaemic after delivery, while Kitzmiller & Cloherty (1978) reported that 65 of 113 IDMs (49%) developed hypoglycaemia despite mean maternal fasting blood glucoses of 105–121 mg dl^{-1}. Although Karlsson & Kjellmer (1972) were unable to correlate maternal blood glucose control with the incidence of hypoglycaemia, few cases of neonatal hypoglycaemia have been noted in several recent series in which physiological maternal glucose levels have been maintained. Jovanovic *et al.* (1981) reported only one case of hypoglycaemia in the offspring of diabetic women whose mean blood glucose was less than 87 mg dl^{-1}. Similarly, Roversi *et al.* (1979) found that only 35 of 240 (15%) infants became hypoglycaemic after birth. In this study, the mean fasting plasma glucose was 70 mg dl^{-1}. Ylinen and colleagues (1981) have also demonstrated that maternal glucose control during late pregnancy may influence the development of neonatal hypoglycaemia. In their series of 104 diabetic women, mean HbA_{1c} levels were higher in women whose offspring became hypoglycaemic after delivery.

Pulmonary development

The precise mechanism by which maternal diabetes affects pulmonary development remains unknown. Experimental animal studies have primarily focused on the effects of hyperglycaemia and hyperinsulinaemia on pulmonary surfactant biosynthesis (Table 8.2). An extensive review of the literature confirms that both of these factors are involved in delayed pulmonary maturation in the IDM (Bourbon & Farrell 1985).

In vitro studies have documented that insulin can interfere with substrate availability for surfactant biosynthesis. In 1975, Smith and colleagues, using monolayers of cultured cells from fetal lungs, demonstrated that insulin stimulates H^3 choline incorporation into phosphatidylcholine (lecithin). More significantly, these investigators noted that when insulin was added to cultures with cortisol present, steroid-enhanced lecithin synthesis was abolished. The incorporation of substrates into lecithin may be in part dependent on the concentration of insulin present. Engle *et al.* (1983) found that low concentrations of insulin could increase glucose incorporation into lecithin, while higher levels resulted in diminished glucose and choline uptake by fetal rat type II alveolar cells. Hyperglycaemia *per se* did not alter *de novo* lecithin synthesis, suggesting that hyperinsulinism is primarily responsible for inhibition of surfactant formation.

Gross and colleagues (1980) have provided morphological evidence that hyperinsulinism may specifically reduce surfactant biosynthesis. Using fetal rat lung explants, these investigators noted a decrease in the number of type II cells and lamellar bodies after prolonged insulin exposure. However, cell membrane phospholipid biosynthesis was increased with excess insulin. It is essential, therefore, to distinguish the effects of hyperinsulinism on surfactant biosynthesis from its actions on total pulmonary phospholipid formation.

Smith (1984) has postulated that insulin interferes with the normal timing of glucocorticoid-induced pulmonary maturation in the fetus. Apparently, cortisol acts on pulmonary fibroblasts to induce synthesis of fibroblast-pneumocyte factor, which then acts on type II cells to stimulate phospholipid synthesis (Post *et al.* 1986). Carlson *et al.* (1984) have shown that insulin blocks cortisol action at the level of the fibroblast by reducing the production of fibroblast-pneumocyte factor. An alternative explanation for insulin's antagonism of cortisol-induced lung lecithin synthesis has been proposed by Rooney *et al.* (1980). In their study of cultures of fetal rat lung cells, dexamethasone-induced stimulation of choline phosphate cytidyltransferase was prevented by insulin administration. This important enzyme is involved in the pathway which eventually converts phosphatidic acid to phosphatidylglycerol (PG).

The elevated levels of myoinositol found in diabetics have also been postulated to alter PG synthesis in the fetal lung. Amniotic fluid PG is a marker of completed pulmonary maturation. The increase in extracellular myoinositol concentration which accompanies hyperglycaemia may enhance phosphatidylinositol biosynthesis while decreasing PG production (Hallman & Wermer 1982).

Derangements in intermediary glucose metabolism caused by hyperinsulinaemia may also impair surfactant synthesis. Stubbs & Stubbs (1978) have suggested that hyperinsulinaemia may shunt glycerol-3-phosphate towards pyruvate and acetyl-CoA, thereby decreasing its availability for phospholipid biosynthesis. Bourbon *et al.* (1982) have demonstrated that hyperinsulinaemia impairs glycogenolysis in fetal rat lung explants. Glycogen breakdown appears to be a prerequisite for normal lipid synthesis in the fetal lung (Singh & Feigelson 1983). Finally, changes in fatty acid metabolism could also play a role in altering lung development in the fetus of the diabetic mother. This subject has recently been discussed in an excellent review (Odom *et al.* 1986).

Clinical studies investigating the effect of maternal diabetes on fetal lung maturation have produced conflicting data. In a series of 805 infants of diabetic mothers delivered over a ten-year period, Robert and co-workers (1976) found the corrected risk for respiratory distress syndrome (RDS) to be nearby six times that of mothers without diabetes mellitus. With the introduction of protocols which have emphasized glucose control and *ante partum* surveillance until lung maturity has been established, RDS has become a less common occurrence in the IDM. Several studies agree that, in well-controlled diabetic women delivered at term, the risk of RDS is no higher than that observed in the general population (Gabbe *et al.* 1977a; Tabsh *et al.* 1982; Dudley & Black

1985). In recent studies which have emphasized rigorous maternal gly-caemic control, RDS has been virtually eliminated (Coustan *et al.* 1980; Jovanovic *et al.* 1981).

The value of the lecithin/sphingomyelin (L/S) ratio has been ques-tioned in diabetic pregnancies. Most series, however, report a low incidence of RDS with a mature L/S ratio. In one study of 93 insulin-dependent patients, an L/S ratio of 2·0 or greater was associated with a 3% risk of RDS, a result no different from that observed in the non-diabetic population (Gabbe *et al.* 1977a). In three of the five cases of RDS, delivery was performed before 37 weeks. Curet *et al.* (1979), using L/S ratios, and Farrell *et al.* (1984), measuring saturated lecithin, found no evidence of delayed maturation in well-controlled diabetic pregnancies. Other investigators have noted higher rates of RDS with an L/S ratio >2·0. In a review of 495 pregnancies complicated by diabetes, O'Brien & Cefalo (1980) found the incidence of RDS with a mature L/S ratio to be 7·9%. Variables which may have affected the findings in these studies include glucose control, severity of disease, presence of birth asphyxia, caesarean delivery rate and, of course, gestational age.

Many obstetricians prefer to rely on the presence of PG before undertaking elective delivery of the diabetic patient. Analysis of amniotic fluid in pregnancies complicated by diabetes mellitus may reveal a marked reduction or absence of PG when compared with normal preg-nancies of a similar gestational age (Cunningham *et al.* 1978; Hallman & Teramo 1979). In one series, four IDMs in whom RDS developed after delivery had L/S ratios between 2·0 and 3·0 but absent PG (Hallman & Teramo 1979). Kulovich & Gluck (1979) have reported that the time of appearance of PG in AF may be delayed significantly in GDM, whereas it may be found earlier than expected in patients with vasculopathy (classes F–R). The appearance of PG in AF has also been correlated with maternal glycaemic control during gestation (Landon *et al.* 1987).

Calcium and magnesium metabolism

Neonatal hypocalcaemia (serum levels below 7 mg dl^{-1}) occurs at an increased rate in the IDM, when one controls for predisposing factors such as prematurity and birth asphyxia (Tsang *et al.* 1972). Hypocalcaemia has been reported in as many as 50% of IDMs during the first few days of life (Tsang *et al.* 1972). Although more recent data suggest that hypocalcaemia occurs less frequently today, it is also possible that some cases go undetected because of inadequate sampling. Whether the current trend towards better maternal glycaemic control explains the apparent decrease in neonatal hypocalcaemia remains unclear.

Hypocalcaemia in the IDM has been associated with a failure to increase parathyroid hormone synthesis following birth (Tsang *et al.* 1975; Cruikshank *et al.* 1980). The reduction in newborn serum calcium concentration cannot be explained by hypersecretion of calcitonin since levels of this hormone are not elevated in the IDM. Whereas reduced parathyroid hormone levels have been observed in diabetic pregnant women, total and ionized calcium levels remain normal during gestation (Cruikshank *et al.* 1980, 1983). However, decreased serum magnesium levels have been documented in diabetic gravid women as well as their infants. Further support for a state of maternal magnesium deficiency rendering the fetus hypomagnesaemic comes from a recent study demonstrating reduced AF magnesium concentrations in insulin-dependent diabetics (Mimouni *et al.* 1987). These findings may be explained by a fall in fetal urinary magnesium excretion which would accompany a relative magnesium-deficient state. Magnesium deficiency may then paradoxically inhibit fetal parathyroid hormone secretion. Several reports indicate that magnesium administration can correct both the hypomagnesaemia and hypocalcaemia observed in the IDM (Tsang *et al.* 1976; Cruikshank *et al.* 1980). Further studies will be necessary to investigate whether adjustments in maternal diet can prevent fetal magnesium deficiency and its sequelae.

Cardiomyopathy

Over four decades ago, Miller & Wilson (1943) recognized that cardiac hypertrophy could be found in association with macrosomia, erythroblastosis and islet cell hyperplasia in the IDM. These authors noted transient cardiomegaly on X-ray in a subset of infants with cyanosis and other signs of heart failure. Subsequent autopsy studies confirmed that cardiomegaly was a common feature in IDMs (Driscoll *et al.* 1960; Naeye 1965).

The frequent findings of macrosomia and poor maternal glycaemic control may indicate that increased cardiac size is yet another by-product of fetal hyperinsulinaemia (Table 8.2). Increased cellular glycogen deposition has not been demonstrated in two autopsy specimens. However, excess insulin could also enhance myocardial protein synthesis (Halliday 1981). Ventricular wall thickness is greater in macrosomic IDMs than in normal non-diabetic macrosomic infants. Therefore, increased body size alone does not explain the finding of cardiomegaly in the IDM (Mace *et al.* 1979).

The nature of the cardiac enlargement remained unknown until Gutgesell *et al.* (1976) described echocardiographic features of three IDMs suffering from congestive heart failure. Hypertrophic subaortic stenosis producing left ventricular outflow obstruction similar to that seen in familial idiopathic hypertrophic subaortic stenosis (IHSS) was documented in each infant studied. The classic finding in IHSS, anterior systolic motion of the mitral valve leading to left ventricular outflow obstruction, was observed in two infants. Importantly, family studies failed to reveal any evidence of cardiomyopathy. In addition, the cardiomyopathy present in these infants was transient as follow-up studies demonstrated complete resolution of symptoms within the first year of life. Way *et al.* (1979) have similarly described 11 cases in which resolution of symptoms generally occurred within the first month of life. These authors noted that complete resolution of septal hypertrophy could be expected within two to twelve months.

Although the incidence of hypertrophic cardiomyopathy in the IDM is unknown, it has been suggested that 10−20% of all IDMs with cardiorespiratory symptoms have features consistent with this diagnosis (Way *et al.* 1979). Walther *et al.* (1985) documented ventricular septal hypertrophy in 18 (43%) of 42 IDMs. Of 13 IDMs experiencing congestive heart failure, seven had marked septal hypertrophy. Gutgesell *et al.* 1980) noted that, among 24 symptomatic IDMs, five have marked septal thickness with echocardiographic features of left outflow obstruction and five had hypertrophy of the right ventricular wall as well. Of 23 asymptomatic IDMs, three had septal hypertrophy, but none had evidence of outflow obstruction. These authors considered septal hypertrophy to be present if the septum was 6 mm or greater. In a prospective echocardiographic study, Mace and colleagues (1979) have reported that the mean septal size in 34 newborn IDMs was 0.6 ± 0.32 cm compared with 0.29 ± 0.06 in 43 normal control infants. In this study, increasing septal size could be correlated with poor maternal glycaemic control.

The development of septal hypertrophy in the fetus of the diabetic mother has been recently described by Veille *et al.* (1987). These investigators employed real-time directed M-mode and 2-D echocardiography to measure intraventricular septal thickness in both diabetic and control fetuses from 20 weeks until term. By 24 weeks' gestation, septal size was found to be greater during systole and diastole in pregnancies complicated by diabetes. Fetal ventricular septal hypertrophy (> 2SD above the mean) was present in 23 (74%) of 31 separate studies. The fetus of a woman with poor glucose control and with marked septal hypertrophy (5·8 mm at 24 weeks) died *in utero*. This study emphasizes the need for further investigations which will establish the haemodynamic consequences of septal hypertrophy in the developing fetus.

Hyperbilirubinaemia and polycythaemia

Hyperbilirubinaemia is frequently observed in the IDM. Neonatal jaundice has been reported in as many as 53% of pregnancies complicated by IDDM (Ylinen *et al.* 1981) and 38% of pregnancies with GDM (Widness *et al.* 1985). Although several mechanisms have been proposed to explain these clinical findings, the pathogenesis of hyperbilirubinaemia remains uncertain. In the past, the jaundice observed in the IDM was often attributed to prematurity. Several studies which have carefully analysed morbidity according to gestational age, however, have rejected this concept (Gabbe *et al.* 1978; Lemons *et al.* 1981). Stevenson and colleagues (1979) have carefully studied bilirubin metabolism in the IDM and report that bilirubin production is significantly increased in these infants when compared with control neonates. By measuring pulmonary excretion of carbon monoxide as an index of bilirubin production, these authors have noted that hyperbilirubinaemia in the IDM cannot be solely explained by increased bilirubin production. They propose that a delay in the clearance of bilirubin is also likely in the jaundiced IDM. Higher prephototherapy bilirubin concentrations in IDMs versus controls also support this concept (Stevenson & Ostrander 1981). Furthermore, hepatic conjugation of bilirubin can be impaired by hypoglycaemia and polycythaemia.

While severe hyperbilirubinaemia may be observed independent of polycythaemia, a common pathway for these complications most likely involves increased red blood cell production stimulated by increased erythropoietin in the IDM. Presumably, the major stimulus for red cell production is a state of relative hypoxia *in utero* as described above in the section on intrauterine fetal deaths. While cord erythropoietin levels are generally normal in IDMs whose mothers demonstrate good glycaemic control during gestation, Shannon *et al.* (1986) and Ylinen *et al.* (1981) found that HbA_{1c} values in late pregnancy were significantly elevated in mothers of hyperbilirubinaemic infants. In summary, enhanced erythropoiesis in the infant of the poorly controlled diabetic woman may be a significant factor contributing to both increased bilirubin production and polycythaemia.

Conclusion

Sixty years ago, Priscilla White, a pioneer in the treatment of pregnancy complicated by diabetes, emphasized that control of maternal diabetes was essential for fetal welfare. Over 30 years ago, Pedersen proposed that fetal hyperglycaemia, a consequence of maternal hyperglycaemia, could stimulate fetal insulin secretion, resulting in fetal macrosomia. It has only been during the past decade that the central role played by hyperglycaemia-induced fetal hyperinsulinaemia in promoting excessive growth has been confirmed. On the other hand, since patients with consistently normal daily glucose profiles and glycosylated haemoglobin values are still at increased risk for the delivery of an LGA infant, we must question whether metabolic aberrations other than hyperglycaemia can also lead to fetal macrosomia. While it appears clear that hyperinsulinaemia contributes to fetal deaths *in utero* and plays an important role in the aetiology of numerous neonatal morbidities such as hypoglycaemia, RDS, cardiomyopathy and polycythaemia, the precise mechanisms are unclear. The process by which maternal diabetes mellitus leads to the development of major congenital malformations also remains to be determined. These uncertainties may be clarified by continued basic research as well as the availability of new techniques such as Doppler ultrasound measurements of umbilical and uterine blood flow and fetal blood sampling. The answers to these questions not only will provide important information to guide our care of the pregnant patient with diabetes mellitus, but are also likely to yield significant insight into the processes of normal fetal growth and development.

References

Akazawas S., Akazawas M. *et al.* (1986) Teratogenic effect of hypoglycemia on early embryogenesis in rat embryo organ culture. *Diabetes,* **35** (suppl. 1), 104A.

Baker L., Egler J.M. *et al.* (1981) Meticulous control of diabetes during organogenesis prevents congenital lumbosacral defects in rats. *Diabetes,* **30**, 955–9.

Ballard J.L., Holroyde J. *et al.* (1984) High malformation rates and decreased mortality in infants of diabetic mothers managed after the first trimester of pregnancy (1956–1978). *Am. J. Obstet. Gynecol.,* **148**, 1111–18.

Bloom S.R. & Johnston D.I. (1972) Failure of glucagon release in infants of diabetic mothers. *Br. Med. J.,* **4**, 453–4.

Bourbon J.R. & Farrell P.M. (1985) Fetal lung development in the diabetic pregnancy. *Pediatr. Res.*, **19**, 253−67.

Bourbon J.R., Rieutort M. *et al.* (1982) Utilization of glycogen for phospholipid synthesis in fetal rat lung. *Biochem. Biophys. Acta*, **712**, 382−9.

Bracero L., Schulman H. *et al.* (1986) Umbilical artery velocimetry in diabetes and pregnancy. *Obstet. Gynecol.*, **68**, 654−8.

Brans Y.W., Shannon D.L. *et al.* (1983a) Maternal diabetes and neonatal macrosomia. II. Neonatal anthropometric measurements. *Early Hum. Dev.*, **8**, 297−305.

Brans Y.W., Shannon D.L. *et al.* (1983b) Maternal diabetes and neonatal macrosomia. III. Neonatal body water estimates. *Early Hum. Dev.*, **8**, 307−16.

Buchanan T.A., Freinkel N. *et al.* (1986) Maternal insulin-hypoglycemia impairs embryo development in the rat: implications for diabetic control in early pregnancy. *Diabetes*, **35** (suppl. 1), 47A.

Carlson K.S., Smith B.T. *et al.* (1984) Insulin acts on the fibroblast to inhibit glucocorticoid stimulation of lung maturation. *J. Appl. Physiol.*, **57**, 1577−9.

Carson B.S., Philipps A.F. *et al.* (1980) Effects of a sustained insulin infusion upon glucose uptake and oxygenation of the ovine fetus. *Pediatr. Res.*, **14**, 147−52.

Chung C.S. & Myrianthopoulos N.C. (1975) Factors affecting risks of congenital malformations. II. Effect of maternal diabetes on congenital malformations. *Birth Defects*, **XI** (10), 23−35.

Cockroft D.L., Coppola P.T. *et al.* (1977) Teratogenic effects of excess glucose on head-fold rat embryos in culture. *Teratology*, **16**, 141−6.

Cockroft D.L., Freinkel L.N. *et al.* (1981) Metabolic factors and organogenesis in diabetic pregnancy. *Clin. Res.*, **29**, 577A.

Coustan D.R., Berkowitz R.L. *et al.* (1980) Tight metabolic control of overt diabetes in pregnancy. *Am. J. Med.*, **68**, 845−52.

Coustan D.R., Imarah J. *et al.* (1984) Prophylactic insulin treatment of gestational diabetes reduces the incidence of macrosomia, operative delivery and birth trauma. *Am. J. Obstet. Gynecol.*, **150**, 836−42.

Cruikshank D.P., Pitkin R.M. *et al.* (1980) Altered maternal calcium homeostasis in diabetic pregnancy. *J. Clin. Endocrinol. Metab.*, **50**, 264−7.

Cruikshank D.P., Pitkin R.M. *et al.* (1983) Calcium metabolism in diabetic mother, fetus and newborn infant. *Am. J. Obstet. Gynecol.*, **145**, 1010−16.

Cunningham M.D., Desai N.S. *et al.* (1978) Amniotic fluid phosphatidylglycerol in diabetic pregnancies. *Am. J. Obstet. Gynecol.*, **131**, 719−24.

Curet L.B., Olson R.W. *et al.* (1979) Effect of diabetes mellitus on amniotic fluid lecithin/sphingomyelin ratio and respiratory distress syndrome. *Am. J. Obstet. Gynecol.*, **135**, 10−13.

Deter R.L. & Hadlock E.P. (1985) Use of ultrasound in the detection of macrosomia: a review. *J. Clin. Ultrasound*, **13**, 519−24.

Driscoll S.G., Benirschke K. *et al.* (1960) Neonatal deaths among infants of diabetic mothers. *Am. J. Dis. Child.*, **100**, 818−30.

Dudley D.K.L. & Black D.M. (1985) Reliability of lecithin/sphingomyelin ratios in diabetic pregnancy. *Obstet. Gynecol.*, **66**, 521−24.

Eliott J.P., Garite T.J. *et al.* (1982) Ultrasonic prediction of fetal macrosomia in diabetic patients. *Obstet. Gynecol.*, **60**, 159−62.

Ely J.T.A. (1981) Major congenital anomalies. *N. Engl. J. Med.*, **305**, 833.

Engle M., Langan S.M. *et al.* (1983) The effects of insulin and hyperglycemia on surfactant phospholipid biosynthesis in organotypic cultures of type II pneumocytes. *Biochem. Biophys. Acta*, **753**, 6−13.

Enzi G., Inelman E.M. *et al.* (1980) Development of adipose tissue in newborns of gestational diabetic and insulin-dependent diabetic mothers. *Diabetes*, **29**, 100−4.

Falluca F., Gargiulo P. *et al.* (1985) Amniotic fluid insulin, C peptide concentrations, and fetal morbidity in infants of diabetic mothers. *Am. J. Obstet. Gynecol.*, **153**, 534−40.

Farquhar J.W. (1959) The child of the diabetic woman. *Arch. Dis. Child.,* **34**, 76−82.

Farrell P.M., Engle M.J. *et al.* (1984) Saturated phospholipids in amniotic fluid of normal and diabetic pregnancies. *Obstet. Gynecol.,* **64**, 77−85.

Freinkel N. (1980) Banting lecture 1980: of pregnancy and progeny. *Diabetes,* **19**, 1023−35.

Freinkel N., Lewis N.J. *et al.* (1984) The honeybee syndrome—implications of the teratogenicity of mannose in rat-embryo culture, *N. Engl. J. Med.,* **310**, 223−30.

Fuhrmann K., Reiher H. *et al.* (1986) Congenital anomalies: etiology, prevention, and prenatal diagnosis. In *Diabetes in Pregnancy. Teratology, Toxicity and Treatment* (Ed. by L. Jovanovic, C.M. Peterson & K. Fuhrmann), pp. 51−71. Praeger, New York.

Gabbe S.G. (1977) Congenital malformations in infants of diabetic mothers. *Obstet. Gynecol. Surv.,* **32**, 125−32.

Gabbe S.G. (1980) Management of diabetes in pregnancy: six decades of experience. In *1980 Yearbook of Obstetrics and Gynecology* (Ed. by R.M. Pitkin), pp. 37−49. Yearbook, Chicago.

Gabbe S.G. (1985) Diabetes in pregnancy. How to manage. *Am. J. Obstet. Gynecol.,* **153**, 824−8.

Gabbe S.G., Lowensohn R.I. *et al.* (1977a) Lecithin/sphingomyelin ratio in pregnancies complicated by diabetes mellitus. *Am. J. Obstet. Gynecol.,* **128**, 757−60.

Gabbe S.G., Mestman J.H. *et al.* (1977b) Management and outcome of pregnancy in diabetes mellitus, Classes B-R. *Am. J. Obstet. Gynecol.,* **129**, 723−32.

Gabbe S.G., Lowensohn R.I. *et al.* (1978) Current patterns of neonatal morbidity and mortality in infants of diabetic mothers. *Diabetes Care,* **1**, 335−9.

Goldman A.S., Baker L. *et al.* (1985) Hyperglycemia-induced teratogenesis is mediated by a functional deficiency of arachidonic acid. *Proc. Natl. Acad. Sci. USA,* **82**, 8227−31.

Gross I., Walker-Smith G.J. *et al.* (1980) The influence of hormones on the biochemical development of fetal rat lung in organ culture. II. Insulin. *Pediatr. Res.,* **14**, 834−8.

Gutgesell H.P., Mullins C.E. *et al.* (1976) Transient hypertrophic subaortic stenosis in infants of diabetic mothers. *J. Pediatr.,* **89**, 120−5.

Gutgesell H.P., Speer M.E. *et al.* (1980) Characterization of the cardiomyopathy in infants of diabetic mothers. *Circulation,* **61**, 441−50.

Halliday H.L. (1981) Hypertrophic cardiomyopathy in infants of poorly controlled diabetic mothers. *Arch. Dis. Child.,* **56**, 258−63.

Hallman M. & Teramo K. (1979) Amniotic fluid phospholipid profile as a predictor of fetal maturity in diabetic pregnancies. *Obstet. Gynecol.,* **54**, 703−7.

Hallman M. & Wermer D. (1982) Effects of maternal insulin or glucose infusion on the fetus: study on lung surfactant phospholipids, plasma myoinisotol, and fetal growth in the rabbit. *Am. J. Obstet. Gynecol.,* **142**, 817−22.

Horii K., Watanabe G. *et al.* (1966) Experimental diabetes in pregnant mice. Prevention of congenital malformations in offspring by insulin. *Diabetes,* **15**, 194−204.

Horton W.E. Jr & Sadler T.W. (1983) Effects of maternal diabetes on early embryogenesis: alterations in morphogenesis produced by the ketone body, β-hydroxybutyrate. *Diabetes,* **32**, 610−15.

Jovanovic L., Druzin M. *et al.* (1981) Effect of euglycemia on the outcome of pregnancy in insulin-dependent diabetic women as compared with normal control subjects. *Am. J. Med.,* **71**, 921−7.

Karlsson K. & Kjellmer I. (1972) The outcome of diabetic pregnancies in relation to the mother's blood sugar level. *Am. J. Obstet. Gynecol.,* **112**, 213−20.

Kitzmiller J.L. & Cloherty J.P. (1978) Diabetic pregnancy and perinatal morbidity. *Am. J. Obstet. Gynecol.,* **131**, 560−80.

Kitzmiller J.L., Phillippe M. *et al.* (1981) Hyperglycemia, hypoxia, and fetal acidosis in Rhesus monkeys. Abstract presented at the 28th Annual Meeting of the Society for Gynecologic Investigation, St Louis, Missouri, March 1981.

Koppe J., Smoremberg-Schoorl M. *et al.* (1983) Diabetes, congenital malformations and

HLA types. In *Intensive Care in the Newborn, Vol. 4* (Ed. by L. Sten, H. Bard & B. Früs-Hansen), pp. 15–28. Masson Publishing, New York.

Kucera J. (1971) Rate and type of congenital anomalies among offspring of diabetic women. *J. Reprod. Med.,* **7**, 61–9.

Kuhl C., Andersen G.E. *et al.* (1982) Metabolic events in infants of diabetic mothers during first 24 hours after birth. *Acta Paediatr. Scand.,* **71**, 19–25.

Kulovich M.V. & Gluck L. (1979) The lung profile. II. Complicated pregnancy. *Am. J. Obstet. Gynecol.,* **135**, 64–70.

Landon M.B., Gabbe S.G. *et al.* (1987) Neonatal morbidity in pregnancy complicated by diabetes mellitus: predictive value of maternal glycemic profiles. *Am. J. Obstet. Gynecol.,* **156**, 1089–95.

Landon M.B., Mintz M.C. *et al.* (1988) Sonographic evaluation of fetal abdominal growth: prediction of the LGA infant in pregnancies complicated by diabetes mellitus. *Am. J. Obstet. Gynecol.* (in press).

Lavin J.P., Lovelace D.R. *et al.* (1983) Clinical experience with one hundred and seven diabetic pregnancies. *Am. J. Obstet. Gynecol,,* **147**, 742–52.

Lemons J.A., Vargas P. *et al.* (1981) Infant of the diabetic mother: review of 225 cases. *Obstet. Gynecol.,* **57**, 187–92.

Leslie R.D.G., Pyke D.A. *et al.* (1978) Haemoglobin A_1 in diabetic pregnancy. *Lancet,* **ii**, 958–9.

Lewis N.I., Arkarawa S. *et al.* (1983) Teratogenesis from β-hydroxybutyrate during organogenesis in rat embryo organ culture and enhancement by subteratogenic glucose. *Diabetes,* **32**, 11A.

Lin C.C., River P. *et al.* (1981) Prenatal assessment of fetal outcome by amniotic fluid C-peptide levels in pregnant diabetic women. *Am. J. Obstet. Gynecol.,* **141**, 671–6.

Mace S. Hirschfeld S.S. *et al.* (1979) Echocardiographic abnormalities in infants of diabetic mothers. *J. Pediatr.,* **95**, 1013–19.

Madsen H. (1986) Fetal oxygenation in diabetic pregnancy. *Dan. Med. Bull.,* **33**, 64–74.

Metzger B.E., Phelps R.L. *et al.* (1980) Effects of gestational diabetes on diurnal profiles of plasma glucose, lipids and individual amino acids. *Diabetes Care,* **3**, 402–9.

Miller E., Hare J.W. *et al.* (1981) Elevated maternal hemoglobin A_{1c} in early pregnancy and major congenital anomalies in infants of diabetic mothers. *N. Engl. J. Med.,* **304**, 1331–4.

Miller H.C. & Wilson H. (1943) Macrosomia, cardiac hypertrophy, erythroblastosis, and hyperplasia of the islands of Langerhans in infants born to diabetic mothers. *J. Pediatr.,* **23**, 251–4.

Milley J.R., Rosenberg A.A. *et al.* (1984) The effect of insulin on ovine fetal oxygen extraction. *Am. J. Obstet. Gynecol.,* **149**, 673–8.

Mills J.L. (1982) Malformations in infants of diabetic mothers. *Teratology,* **25**, 385–94.

Mills J.L. (1984) A prospective study of fetal losses in diabetic and control pregnancies from the third week post conception. *Diabetes,* **33** (suppl. 1), 46A.

Mills J.L. (1987) A controlled prospective study of glycemic control and malformations. The diabetes in early pregnancy study (DIEP). Abstract presented at the 47th Scientific Sessions Meeting of the American Diabetes Association, Indianapolis, Indiana, June 7–9, 1987.

Mills J.L. & Withiam M.J. (1986) Diabetes, pregnancy and malformations: an epidemiologic perspective. In *Diabetes and Pregnancy. Teratology, Toxicity, and Treatment* (Ed. by L. Jovanovic, C.M. Peterson & K. Fuhrmann), pp. 3–14. Praeger, New York.

Mills J.L., Baker L. *et al.* (1979) Malformations in infants of diabetic mothers occur before the seventh gestational week. Implications for treatment. *Diabetes,* **28**, 292–3.

Milner G.R., deGasparo M. *et al.* (1979) Effects of glucose and amino acids on insulin, glucagon, and zyniogen granule size of foetal rat pancreas grown in organ culture. *J. Endocrinol.,* **82**, 179–89.

Milner R.D. & Hill D.J. (1984) Fetal growth control: the role of insulin and related peptides. *Clin. Endocrinol.*, **21**, 415−33.

Milner R.D.G., Wirdnam P.K. *et al.* (1981) Quantitative morphology of B, A, D, and PP cells in infants of diabetic mothers. *Diabetes*, **30**, 271−4.

Mimouni F., Miodovnik M. *et al.* (1987) Decreased amniotic fluid magnesium concentration in diabetic pregnancy. *Obstet. Gynecol.*, **69**, 12−15.

Miodovnik M., Lavin J.P. *et al.* (1982) Effect of maternal ketoacidemia on the pregnant ewe and the fetus. *Am. J. Obstet. Gynecol.*, **144**, 585−93.

Miodovnik M., Skillman C. *et al.* (1985) Elevated maternal glycohemoglobin in early pregnancy and spontaneous abortion among insulin-dependent diabetic women. *Am. J. Obstet. Gynecol.*, **153**, 439−42

Miodovnik M., Mimouni F. *et al.* (1986) Glycemic control and spontaneous abortion in insulin-dependent diabetic women. *Obstet. Gynecol.*, **68**, 366−9.

Modanlou H.D., Komatsu G. *et al.* (1982) Large-for-gestational age neonates: anthropometric reasons for shoulder dystocia. *Obstet. Gynecol.*, **60**, 417−23.

Naeye R.L. (1965) Infants of diabetic mothers: a quantitative morphologic study. *Pediatrics*, **35**, 980−8.

Navarette V.N., Paniagua H.E. *et al.* (1970) The significance of metabolic adjustment before a new pregnancy. Prophylaxis of congenital malformations. *Am. J. Obstet. Gynecol.*, **107**, 250−3.

Nyland L., Lunell N.-O. *et al.* (1982) Uteroplacental blood flow in diabetic pregnancy: measurements with indium 113 m and a computer-linked gamma camera. *Am. J. Obstet. Gynecol.*, **144**, 298−302.

O'Brien W.F. & Cefalo R.C. (1980) Clinical applicability of amniotic fluid tests for fetal lung maturity. *Am. J. Obstet. Gynecol.*, **136**, 135−44.

Odom M.J., MacDonald P.C. *et al.* (1986) Diabetes and fetal lung maturation. Suppl 7. In *Williams Obstetrics* (Ed. by J. Pritchard, P.C. MacDonald & N. Gant). Appleton Century Crofts, Connecticut.

Ogata E.S., Sabbagha R. *et al.* (1980) Serial ultrasonography to assess evolving fetal macrosomia. Studies in 23 pregnant diabetic women. *JAMA*, **243**, 2405−8.

Osler M. & Pedersen J. (1960) The body composition of newborn infants of diabetic mothers. *Pediatrics*, **26**, 985−92.

Pedersen J. (1954) Weight and length at birth of infants of diabetic mothers. *Acta Endocrinol.*, **16**, 330−42.

Pedersen J. & Molsted-Pedersen L. (1979a) Congenital malformations: the possible role of diabetes care outside pregnancy. In *Pregnancy Metabolism, Diabetes and the Fetus*, Ciba Foundation Symposium 63, pp. 265−281. Excerpta Medica, Amsterdam.

Pedersen J.E. & Molsted-Pedersen L. (1979b) Early growth retardation in diabetic pregnancy. *Br. Med. J.*, **1**, 18−19.

Persson B., Stangenberg M. *et al.* (1985) Gestational diabetes mellitus. Comparative evaluation of two treatment regimens, diet versus insulin and diet. *Diabetes*, **34** (Suppl. 2), 101−5.

Persson B., Pschera H. *et al.* (1986) Amino acid concentrations in maternal plasma and amniotic fluid in relation to fetal insulin secretion during the last trimester of pregnancy in gestational and type I diabetic women and women with small-for-gestational age infants. *Am. J. Perinatol.*, **3**, 98−103.

Pettit D.J., Baird H.R. *et al.* (1983) Excessive obesity in offspring of Pima Indian women with diabetes during pregnancy. *N. Engl. J. Med.*, **308**, 242−5.

Phelps R.L., Freinkel N. *et al.* (1978) Carbohydrate metabolism in pregnancy. XV. Plasma C-peptide during intravenous glucose tolerance in neonates from normal and insulin-treated diabetic mothers. *J. Clin. Endocrin. Metab.*, **46**, 61−8.

Phillips A.F. & Dubin J.W. *et al.* (1982) Arterial hypoxemia and hyperinsulinemia in the chronically hyperglycemic fetal lamb. *Pediatr. Res.*, **16**, 653−8.

Pinter E. & Reece E.A. (1986) Arachidonic acid prevents hyperglycemia-associated yolk sac damage and embryopathy. *Am. J. Obstet. Gynecol.*, **155**, 691–702.

Pinter E., Reece E.A. *et al.* (1986) Yolk sac failure in embryopathy due to hyperglycemia: ultrastructural analysis of yolk sac differentiation associated with embryopathy in rat conceptuses under hyperglycemic conditions. *Teratology*, **33**, 73–84.

Post M., Barsoumian A. *et al.* (1986) The cellular mechanisms of glucocorticoid acceleration of fetal lung maturation. *J. Biol. Chem.*, **261**, 2179–84.

Quissell B.J. & Bonds D.R. (1981) The effects of chronic fetal insulin infusion upon fetal oxygenation. *Clin. Res.*, **28**, 125A.

Reece E.A. & Hobbins J.C. (1986) Diabetic embryopathy: pathogenesis, prenatal diagnosis and prevention. *Obstet. Gynecol. Surv.*, **41**, 325–35.

Reiher H., Fuhrmann K. *et al.* (1983) Age-dependent insulin secretion of the endocrine pancreas *in vitro* from fetuses of diabetic and nondiabetic patients, *Diabetes Care*, **6**, 446–51.

Resnik R. (1980) Management of shoulder girdle dystocia. *Clin. Obstet. Gynecol.*, **23**, 559–64.

Robert M.F., Neff R.K. *et al.* (1976) Association between maternal diabetes and the respiratory distress syndrome in the newborn. *N. Engl. J. Med.*, **294**, 357–60.

Rooney S.A., Ingleson L.D. *et al.* (1980) Insulin antagonism of dexamethasone induced stimulation of cholineophosphate cytidyltransferase in fetal rat lung in organ culture. *Lung*, **158**, 151–5.

Roversi G.D., Gargiulo M. *et al.* (1979) A new approach to the treatment of diabetic pregnant women. *Am. J. Obstet. Gynecol.*, **135**, 567–76.

Sadler T.W. & Horton W.E. Jr (1986) Mechanisms of diabetes-induced congenital malformations as studied in mammalian embryo culture. In *Diabetes in Pregnancy, Teratology, Toxicity and Treatment* (Ed. by L. Jovanovic, C.M. Peterson & K. Fuhrmann), pp. 51–71. Praeger, New York.

Sepe S.J., Connell F.A. *et al.* (1985) Gestational diabetes: incidence, maternal characteristics, and perinatal outcome. *Diabetes*, **34** (suppl 2), 13–16.

Shannon K., Davis J.C. *et al.* (1986) Erythropoiesis in infants of diabetic mothers. *Pediatr. Res.*, **20**, 161–5.

Shelley J.H., Bassett J.M. *et al.* (1975) Control of carbohydrate metabolism in the fetus and newborn. *Br. Med. Bull.*, **31**, 37–43.

Simpson J.L., Elias S. *et al.* (1983) Diabetes in pregnancy, Northwestern University Series (1977–1981). I. Prospective study of anomalies in offspring of mothers with diabetes mellitus. *Am. J. Obstet. Gynecol.*, **146**, 263–70.

Singh M. & Feigelson M. (1983) Effects of maternal diabetes on the development of carbohydrate metabolizing enzymes, glycogen deposition and surface active phospholipids in the fetal rat lung. *Biol. Neonate*, **43**, 33–42.

Smith B.T. (1984) Pulmonary surfactant during fetal development and neonatal adaptation: hormonal control. In *Pulmonary Surfactant* (Ed. by B. Robertson, L.M.G. Van Golde & J.J. Batenburg), pp. 357–81. Elsevier, Amsterdam.

Smith B.T., Giroud C.J.P. *et al.* (1975) Insulin antagonism of cortisol action on lecithin synthesis by cultured fetal lung cells. *J. Pediatr.*, **87**, 953–5.

Soler N.G., Soler S.M. *et al.* (1978) Neonatal morbidity among infants of diabetic mothers. *Diabetes Care*, **1**, 340–50.

Sosenko I.R., Kitzmiller J.L. *et al.* (1979) The infant of the diabetic mother—correlation of increased cord C-peptide levels with macrosomia and hypoglycemia. *N. Engl. J. Med.*, **301**, 859–62.

Spellacy W.N., Miller S. *et al.* (1985) Macrosomia—maternal characteristics and infant complications. *Obstet. Gynecol.*, **66**, 185–61.

Spiers P.S. (1982) Does growth retardation predispose the fetus to congenital malformation? *Lancet*, **i**, 312–14.

Steel J.M., Johnstone S.D. *et al.* (1984) Early assessment of gestation in diabetics. *Lancet*, **ii**, 975–6.

Stevenson D.K. & Ostrander C.R. (1981) Pulmonary excretion of carbon monoxide as an index of bilirubin production. IIa. Evidence for possible delayed clearance of bilirubin in infants of diabetic mothers. *J. Pediatr.*, **98**, 822−4.

Stevenson D.K., Bartoletti A.L. *et al.* (1979) Pulmonary excretion of carbon monoxide in the human infant as an index of bilirubin production. II. Infants of diabetic mothers. *J. Pediatr.*, **94**, 956−8.

Stubbs W. & Stubbs S.M. (1978) Hyperinsulinemia, diabetes mellitus, and respiratory distress of the newborn: a common link? *Lancet*, **i**, 308−9.

Susa J.B., McCormick K.L. *et al.* (1979) Chronic hyperinsulinemia in the fetal Rhesus monkey. *Diabetes*, **28**, 1058−68.

Tabsh K.M.A., Brinkman C.R. *et al.* (1982) Lecithin/sphingomyelin ratio in pregnancies complicated by insulin-dependent diabetes mellitus. *Obstet. Gynecol.*, **59**, 353−8.

Tchobroutsky C., Breart G.L. *et al.* (1985) Correlation between fetal defects and early growth delay observed by ultrasound. *Lancet*, **i**, 706−7.

Tsang R.C., Kleinman L.I. *et al.* (1972) Hypocalcemia in infants of diabetic mothers. *J. Pediatr.*, **80**, 384−95.

Tsang R.C., Chen I.-W. *et al.* (1975) Parathyroid function in infants of diabetic mothers. *J. Pediatr.*, **86**, 399−404.

Tsang R.C., Strub R. *et al.* (1976) Hypomagnesemia in infants of diabetic mothers. Perinatal studies. *J. Pediatr.*, **89**, 115−19.

Veille J.C., Sivakoff M. *et al.* (1987) Fetal intraventricular septal thickness as assessed by 2-D directed M-mode echocardiography: comparison between normal and diabetic pregnancies. Presented at the Society of Perinatal Obstetricians, February 1987.

Walther F.J., Siassi B. *et al.* (1985) Cardiac output in infants of insulin-dependent diabetic mothers. *J. Pediatr.*, **107**: 109−14.

Watanabe G. & Ingalls T.H. (1963) Congenital malformations in the offspring of alloxan-diabetic mice. *Diabetes*, **12**, 66−72.

Way G.L., Wolfe R.R. *et al.* (1979) The natural history of hypertrophic cardiomyopathy in infants of diabetic mothers. *J. Pediatr.*, **95**, 1020−5.

Weiss P.A.M., Hofinan H. *et al.* (1984) Gestational diabetes and screening during pregnancy. *Obstet. Gynecol.*, **63**, 776−80.

Widness J.A., Cowett R.M. *et al.* (1985) Neonatal morbidities in infants of mothers with glucose intolerance in pregnancy. *Diabetes*, **34** (suppl. 2), 61−5.

Widness J.A., Teramo K.A. *et al.* (1987) Direct relationship of fetal erythropoietin and delivery to maternal glycohemoglobin levels in diabetic pregnancy. Presented at the Society of Perinatal Obstetricians, February 1987.

Willman S.P., Leveno K.J. *et al.* (1986) Glucose threshold for macrosomia in pregnancy complicated by diabetes. *Am. J. Obstet. Gynecol.*, **154**, 470−5.

Wladmiroff J.W., Bloemsa C.A. *et al.* (1978) Ultrasonic diagnosis of the large-for-dates infant. *Obstet. Gynecol.*, **52**, 285−8.

Ylinen K., Raivio K. *et al.* (1981) Haemoglobin A_{1c} predicts the perinatal outcome in insulin-dependent diabetic pregnancies. *Br. J. Obstet. Gynaecol.*, **88**, 961−7.

Ylinen K., Aula P. *et al.* (1984) Risk of minor and major fetal malformations in diabetics with high haemoglobin A_{1c} values in early pregnancy. *Br. Med. J.*, **289**, 345−6.

9

The Effects of Autoimmune Disease on the Fetus

N. KOCHENOUR

The immune system is a complex, integrated system whose primary function is to protect the individual from infection. Normally, the immune system discriminates between foreign substances, which it attempts to destroy, and the individual's own tissues, which it tolerates. Occasionally, this system breaks down and an individual reacts against his or her own tissues. This process is termed autoimmunity. Generally, it is characterized by immunologically mediated mechanisms, either humoral or cellular, that initiate inflammation and result in the destruction of healthy tissue. Pregnancy provides a unique situation for this process, involving not only the host but also her fetus. The purpose of this chapter is to describe the effects of autoimmune disease on pregnancy, particularly on the developing fetus. Before discussing specific autoimmune conditions. I will briefly review the normal immune system and the immune response.

The immune system

Components of the immune system

The primary effector cell of the immune system is the lymphocyte. Lymphocytes can generally be classified into two categories based upon their tissue of origin. T- (thymus-derived) lymphocytes are responsible for cell-mediated immunity and B- (bursa-derived) lymphocytes are responsible for the production of antibody. T-lymphocytes include those cells responsible for transferring delayed hypersensitivity, those involved in the cellular killing of target cells (cytotoxic), and those responsible for facilitating (helper) or for suppressing (suppressor) the immune response.

Antibodies are serum glycoproteins that are produced by mature B-lymphocytes (plasma cells), which have been transformed from immature lymphocytes in response to a challenge by an immunogen. An immunogen is a substance that can induce the formation of the components of the immune system. Although this term is frequently used interchangeably with antigen, strictly speaking, an antigen is a substance that reacts with the components of the immune system. Haptens are low molecular weight substances which are antigens in that they react with the antibodies once they are formed, but they are not immunogens because they cannot induce an antibody response.

There are five classes of antibodies (IgA, IgD, IgE, IgG, IgM). Within these classes are several subclasses, including four subclasses of IgG and two subclasses each of IgA and IgM. The basic structure of an antibody consists of four chains of amino acids covalently joined by interchain and intrachain disulphide bonds (Fig. 9.1). The molecule consists of two identical short or light (L) chains and two identical long or heavy (H) chains. Each class and subclass of antibody has a unique type of H chain. Structural analysis of immunoglobulins has shown that, under controlled conditions, limited papain digestion of the IgG molecule cleaves it into three fragments, two of which are identical. The two identical fragments contain the antigen-binding capacity and are termed antibody-combining fragments (Fab fragments). The other piece crystallizes when separated and is termed the crystalline fragment (Fc fragment). The Fab portion contains the recognition site for antigen and confers specificity, whereas the Fc portion is responsible for complement activation and for Fc receptor recognition by polymorphonuclear cells, mast cells, platelets, and trophoblasts. This portion is also involved in most of the antibodies' interaction with non-specific effector systems. IgG, the major class of antibodies in the immune response, comprises 80–85% of circulating immunoglobulins and is responsible for most of the functions attributed to antibodies, such as agglutination, precipitation and complement activation. As a result of selective transport across the trophoblast, IgG is the major maternal antibody found in the fetus. Although the predominant IgG in serum is IgG1, individual responses to different immunogens are variable and certain immunogens may specifically induce one subclass rather than another.

Antibodies are an integral part of a number of biological reactions. Antibodies react with soluble antigen molecules to produce immune complexes. When there is a large excess of either antibody or antigen, these complexes are usually soluble. If the ratios are such that antibody-mediated cross-linking can occur between antigen molecules, a visible precipitate will form. When the antigen is particulate, such as erythrocytes or bacteria, agglutination can occur in the same manner. Antibody can

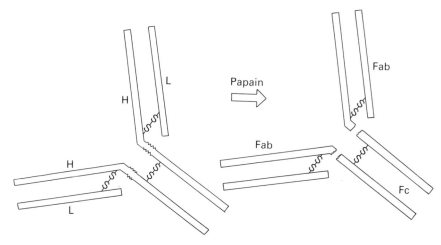

Fig. 9.1. Schematic diagram of the basic structure of an antibody. The molecule consists of four chains, two light (L) and two heavy (H), held together by disulphide linkages. Limited papain digestion of IgG results in two identical fragments (Fab) containing the antigen-binding activity and a third fragment (Fc), which crystallizes when separated from the Fab fragments.

also activate complement. The complement system consists of a group of plasma proteins that are present in inactive forms and which, when the initial component is activated, sequentially activate. This activated cascade results in a number of biological phenomena, including lysis and the generation of several products which are opsonic, chemotactic or anaphylactic. There are two pathways by which the complement cascade can be activated. The classical pathway is initiated by an antibody–antigen complex, while the alternate pathway can be activated by a number of naturally occurring substances, including endotoxin and cobra venom factor.

The immune response

The immune response to an antigenic challenge has classically been divided into two phases, the primary and the secondary responses. Following exposure to a new antigen, there is a lag period of approximately five days during which no antibody is detectable. The primary response is usually characterized by IgM and a small amount of IgG antibody. As a result of this exposure to an antigen, the individual has generated a number of memory cells and, if exposed to the same antigen at a later time, is able to produce a larger amount of antibody more quickly than during the primary response. The amount of IgM produced in a secondary response is approximately the same as during a primary response; however, IgG is produced in much larger quantities and is the predominant antibody of the secondary response. Very few antigens are capable of stimulating B-lymphocytes directly to produce antibody but, rather, require the interaction of several cell populations including helper T-cells and antigen-presenting cells. In order for an antigen to induce a B-lymphocyte to produce antibody, the antigen must first be processed. Circulating antigen is cleared by the cells of the reticuloendothelial system, where lysosomal enzymes degrade the antigen. Remnants of the antigenic determinant, along with HLA-D/DR determinants, are presented to helper lymphocytes to initiate the immune response.

The major histocompatibility antigens that the human fetus and other grafts express are called HLA determinants: H for human, L for leucocyte and A for antigens. HLA antigens are expressed on the surface of all nucleated cells. These antigens are genetically determined by four different genes, termed HLA-A, HLA-B, HLA-C and HLA-D/DR, which are located on human chromosome 6 in a region called the major histocompatibility complex (MHC). The products of these genes are extremely polymorphic so that the alleles for 65 to 75 different antigens have been identified at these loci. These markers are inherited in a codominant fashion so that a child will inherit four different alleles from each parent. There are also Ir genes within the MHC that control the quality and quantity of an immune response. Whenever a population first encounters a disease, there are usually some people who succumb rapidly, some who recover from relatively severe symptoms and some who contract mild disease and recover rapidly. It has been postulated that there is a genetic aspect of this resistance and susceptibility, and that it may be related to the Ir genes (Rote 1985). Whether or not a Rh-negative individual will be immunized with Rh-positive erythrocytes may also be under Ir gene control.

Autoimmune diseases

Autoimmune thrombocytopenic purpura

Autoimmune thrombocytopenic purpura (ATP) is the most common autoimmune disorder encountered during pregnancy. Thrombocytopenia is defined as a platelet count $<150\,000$ mm^{-3}. The diagnosis of ATP is made according to established criteria (Baldini 1966), which include a normal haematocrit, haemoglobin and white blood cell count, unless there has been a recent haemorrhage, a normal bone marrow with adequate or increased megakaryocytes, a blood smear showing an increased percentage of large platelets, normal clotting studies and no other obvious cause for the thrombocytopenia. The presence of free or bound platelet-associated antibodies serves to support the diagnosis of ATP. The condition may be classified on the basis of acuity. The acute disorder, most commonly seen in children, often follows a viral illness. The intermittent form can occur in either children or adults and is characterized by intervals when the platelet count is normal. The chronic form most commonly affects adults and is long-lasting. As with most autoimmune diseases, it is more common in women than in men.

Although the precipitating event responsible for ATP is not known, a genetic predisposition is suspected (Laster *et al.* 1982) and a recent viral infection has been implicated in some patients (Lurhuma *et al.* 1977). While it is clear that humoral immunity plays a critical role in the pathogenesis of ATP, the role of cell-mediated immunity is uncertain (McMillan 1981). Most patients have an increased amount of immunoglobulin directed towards platelet-associated antigens present on the surface of their platelets. This leads to rapid platelet clearance by the reticuloendothelial system. The antibody is usually of the IgG class and has been shown to be synthesized in the spleen (Karpatkin *et al.* 1972) and bone marrow (McMillan *et al.* 1976) of patients with ATP. Most evidence suggests that antiplatelet IgG binds directly to platelet antigens. Circulating immune complexes have also been demonstrated and complement (C3) has been implicated in the pathogenesis of ATP in some patients (Hauch & Rosse 1977; Cines & Schreiber 1979). Most patients with ATP have increased levels of platelet-associated IgG. Another group of patients has activated C3, causing elevated levels of both IgG and C3 and a third group has normal levels of platelet-associated IgG but elevated levels of platelet-associated C3 (Myers *et al.* 1982).

Early quantitative assays for measuring platelet-associated IgG were impractical for routine use by clinical laboratories. Recently, radiolabelled Coombs' antiglobulin (Cines & Schreiber 1979) and enzyme-linked immunosorbent assays (ELISAs) (Rote *et al.* 1983) have been developed. In the direct test, the patient's platelets are tested and, in the indirect test, the plasma or serum is tested. The direct assay generally correlates better with the patient's clinical picture than the indirect test.

Corticosteroids represent the cornerstone of therapy for ATP and are used initially in the absence of contraindications. Prednisone (or its equivalent) in the dose of $1-2$ mg/kg daily in divided doses will result in an increase in platelet count in 70 to 90% of patients and approximately 20 to 25% will achieve complete remission (Shulman & Jordan 1982). A favourable response, if it occurs, is usually apparent by 21 days. If remission is achieved, the high initial dose should be gradually tapered to one that will prevent clinical bleeding and maintain platelets above 50 000 mm^{-3}. It appears that corticosteroids function therapeutically in patients with ATP through a number of mechanisms. Corticosteroids decrease antiplatelet antibody production by the spleen, bone marrow, liver and other tissues of the reticuloendothelial system (McMillan *et al.* 1974), interfere with the interaction between antiplatelet antibody and the platelet surface (McMillan *et al.* 1974), decrease the clearance of antibody or complement-coated platelets by macrophages in the liver or spleen (Handin & Stossel 1975) and improve normal capillary fragility (Fallon *et al.* 1952).

Splenectomy is frequently indicated in patients with ATP when they have not responded initially to corticosteroid therapy, when too high doses of corticosteroids are required to maintain adequate platelet counts, or when frequent exacerbations justify an attempt at long-term remission through surgery. The platelet count usually increases rapidly following surgery and is often normal within one to two weeks. Significant improvement is achieved in 70 to 90% of patients and permanent remission in about 45% (Shulman & Jordan 1982).

Immunosuppressive agents, such as cyclophosphamide, the vinca alkaloids and azathioprine, have been used for the treatment of patients with ATP who are refractory to corticosteroids and splenectomy. In general they have been effective in about one-third of treated patients (Karpatkin 1980; McMillan 1981).

The effective use of high-dose intravenous IgG in the treatment of ATP in childhood (Imbach *et al.* 1981) was followed by similar reports in adult patients (Fehr *et al.* 1982; Newland *et al.* 1983). Immunoglobulin in a dose of 0·4 g kg^{-1} day^{-1} for a period of five days has been associated with an increase in platelet counts to normal values in a high proportion of patients within four to five days. Although the exact mechanism of action of this therapy is not known, interference with the Fc-receptor binding of immune particles appears to be a likely explanation for at least part of its action. The number of patients treated by this regimen is limited; nevertheless, reported side-effects have been minimal.

Although two published reports indicated an exacerbation of ATP during pregnancy (Zilliacus 1964; Laros & Sweet 1975), the majority of the literature supports the thesis that the overall course and severity of ATP is not significantly affected by pregnancy (Peterson & Larson 1954; Tancer 1960; Carloss *et al.* 1980). Some authors have reported a tendency towards thrombocytopenia (Laros & Sweet 1975; Handin 1981) and it has been postulated that pregnancy enhances phagocytosis by accelerating the clearance of antibody-coated platelets (Handin 1981). The principal maternal risk is associated with bleeding from the episiotomy, lacerations of the birth canal or caesarean delivery. If a surgical delivery is indicated, platelet transfusions are utilized to minimize maternal haemorrhage if the platelet count is less than 50 000 mm^{-3}.

Because the human placenta has receptors for the Fc portion of the IgG molecule and actively transports IgG antibodies of all types, the most serious clinical problem in the management of pregnant patients with ATP involves the transplacental transfer of the maternal antiplatelet antibody, which can result in thrombocytopenia in the fetuses and infants of these women. Even in women who have had a splenectomy for their disease, high levels of antibodies can cause shortened platelet survival and thrombocytopenia in themselves and their fetuses. The risk of spontaneous abortion in pregnant women with ATP has been reported to be as high as 33% (Shenker & Polishuk 1968). Neonatal thrombocytopenia has been reported in 40 to 60% of the infants born to women with ATP (Peterson & Larson 1954; Tancer 1960; Territo *et al.* 1973: Laros & Sweet 1975). The major controversial issue in the management of ATP has been the management of labour and delivery. The debate centres on the magnitude of the risk of labour and vaginal delivery to the thrombocytopenic fetus and on the methods of predicting the fetal platelet count.

The most feared perinatal complication is intracranial haemorrhage, a condition considered to be more likely in the thrombocytopenic fetus undergoing vaginal delivery. The evidence for that assumption is scanty. While the incidence of intracranial haemorrhage is increased in thrombocytopenic fetuses, it is a rare event (Kelton 1983). A significant number of fetal deaths in women with ATP occur before the onset of labour (O'Reilly & Taber 1978) and are not always due to detectable haemorrhage. Nevertheless, it appears that, at least in the neonate, the greater the degree of thrombocytopenia, the greater the risk of serious haemorrhage. Scott *et al.* (1980) retrospectively analysed data from 96 women with ATP in a total of 113 pregnancies. These data included the authors' series plus a review of the literature. There were 11 instances of serious haemorrhage in the 39 infants (28%) with platelet counts below 50 000 mm^{-3}. There were no cases of severe bleeding in infants with a platelet count above 50 000 mm^{-3}.

Considerable effort has been directed toward identification of the fetus at risk, and delivery of the severely affected fetus by a caesarean section has been advocated. Knowledge of the fetal platelet count is essential if this plan of management is to be considered. Unfortunately, a reliable method of predicting the fetal platelet count has been elusive. In a prospective study (Territo *et al.* 1973), 27% of women with a platelet count greater than 100 000 mm^{-3} delivered infants with platelet counts less than 50 000 mm^{-3}. Others (Scott *et al.* 1980 — see Fig. 9.2; Cines *et al.* 1982; Kelton *et al.* 1982) have also demonstrated that the maternal platelet count is an unreliable predictor of fetal or neonatal platelet count. This discrepancy between maternal and fetal platelet counts is even greater than in patients who have had a previous splenectomy. There have been conflicting reports concerning the reliability of maternal antiplatelet antibody measurement as a predictor of neonatal platelet count. Kelton *et al.* (1982) found that the measurement of maternal platelet-associated IgG levels can be used to predict neonatal thrombocytopenia, but they did not measure circulating maternal antiplatelet antibody. Cines *et al.* (1982) observed that the level of maternal platelet-associated IgG did not identify the neonates at risk for thrombocytopenia whereas the level of maternal circulating antiplatelet antibody correlated with both the presence and extent of neonatal thrombocytopenia. J.R. Scott *et al.* (1983) found no consistent relationship between circulating maternal or cord antiplatelet antibody levels and neonatal thrombocytopenia.

Although it has been reported that maternal treatment with corticosteroids during pregnancy is of value in maintaining an adequate fetal platelet count at the time of delivery (Karpatkin *et al.* 1981), experience with the disease indicates that such protection is incomplete in some cases and unnecessary in others (Logaridis *et al.* 1983). A twin gestation (Scott *et al.* 1980) in which one infant was thrombocytopenic and the other was not raises the question of whether any maternal clinical characteristic or laboratory test will reliably predict fetal platelet count.

Fetal scalp platelet count obtained early in labour has been recommended (Ayromlooi 1978; Scott *et al.* 1980) as a method of reliably determining the fetal platelet count to assess the safety of vaginal delivery. Early in labour or at the time of amniotomy for the induction of labour, scalp blood is obtained as it would be for scalp blood pH determination. If the fetal platelet count is below 50 000 mm^{-3}, a caesarean delivery is

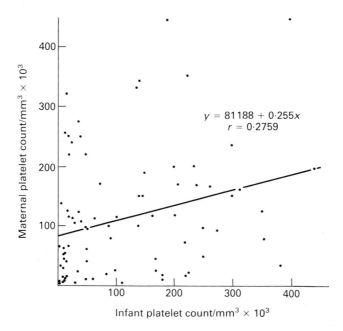

$$y = 81\,188 + 0{\cdot}255x$$
$$r = 0{\cdot}2759$$

Fig. 9.2. Relationship between maternal platelet count at delivery and infant platelet count in women with ATP (Scott *et al.* 1980).

performed; if above $50\,000$ mm^{-3}, labour is continued and caesarean delivery performed for obstetric indications only. A disadvantage of this procedure is that it can only be performed through a dilated cervix after rupture of the membranes. Another alternative for determining the fetal platelet count is direct puncture of the umbilical cord under ultrasound guidance (Daffos *et al.* 1984). Direct fetal platelet transfusions are also possible by this method (Daffos *et al.* 1984). Platelet transfusion in patients with ATP is a temporary measure, useful therapeutically in life-threatening situations and prophylactically as part of the preoperative preparation. The survival of transfused platelets in patients with ATP is variably shortened to between 48 and 230 minutes (Harker & Finch 1969). Repeated fetal platelet transfusions for patients with ATP does not seem to be very practical, although it may be an alternative in fetal isoimmune thrombocytopenia where platelet-specific antigens are identified and platelets free of that antigen can be infused.

The recent introduction of high-dose intravenous IgG therapy in the management of ATP has raised hopes that the effect of the immunoglobulin would extend transplacentally to the fetus. In the pregnant patients with ATP who have been treated and reported to date

(Mizunuma *et al.* 1984; Tchernia *et al.* 1984; Lavery *et al.* 1985), the effect on maternal platelet count has been similar to that in the non-pregnant patient; however, the fetal response has not been as predictable (Davies *et al.* 1986; Pappas 1986).

Antiphospholipid antibodies — lupus anticoagulant and anticardiolipin

Two antiphospholipid autoantibodies, lupus anticoagulant (LAC) and anticardiolipin (ACA), have recently been recognized to be associated with first-trimester spontaneous abortions, intrauterine growth retardation (IUGR), and second- and early third-trimester fetal death. These two closely related autoantibodies have been found in patients with systemic lupus erythematosus (SLE) or other autoimmune disorders, and in patients with no apparent disease. The fetal loss rate is very high, whether or not maternal clinical autoimmune disease is present. The antibodies are usually of the IgG type but may also be IgM.

Lupus anticoagulant prolongs phospholipid-dependent coagulation tests by binding to the phospholipid portion of the prothrombin–prothrombinase complex (Thiagarajan *et al.* 1980; Hougie 1985) and it is this action of the immunoglobulin that forms the basis of its detection and measurement. The presence of LAC is suggested by prolongation of the activated partial thromboplastin time (APTT) or by other phospholipid-dependent coagulation tests. A factor deficiency as an explanation for the prolongation of the coagulation test is excluded by the failure of LAC-containing plasma to 'correct' to a near normal value with the addition of an equal volume of normal plasma. Other phospholipid-dependent coagulation assays, such as the kaolin clotting time (KCT), do not use added phospholipid and are more sensitive than the APTT for detecting LAC (Exner *et al.* 1978).

Anticardiolipin antibodies are identified by immunoassays, such as an enzyme-linked immunoassay (ELISA) or a radioimmunoassay. Harris *et al.* (1984) have reported a close correlation between the degree of prolongation of the coagulation assays used to detect LAC and the levels of ACA by immunoassay, suggesting that LAC and ACA may be the same immunoglobulin. Others (Branch *et al.* 1985) have not found such a close correlation, and there are several reports of patients with one or the other antibody but not both (Harris *et al.* 1983; Branch *et al.* 1985; Lockshin *et al.* 1985).

Lupus anticoagulant is found in 5% to 15% of patients with SLE;

conversely, about 40% of individuals with LAC have evidence of SLE (Schleider *et al.* 1976). It is present in about 40% of patients with a biologically false positive test for syphilis (BFP-STS) (Johansson & Lassus 1974). In addition to recurrent pregnancy loss, a number of other clinical features have been associated with the antiphospholipid activity of this autoantibody. Boey *et al.* (1983) reported thrombotic episodes in 18 of 31 patients with SLE and other connective-tissue disorders plus LAC, but in only 3 of 29 such patients without LAC. More than 50% of the 35 patients with LAC studied by Elias & Eldor (1984) had thrombotic episodes, 6 of them with pulmonary embolism. Other clinical conditions associated with LAC include idiopathic thrombocytopenia (Hughes *et al.* 1984) and chorea gravidarum (Lubbe & Walker 1983). Absence of any identifiable disorder apart from recurrent pregnancy loss is not uncommon. Numerous retrospective studies have demonstrated a high frequency of pregnancy loss in women with LAC. The literature documents 242 previous, untreated pregnancies in 65 women with LAC (Branch 1987). Of these pregnancies, 220 (91%) were lost as spontaneous abortions or fetal deaths. About 30−40% of pregnancy losses in these women occur after 13 weeks' gestation. There are only six published cases of viable liveborns delivered of untreated women who were documented to have LAC prior to or early in pregnancy (Branch 1987).

Anticardiolipin antibodies in patients with SLE and other autoimmune disorders are responsible for the BFP-STS (Catterall 1973). Patients with BFP-STS usually have low-titre positive VDRL tests, in contrast to patients with untreated syphilis who have high VDRL titres (Fiumara 1963). Harris *et al.* (1985), using the solid phase radioimmunoassay to detect ACA, have found that BFP-STS patients usually have very high ACA levels. They found several VDRL-negative patients with high ACA levels and, conversely, several patients with untreated syphilis and high VDRL titres who had normal ACA levels. These findings suggest that the ACA antibodies in patients with syphilis vary in specificity from those with SLE and other autoimmune diseases. As previously noted, lupus anticoagulant has been identified in a high percentage of patients with BFP-STS, but not in patients with syphilis (Johansson & Lassus 1974). Although less well studied, the fetal death rate among women with ACA is also high. Lockshin *et al.* (1985), in a study of 21 pregnant patients with SLE, found ACA to be the most sensitive predictor of fetal distress or fetal death. Among the nine patients with significant levels of ACA, there were one first-trimester spontaneous abortion, three fetal deaths and five cases of abnormal *ante partum* fetal heart rate testing.

The 12 women without ACA had neither fetal death nor abnormal *ante partum* fetal heart rate testing. Derue *et al.* (1985) studied antiphospholipid antibody levels in women with SLE and found that ACA and LAC were significantly associated with a history of one or more pregnancy losses. Sixteen of the 23 patients with pregnancy losses had elevated levels of ACA. Seventeen of the patients with pregnancy losses also had LAC. The authors did not distinguish those patients with one or the other autoantibody.

A number of immunopathological mechanisms have been postulated for the action of antiphospholipid antibodies, especially LAC, which has been more extensively investigated. These mechanisms, all antibody-mediated, include inhibition of protein C activation on endothelial phospholipids (Cariou *et al.* 1986), of prekallikrein activity (Sanfelippo & Drayna 1982), of endothelial plasminogen activator release (Angles-Cano *et al.* 1979) and of endothelial prostacyclin synthetase activity (Carreras *et al.* 1981a). At present, the most attractive hypothesis involves antibody mediated inhibition of prostacyclin (PGI_2) production. Prostacyclin, produced and released by vascular endothelium, is a potent vasodilator and inhibitor of platelet aggregation (Moncada *et al.* 1977), felt to be important in the maintenance of normal vascular patency (Moncada & Vane 1978). Thromboxane A2, a prostaglandin produced by platelets, is a vasoconstrictor and promotes platelet aggregation. Plasma from patients with LAC has been shown to inhibit the production of PGI_2 (Carreras *et al.* 1981a, b; De Castellarnau *et al.* 1983) by vascular endothelium. In this situation, thromboxane A2 would predominate, predisposing to vasoconstriction, platelet aggregation and intravascular thrombosis. It has been postulated that LAC inhibits PGI_2 production by binding to endothelial cell membranes and interfering with the release of the phospholipid precursors of prostaglandin production (Carreras *et al.* 1981b). Interestingly, decreased PGI_2 production by both maternal and fetal vascular tissues has also been demonstrated in pregnancies complicated by pre-eclampsia and chronic placental insufficiency syndromes (Remuzzi *et al.* 1980). In addition to the inhibition of PGI_2 production by vascular endothelium, LAC also interacts with the phospholipid fraction of platelets (Thiagarajan *et al.* 1980) (Fig. 9.3).

Successful treatment of pregnant patients with LAC was first reported by Lubbe *et al.* (1983) and subsequently by Farquharson *et al.* (1984) and Branch *et al.* (1986). Each group used a combination of prednisone and low-dose aspirin therapy. Prednisone is given because doses of $40-60$ mg day^{-1} have been shown to suppress the production or activity

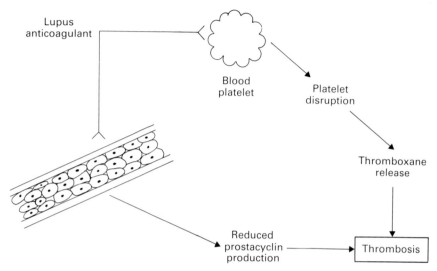

Fig. 9.3. Schematic diagram of proposed mechanism of activity of lupus anticoagulant (LAC) *in vivo*.

of LAC, as measured by a lowered APTT (Conley & Hartman 1952; Exner *et al.* 1978). The optimal dose of aspirin for preventing platelet aggregation and restoring a normal prostacyclin–thromboxane balance is 40–80 mg day^{-1} (Weksler *et al.* 1983). Six women who previously had had a total of 14 pregnancies all ending in intrauterine death were treated with 40–60 mg day^{-1} of prednisone and 75 mg day^{-1} of aspirin (Lubbe *et al.* 1983). Correction of APTT values occurred in five of the six patients and was accompanied by a live birth in all five. In the sixth patient intrauterine death occurred at 16 weeks, when the APTT was only partly corrected. Farquharson *et al.* (1984) reported the successful therapy of two patients with a modification of Lubbe's regimen. Living children were born to five of the eight patients who were treated with prednisone and low-dose aspirin by Branch *et al.* (1985). Unlike the previous investigators, they did not find that suppression of the APTT to the normal range ensured a live birth. On the other hand, persistently elevated APTT did not invariably result in fetal death. Three of their eight patients — those who did not receive prednisone and aspirin until after the 16th week of gestation — experienced severe pre-eclampsia that necessitated preterm delivery between 27·5 and 33 weeks of gestation. Intrauterine fetal growth retardation was confirmed in each instance by the delivery of an infant who was small for gestational age (< 10th percentile). In each of these cases, the placenta was also small and, on histological evaluation, was found to have extensive infarction. Two patients who had infants who survived began treatment before the sixth week of pregnancy, but one had a persistently elevated APTT in spite of a daily dose of 50 mg of prednisone. The infants of both of these women were appropriately grown for gestational age, and the placentas were normal in size and histology.

The optimum therapy for patients with antiphospholipid antibodies is not known. Data on the treatment of patients with ACA antibodies are scarce. Whether or not all patients with either or both of these antibodies need to be treated and how early in pregnancy therapy must be started are not clear. Further investigation is required before these questions can be answered; however, several generalizations can be made. Patients with the antiphospholipid antibodies ACA or LAC have a high rate of pregnancy loss. Treatment with corticosteroids and low-dose aspirin improves the pregnancy outcome but does not always eliminate the effects of the condition. Women with SLE, a BFP-STS, a history of thrombotic episodes, a history of unexplained fetal death or a history of IUGR who are pregnant or considering pregnancy should be screened for the presence of antiphospholipid antibodies.

Antibodies against ribonucleoprotein antigens

The neonatal lupus syndrome is a rare condition characterized by congenital heart block, transient cutaneous lupus or both. Congenital heart block is the only aspect of the lupus neonatal syndrome that is life-threatening. It may result in fetal death, but is more commonly reported to result in neonatal cardiac morbidity or mortality. The typical antenatal presentation is that of a fixed fetal heart rate of 50–60 beats per minute, often with 'non-immune' hydrops. Mothers of these infants may have connective tissue disease or may be asymptomatic.

A maternal immunological abnormality to explain the congenital heart block which was detected in three successive live births from one mother was first postulated by Wallgren & Agoria in 1960. An association between neonatal heart block and maternal systemic lupus erythematosus was subsequently confirmed (Chameides *et al.* 1977; McCue *et al.* 1977). In 1981, Franco *et al.* first reported a more specific association between neonatal lupus syndrome and maternal antinuclear antibodies directed against the Ro(SSA) and La(SSB) (soluble tissue ribonucleoprotein antigens) in three maternal/infant pairs. The SSA antigen is a soluble nuclear antigen; the Ro antigen is a soluble cytoplasmic antigen. The antigens

Ro and La were described independently but subsequent studies have demonstrated that they are immunologically identical (Alspaugh & Maddison 1979). Anti-Ro(SSA) and anti-La(SSB) are IgG antibodies to these soluble tissue ribonucleoprotein antigens. The prevalence of anti-Ro(SSA) is over 40% in patients with Sjögren's syndrome, 25–30% in those with systemic lupus erythematosus and about 5% in those with rheumatoid arthritis, but the antibody was found in only 6 of 5000 persons without connective tissue disease (Maddison *et al.* 1979: Alexander & Provost 1981).

Scott (1984) studied the relationship between congenital heart block and maternal connective tissue disease by antibody screening of serum samples obtained in connection with 45 cases of isolated congenital complete heart block. Of the 41 mothers from whom serum was available, 17 had connective tissue disease and 24 were healthy. Thirty-four of these mothers had anti-Ro(SSA) and 17 had anti-La(SSB). Anti-Ro(SSA) was found in seven of eight serum samples collected from affected children when they were less than 3 months old but in none of 13 samples obtained when the children were older. In the anti-Ro(SSA) positive group, the diagnosis of congenital heart block was made within 3 months before or after birth in 36 of 38 cases, whereas in the anti-Ro(SSA) negative group the diagnosis was made after 1 year of age in 6 of 7 infants. Whether anti-Ro(SSA) is responsible for the condition, is involved with another factor in the pathological process of congenital complete heart block or merely serves as a marker is not clear. Not all children born to women with anti-Ro(SSA) have congenital heart block. Tissue-antigen variation in the child may be relevant, since only one member of dizygous twins born to a mother with anti-Ro(SSA) in her serum was affected (J.S. Scott *et al.* 1983). It may be that the pathological changes can be of various degrees, producing heart block only if severe. One woman with systemic lupus erythematosus had two children with heart block and two apparently healthy children with incomplete right bundle-branch block (Stephensen *et al.* 1981).

The cardiac histopathological features in infants with complete heart block have been described as interruption of the conduction system by fibrosis, fibrotic replacement of the sinoatrial and atrioventricular nodes, and calcification suggestive of earlier inflammation (Kephart *et al.* 1981). Although the sinus node is found by 6–8 weeks of fetal age (McCue *et al.* 1977), fetuses who develop congenital complete heart block may have normal cardiac rate and rhythm as late as several months after birth, or the rhythm disturbance may develop as early as 16 weeks of gestation (Lee & Watson 1984). This suggests that the immunological damage may occur early, develop slowly or appear late. Litsey *et al.* (1985) demonstrated, by an immunofluorescent technique, antibody deposition in atrial tissue of an infant with fatal congenital heart block in whom antinuclear and anti-Ro(SSA) antibodies were present at birth. Taylor *et al.* (1986) found IgG antibody reactive with fetal heart tissue in the serum of 21 of 41 mothers who gave birth to infants with isolated complete congenital heart block. The antibodies reacted with all myocardial tissue and were not directed specifically to the conduction tissue. In the two hearts from babies with congenital complete heart block that were examined by the immunoperoxidase technique, staining was positive for all components of the complement system and for IgG and IgM. A diffuse cytoplasmic pattern of staining was evident in all cardiac tissues, including nodal tissue, the bundle of His, Purkinje's fibres and muscle.

The current postdelivery mortality in infants with congenital complete heart block is about 25%. There is, at present, no successful *in utero* therapy. Since the fetal cardiac conduction system is destroyed, the administration of medications to the mother in an effort to increase the fetal heart rate will be unsuccessful. In the fetus with severe hydrops, the only hope for improving the cardiac output is to increase the contractility of the heart with medications or provide electrical pacing of the heart to increase the heart rate. Although some have advocated the use of maternally administered digitalis in the presence of fetal ascites (Levy 1985), there is no evidence that this therapy is beneficial. No successful cases of *in utero* pacing have been reported to date.

Although anti-Ro(SSA) antibody is associated with maternal systemic lupus erythematosus, Sjögren's syndrome and rheumatoid arthritis, many mothers delivering infants with neonatal lupus are asymptomatic. Many such women will develop connective tissue disease at a later date. In one woman, lupus erythematosus became clinically and serologically evident 16 years following the delivery of the first of three infants with heart block (Kasinath & Katz 1982). The risk of a woman who has anti-Ro(SSA) antibodies delivering an infant with congenital heart block is not known. Nevertheless, if this antibody is known to be present, patients should be counselled that their risk is increased. Women with systemic lupus erythematosus, Sjögren's syndrome or rheumatoid arthritis and those with symptoms suggestive of connective tissue disease who are considering becoming pregnant should be screened for anti-Ro(SSA) antibodies. A recent case report (Barclay *et al.* 1987) documents a successful pregnancy following steroid therapy and plasma exchange in a patient with anti-Ro(SSA) antibodies. She had four previous pregnancy losses, one documented to be due to congenital heart block.

Systemic lupus erythematosus

Systemic lupus erythematosus (SLE) is a chronic, multisystem auto-immune disease of undetermined cause afflicting predominantly women in their childbearing years. Theories regarding its aetiology have involved the role of viruses, histocompatibility loci such as HLA-DR, and oestrogen-mediated inhibition of suppressor cell function (Lahita *et al.* 1982). Whatever the cause, the disease results in a pathological population of B-lymphocytes which produce autoantibodies. This hyperactivity may reflect either a primary B-cell defect or a deficiency in regulator function.

The disease may be easily overlooked because it frequently begins with mild symptoms, has protean manifestations and is characterized by periods of exacerbation and remission. To standardize the diagnosis of SLE, the American Rheumatism Association has outlined criteria. These guidelines, along with a proposed set of revisions (Tan *et al.* 1982) are listed in Table 9.1. If four or more of the signs and symptoms are present, SLE is likely. The diagnosis of SLE is supported by the presence of antinuclear antibodies in high titre, lowered serum complement levels or a decrease in the absolute number and total proportion of T- and B-cells (Budman & Steinberg 1977).

The manifestations of SLE vary but arthritis or arthralgia is present in approximately 90% of patients. Dermatological manifestations are seen in 70–80%, renal disease in 46%, haematological abnormalities in 50% and cardiovascular disease in 30–50% (Budman & Steinberg 1977).

Although there is not unanimous agreement as to the effect of pregnancy on the frequency of exacerbations or the worsening of the condition, it is currently believed that, in a pregnancy conceived during a period of remission, the disease is likely to remain quiescent and that, in general, the clinical course of the disease is not adversely influenced by pregnancy. SLE affects the fetoplacental unit before and after its clinical recognition. Spontaneous abortion occurs in 5–40% of pregnancies and premature delivery has been reported in 16–37% of pregnancies following the diagnosis of SLE (Syrop & Varner 1983). Estes & Larson (1965) reported an increased risk of fetal death late in pregnancy, and estimates of stillbirths range from 12 to 30% (Donoldson & DeAlvarez 1962; Mund *et al.* 1963). The severity of lupus renal disease has been shown to be an important determinant in pregnancy outcome. Houser *et*

Table 9.1. Diagnosis of systemic lupus erythematosus (SLE). For each set of criteria, four or more are required for the diagnosis of SLE

1971 Criteria	Proposed 1982 revision
1 Facial erythema, butterfly rash	1 Malar rash
2 Discoid lupus	2 Discoid lupus
3 Raynaud's phenomenon	3 Photosensitivity
4 Alopecia	4 Oral ulcers
5 Photosensitivity	5 Arthritis
6 Oral or nasopharyngeal ulceration	6 Antibodies to DNA Sm or LE cells or BFP-STS
7 Arthritis without deformity	7 Proteinuria > 0.5 g day^{-1} or cellular casts
8 LE cells	8 Pleuritis and pericarditis
9 Chronic BFP-STS	9 Psychosis or seizures
10 Profuse proteinuria, $3 \cdot 5$ g 24 hr^{-1}	10 Haemolytic anaemia or leucopenia or thrombocytopenia
11 Cellular casts	
12 Pluritis and pericarditis	
13 Psychosis and/or convulsions	
14 Haemolytic anaemia or leucopenia or thrombocytopenia	

al. (1980) found, in patients with previously documented lupus nephropathy, that all ten pregnancies without clinical renal disease or active SLE at conception delivered at term and experienced a benign neonatal course. A maternal serum creatinine of $1 \cdot 5$ mg dl^{-1} or greater is associated with a fetal loss rate of 50% (Hayslett & Lynn 1980). A creatinine clearance of less than 100 ml min^{-1} was found in 12 patients reported by Fine *et al.* (1981) and was accompanied by a perinatal loss of 45%. In their series, the presence of both proteinuria and a reduction in glomerular filtration rate in the same patient produced a perinatal wastage of 80%. Varner *et al.* (1983) showed that patients who experience the onset of SLE during gestation have a high incidence of thrombocytopenia and/or nephrotic syndrome. In their series, eight patients had their disease initially diagnosed during pregnancy and this group experienced a 50% perinatal mortality.

The mainstay of therapy in active SLE is corticosteroids. An initial regimen of prednisone in the range of $60-100$ mg daily induces remission in most patients. With a satisfactory response, the dosage can usually be tapered gradually over several weeks to $10-15$ mg daily. A difficulty in the management of SLE in pregnancy has been the decision of whether the corticosteroid dose can be decreased and, if so, when and by how much. In some patients, clinical parameters, such as the amount of proteinuria or the platelet count, provide a guide to the activity of the disease. In others, especially those in remission, satisfactory clinical parameters are not always readily available. It has been suggested that serum complement levels may be beneficial in the assessment of fetal as well as maternal prognosis in pregnancies complicated by SLE. DeVoe & Taylor (1979) in a prospective study of pregnancy in 13 patients with SLE found that serum complement component (C3 and C4) levels correlated with perinatal outcome. Even in women in remission at the onset of pregnancy, low levels of serum complement were associated with a poor pregnancy outcome. These authors suggested that serial determinations of serum complement components may aid in the management of lupus-complicated pregnancies. Not all investigators have, however, found a good correlation between serum complement levels and clinical disease activity (Varner *et al.* 1983).

Recently, the presence of specific antibodies has been correlated with perinatal outcome in patients with SLE. As previously noted, the presence of ACA has been associated with fetal loss in patients with SLE (Derue *et al.* 1985; Lockshin *et al.* 1985), LAC is associated with a high rate of pregnancy wastage and the presence of anti-Ro(SSA) antibody has been associated with congenital complete heart block. Much of the medical literature dealing with the course and outcome of pregnancy in patients with SLE is biased by patient selection. Series reported prior to the establishment of criteria for the diagnosis of SLE are likely to include only the patients with severe disease. Similarly, it is likely that reports from medical centres in urban areas are biased because they include only patients with severe disease, whereas patients with milder manifestations of SLE are cared for by their local physicians. Although these reports are helpful in identifying subpopulations of patients at risk, they overestimate the overall influence of SLE on pregnancy outcome and are not very helpful in the preconceptual counselling of patients with milder disease. A more rational approach to individual patients will be possible as individual antibodies are found to be associated with specific consequences. Individual patients can then be given a more realistic appraisal of their prospects for a successful pregnancy and, in some cases, specific antibody levels may serve as a more effective guide to therapy.

Myasthenia gravis

Myasthenia gravis, a chronic autoimmune disease involving the neuro-muscular endplate, is seen most frequently in women in the mid-reproductive years. The disease is characterized by progressive fatigue and weakness, typically of the extraocular, facial, pharyngeal and respiratory muscles. Antibodies to human acetylcholine receptors (AChR) are detectable in up to 90% of patients with myasthenia gravis (Lindstrom 1977). These are usually IgG but have occasionally been IgM. The serum concentration of anti-AChR antibodies correlates poorly with the severity of the muscular weakness (Roses *et al.* 1981); rather, it is the ability of this antibody to induce accelerated degradation and blockade of the AChR of skeletal muscle that corresponds to the clinical severity of the disease (Drachman *et al.* 1982). In addition to the presence of anti-AChR antibodies, evidence supporting the immunological aetiology of this condition includes: (i) an association with HLA-B8 antigen (Newsom-Davis & Vincent 1982); (ii) familial occurrence; (iii) an increased incidence of other autoantibodies (Hokkanen 1969); (iv) the presence of a thymoma, thymic hyperplasia or other autoimmune diseases (Osserman & Genkins 1971); (v) abnormal T-cells that respond to corticosteroids; (vi) the presence of immune complexes at the neuromuscular junction in skeletal biopsies from patients with myasthenia gravis (Engle 1980); and (vii) the occurrence of transient neonatal disease.

Treatment modalities for myasthenia gravis include anticholinesterase medications, corticosteroids, thymectomy, plasmaphaeresis and immunosuppressant drugs. Plasmaphaeresis is usually utilized only in the case of myasthenic crisis, defined as an exacerbation of symptoms that requires mechanical ventilation. The role of thymectomy in the management of myasthenia gravis is controversial (Buckingham *et al.* 1976; Grob *et al.* 1981; Olanow *et al.* 1982).

The clinical course during pregnancy is variable. However, there is a tendency for exacerbation and crisis, especially during the puerperium. In a literature review series of 314 pregnancies in 217 myasthenic mothers (Plauche 1983), there were exacerbations during 41% of the pregnancies and in 31% during the puerperium. *Post partum* exacerbations in this series were particularly sudden and severe. Ten of the women died. Myasthenic medication requires frequent adjustment during pregnancy. After a retrospective study of pregnancy in patients with myasthenia gravis, Eden & Gall (1983) suggested that thymectomy early in the course of the disease may exert a beneficial effect on myasthenia gravis in pregnancy.

Since the majority of the antibodies produced in patients with myasthenia gravis are IgG, they can be expected to cross the placenta. In spite of this, the apparent fetal effects of these antibodies are small. Myasthenic mothers usually report normal fetal movement. Nevertheless, arthrogryposis has been described in several infants of myasthenic mothers (Holmes *et al.* 1980). Polyhydramnios, which might be expected on the basis of decreased fetal swallowing, has not been a reported feature of this disease. The ability of alphafetoprotein to inhibit anti-AChR antibody could explain the rarity of myasthenia *in utero*, since the fetus has high serum alphafetoprotein levels (Brenner *et al.* 1980). The overall perinatal morbidity and mortality does, however, appear to be increased. Plauche (1983) in a summary of 12 reports from the medical literature found a 41% prematurity or low birthweight delivery rate in 46 pregnancies in women with myasthenia gravis. In his larger review series of 314 pregnancies, there were 22 perinatal deaths (8 stillbirths and 14 neonatal deaths) giving a perinatal mortality of 82 per 1000 live births.

Neonatal myasthenic symptoms characterized by flat facies, weak suckling, feeble cry and respiratory distress, all of which respond to anticholinesterase medications, develop in 10−20% of infants born to women with myasthenia gravis (Namba *et al.* 1970; Donaldson *et al.* 1981). The disorder usually begins 12−48 hours after birth and may last 10 days to 15 weeks (mean 3 weeks) (Scott 1977). The delay in onset of symptoms in the newborn has been attributed to falling levels of protective alphafetoprotein and the presence of residual anticholinesterase drug from the mother. In contrast to the adult, where the antibody titre does not correlate well with the severity of clinical disease, in the small number of cases reported since the development of assays for anti-AChR antibodies the maternal antibody titre has closely reflected the extent of neonatal disease (Donaldson *et al.* 1981). Mothers whose antibody titres are especially high may be at particular risk of having infants affected *in utero* as well as in the newborn period (Barlow 1981).

Herpes gestationis

Herpes gestationis (HG) is a rare, recurrent, pruritic vesiculobullous skin disease of pregnancy. Because it is not of viral aetiology and its name has led to some confusion, it has been suggested that a more appropriate name for this condition would be pemphigoid gestationis. The disease is mediated by an IgG immunoglobulin that has the propensity to localize in the basement membrane zone of the skin. The disease often begins with prodromal symptoms of malaise, fever, nausea, headaches, burning and pruritus. The earliest skin lesions consist of erythema and urticarial oedema, accompanied by intense pruritus. The oedematous plaques, which have a predilection for the abdomen, commonly assume geographic configurations. Usually within a few days, papules, vesicles and large tense bullae develop. The blister location in HG is subepidermal. When fully developed, the eruption may involve the abdomen, buttocks, back, forearms, genitalia and virtually any other area, although mucous membrane involvement is rare. When fresh bullae are present, they are usually tense; this is a clinical characteristic of subepidermal blisters. With age, the bullae become more flaccid and, after rupturing, leave denuded areas covered with crusts. Barring significant secondary bacterial infection, the lesions usually heal without scar, though marked post-inflammatory hyperpigmentation may occur. Usually this fades slowly with time.

The onset of the disease is usually in the second trimester of pregnancy but may occur earlier, especially in women affected by the disease in an earlier pregnancy (Carruthers 1978). It can also occur later and has been reported beginning in the immediate *post partum* period. In three of 93 episodes of HG, the onset was after the third *post partum* day (Kolodny 1969). It is a disease of varying intensity. Even in the same patient, the disease often waxes and wanes in activity over its time course. The disease usually recurs in subsequent pregnancies, with a tendency for earlier onset and more severe manifestations (Hertz *et al.* 1976). Recurrences have been precipitated by menstruation (Carruthers 1978) and oral contraceptives (Gordon 1967). The majority of affected women require systemic corticosteroid therapy (Lawley *et al.* 1978; Foidart *et al.* 1981).

Skin biopsy is important in confirming the diagnosis. Direct immunofluorescence light microscopy provides the usual laboratory confirmation of the disease. The most diagnostic finding is the deposition of C3 with or without IgG along the basement membrane zone (Harrington & Bleehen 1979; Holmes *et al.* 1982). HG is mediated by a circulating humoral factor, designated 'HG factor' when first reported by Provost & Tomasi (1973). This factor has subsequently been identified as an IgG immunoglobulin. Generally, the titre of HG factor is unrelated to disease activity. In contrast to the circulating IgG in bullous pemphigoid, which is present in sufficiently high titres to be identified by indirect immunofluorescent techniques, the IgG in HG appears in such low titres that routine immunofluorescent microscopy will not detect it. Instead, complement indirect immunofluorescence must be used. In this procedure, the serum of a patient with HG is incubated with an epithelial substrate, rinsed, covered with complement (C3), rinsed again, and finally stained with fluorescein-conjugated anti-C3 antibody. Holmes & Black (1980) have reported an association of HG with other autoimmune diseases. Recently, attention has been focused on an association of HG with specific HLA types. An increased incidence of HLA-B8 (79%) and HLA-DR3 (80%) has been reported (Holmes *et al.* 1983) and Shornick *et al.* (1981) reported an increased incidence of HLA-DR3 and DR4 in patients with a history of HG, compared with control subjects. Reunala *et al.* (1977) suggested that a high titre of anti-HLA antibodies may play a role in the pathogenesis of this condition. Subsequently, several investigators (Eberst *et al.* 1981; Shornick *et al.* 1982) reported increased antibodies to both maternal and paternal HLA antigens in serum of patients with HG.

Although there is no evidence for the disease being associated with an increase in maternal mortality, the fetal risk is more controversial. Kolodny (1969), in a report of several cases and a literature review, found no evidence for increase fetal morbidity or mortality. A later study of 28 cases confirmed the previous findings (Shornick *et al.* 1983). Other investigators (Lawley *et al.* 1978; Holmes & Black 1984), however, have demonstrated an increased fetal risk. Lawley *et al.* (1978), in a series of 39 cases, found a 23% incidence of premature delivery and an 8% incidence of stillbirth. Holmes & Black (1984) found a 26% incidence of low birthweight infants ($< 2 \cdot 5$ kg) and a 26% incidence of small-for-gestational-age infants ($<$ 10th centile) in a study of 50 pregnancies which progressed to parturition in women with HG.

Passive transfer of the anti-basement membrane antibodies to the fetus has been documented. These antibodies have been found in cord blood (Katz *et al.* 1976) and in the blood of newborns, both with (Lawley *et al.* 1978) and without (Reunala *et al.* 1977) skin lesions. Complement (C3) deposition has been found in the basement zone of affected (Lawley *et al.* 1978) and unaffected (Katz *et al.* 1976) infants born to women with HG. The incidence of clinical skin lesions developing in the infants of women with HG is low (Lawley *et al.* 1978).

Autoimmune thyroid disease

Graves' disease is an autoimmune disorder characterized by the production of thyroid-stimulating antibodies (TSAb) directed against receptors for thyroid-stimulating hormone (TSH-R) on the thyroid cell. Classically, the syndrome consists of the triad of goitre, exophthalmos and hyper-thyroidism. Hashimoto's disease is a form of chronic thyroiditis in which patients are usually euthyroid or slowly progress to hypothyroidism. Some patients, however, develop signs and symptoms of hyperthyroidism. Almost all patients with Hashimoto's disease have thyroid autoantibodies.

Clinical experience has demonstrated that these thyroid syndromes rarely present in their pure form. Goitrous and atrophic thyroiditis merge in a continuous spectrum. The term autoimmune thyroid disease (AITD) has been used to encompass all variants of Hashimoto's thyroiditis and Graves' disease and their incomplete forms. In addition to TSAb, a number of other thyroid-directed immunoglobulins have been detected in patients with AITD: long-acting thyroid stimulator (LATS), long-acting thyroid stimulator protector (LATS-P), human thyroid stimulator (HTS), thyroid growth-blocking antibodies (TBA) and human adenylcyclase stimulator (H-TACS). The unifying concept for AITD is based on the coexistence of these separate classes of autoantibodies: some are cytotoxic, some are stimulatory and others block the TSH receptors (Doniach *et al.* 1982). If a patient has mostly microsomal and thyroglobulin antibodies, the resultant condition will be Hashimoto's disease. If TSH-R blocking antibodies are present, the gland will atrophy. Patients who have only TSAb will develop non-goitrous Graves' thyrotoxicosis or non-toxic diffuse thyroid enlargement. The majority of patients with Graves' disease have a mixture of thyroid-stimulating antibodies as well as other autoantibodies. A few patients with Hashimoto's disease have a mixture of thyroid-stimulating antibodies plus the typical cytotoxic antibodies.

Maternal thyroid function is normal during pregnancy. An increase in the serum concentration of T4 occurs early in the first trimester because of an increased binding capacity of thyroid-binding globulin (TBG) secondary to a rise in serum oestrogen levels. Although there is a slight rise in maternal free T4 values during pregnancy, the level remains within the normal range for non-pregnant women. The fetal thyroid develops independently of maternal influence (Fisher & Klein 1981). Maternal TSH does not cross the placenta and the placental transfer of T3 and T4 is minimal in the human. Autoantibodies produced in women with AITD do, however, frequently cross the placenta and can result in fetal thyroid dysfunction. In pregnancies complicated by Graves' disease, TSAbs readily cross the placenta to stimulate the fetal thyroid gland.

The clinical spectrum of *in utero* Graves' disease is broad. Fetal death and preterm delivery are increased. A few affected newborns show widespread evidence of autoimmune disease with generalized hypertrophy of lymphatic tissue and thrombocytopenia. In others, the disease is apparent at birth with goitre or exophthalmos, or both, which may be accompanied by signs and symptoms of hypermetabolism (Hollingsworth & Alexander 1983). The half-life of thyroid-stimulating immunoglobulins has been estimated to range from 5 to 14 days. Most neonates with hyperthyroidism have a transient disorder lasting 1–5 months (Wilroy & Etteldorf 1971), although occasionally the condition persists for much longer. The presence of thyroid growth-blocking antibodies (TBA) has been demonstrated in primary myxoedema (Endo *et al.* 1978). Placental passage of such blocking antibodies would explain a report by Goldsmith *et al.* (1973) in which a patient with treated primary myxoedema gave birth to five babies all of whom had temporary hypothyroidism.

The complicated interaction of circulating autoantibodies in thyroid disorders during pregnancy can be illustrated by several clinical observations: (i) high maternal titres of TSAb are more likely to be associated with neonatal hyperthyroidism than low titres; (ii) LATS titres may be negative in mothers with positive TSAb assays; (iii) newborn infants with hyperthyroidism may have persistent hyperthyroidism long after the biological half-life of transplacental TSAb; (iv) infants with neonatal Graves' disease have been born to women with no history of thyroid disease; and (v) delayed-onset neonatal hyperthyroidism has been reported in two infants of a mother with Hashimoto's disease who was negative for LATS and LATS-P but whose serum had a TSAb inhibitor (Hollingsworth & Alexander 1983). The maternal–fetal thyroid relationships and the placental transfer of autoantibodies and thyroid medications are illustrated in Fig. 9.4.

Although in normal pregnancies the fetal thyroid develops independently of maternal influence, the fetuses in pregnancies complicated by AITD are at risk for hyperthyroidism due to transplacentally acquired autoantibodies or hypothyroidism secondary to transplacental passage of antithyroid medication. The perinatal morbidity and mortality associated with fetal hyper- and hypothyroxinaemia is not well established. Montoro & Mestman (1981) reported that, among 19 untreated cases of maternal Graves' disease with hyperthyroidism, there were 15 premature deliveries, 5 perinatal deaths and 5 cases of serious neonatal morbidity. The first two pregnancies in a woman previously made hypothyroid by partial thyroidectomy for hyperthyroidism resulted in a late fetal death with features compatible with hyperthyroidism and an infant with skull deformities thought to be due to uncontrolled fetal hyperthyroidism as evidenced by persistent fetal tachycardia and an elevated neonatal thyroxine level. During two subsequent pregnancies, the mother received antithyroid medication to control the fetal thyroid and both infants were

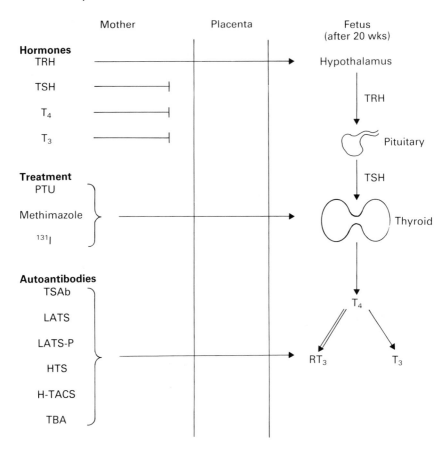

Fig. 9.4. Maternal–fetal thyroid relationships and the placental transfer of medications and autoantibodies to the fetus.

euthyroid at birth (Cove & Johnson 1985). The fetal hyperthyroidism was presumably due to the transplacental passage of thyroid-stimulating immunoglobulins, which may persist for years after thyroidectomy or radioiodine therapy.

The first choice of therapy for pregnant patients with hyperthyroidism is an antithyroid medication such as propylthiouracil (PTU) or methimazole (Tapazole). Although no prospective randomized studies have been performed comparing these medications, many prefer PTU because of several instances of aplasia cutis of the scalp in infants born to mothers treated with methimazole (Mujtaba & Burrow 1975). Even modest doses of PTU ingested by mothers significantly reduce serum thyroxine in newborns (Cheron *et al.* 1981). Although the maternal dose of PTU is not well correlated with the suppressant effect on the fetal thyroid (Cheron *et al.* 1981), there is a strong negative correlation between the maternal serum concentration of PTU during the late third trimester and cord thyroxine levels (Gardner *et al.* 1986). Even when low maternal doses of PTU are used and the infants are clinically euthyroid, they have biochemical evidence of mild, usually transient, hypothyroidism.

The long-term effects, if any, of fetal hypothyroxinaemia are not known. Both untreated fetal hyperthyroidism and hypothyroidism secondary to transplacentally acquired antithyroid medications have been associated with decreased intellectual performance in children. Hollingsworth *et al.* (1980), in an 11-year follow-up of 26 pregnancies in 20 women with Graves' disease, found that 27% of 24 surviving children had persistent neurological problems or hyperactivity, even when euthyroid. Burrow *et al.* (1978) reported the findings of long-term follow-up on a group of children exposed *in utero* to PTU. Although the median IQ for the total group of children was 100, 11 children who had been exposed to 300 mg PTU or more had a mean IQ of 85±8SD, 5 children having IQs less than 80.

Until very recently, assessment of fetal thyroid function *in utero* has been extremely difficult. Although it is possible to measure thyroid hormone levels in amniotic fluid throughout pregnancy, this has not proved to be a satisfactory method of diagnosing fetal hypo- or hyperthyroidism (Hollingsworth & Alexander 1983; Pekonen *et al.* 1984). Several biophysical methods of fetal assessment may provide clues to fetal thyroid dysfunction but are not, in themselves, diagnostic. The hyperthyroid fetus may have intrauterine growth retardation. The fetal heart rate may be abnormally slow in hypothyroidism and fast in the hyperthyroid fetus (Maxwell *et al.* 1980). Both fetal biophysical parameters (Cove & Johnson 1985) and maternal thyroid hormone levels (Momotani *et al.* 1986) have been utilized to guide the therapy in pregnant patients with hyperthyroidism. It is clear, however, that optimal management can only be achieved when both maternal and fetal thyroid function can be accurately assessed. The development of the technique of fetal blood sampling provides access to the fetal circulation so that fetal levels of TSH and thyroid hormones can be measured directly. We have evaluated fetal thyroid function in a pregnancy during which the mother was given ^{131}I early in pregnancy. Because of the risks associated with fetal thyroid dysfunction, assessment of fetal thyroid function by fetal blood sampling is indicated in those pregnancies at risk.

Summary

Autoimmunity is now clearly recognized as being important in many diseases. As we have seen, when these conditions are present during pregnancy, the fetus is frequently involved. Sometimes the autoimmune response is very specific, with one autoantibody directed against a specific organ, as in myasthenia gravis. In other instances, such as autoimmune thyroid disease, a number of autoantibodies are directed at one organ. In systemic lupus erythematosus, the autoimmune response is very broad and involves several different organs. Nevertheless, within this syndrome, specific autoantibodies, such as the antiphospholipid antibodies LAC and ACA and anti-Ro(SSA) and their targets, have been characterized. Therapy is most commonly directed at decreasing the production of the antibody (SLE, ATP) and occasionally at decreasing its end-organ effect (myasthenia gravis, LAC). Because the maternal disease activity is frequently not well correlated with the fetal effects (ATP, AITD, SLE), methods of assessing the fetal status are important. Some autoimmune diseases, such as scleroderma, dermatomyositis and rheumatoid arthritis, have not been discussed because their fetal effects, if any, are either not known or not well substantiated.

References

Alexander E.L. & Provost T.T. (1981) Ro(SSA) and LA(SSB) antibodies. *Springer Semin. Immunopathol.*, **4**, 253–73.

Alspaugh M. & Maddison P. (1979) Resolution of the identity of certain antigen–antibody systems in systemic lupus erythematosus and Sjögren's syndrome: an interlaboratory collaboration. *Arthritis Rheum.*, **22**, 796–8.

Angles-Cano E., Sultan Y. & Clauvel J.P. (1979) Predisposing factors to thrombosis in systemic lupus erythematosus. *J. Lab. Clin. Med.*, **94**, 312–23.

Ayromlooi J. (1978) A new approach to the management of immunologic thrombocytopenic purpura in pregnancy. *Am. J. Obstet. Gynecol.*, **130**, 235–6.

Baldini M. (1966) Idiopathic thrombocytopenic purpura. *N. Engl. J. Med.*, **274**, 1245–51.

Barclay C., French M., Ross L. & Sokol R. (1987) Successful pregnancy following steroid therapy and plasma exchange in a woman with anti-Ro(SS-A) antibodies. Case report. *Br. J. Obstet. Gynaec.*, **94**, 369–71.

Barlow C.F. (1981) Neonatal myasthenia gravis. *Am. J. Dis. Child.*, **135**, 209.

Boey M.I., Colaco C.B., Gharavi A.E., Elkon K.B., Loizou S. & Hughes G.R.V. (1983) Thrombosis in systemic lupus erythematosus: striking association with the presence of circulating lupus anticoagulant. *Br. Med. J.*, **287**, 1021–3.

Branch D.W. (1987) Immunologic disease and fetal death. *Clin. Obstet. Gynecol.*, **30**, 295–311.

Branch D.W., Scott J.R., Kochenour N.K. & Hershgold E. (1985) Obstetric complications associated with the lupus anticoagulant. *N. Engl. J. Med.*, **313**, 1322–6.

Branch D.W., Rote N.S., & Scott J.R. (1986) The demonstration of lupus anticoagulant by an enzyme-linked immunoadsorbent assay. *Clin. Immunol. Immunopathol.*, **39**, 298–307.

Brenner T., Beyth U. & Abramsky O. (1980) Inhibitory effect of alpha fetoprotein on the binding of myasthenia gravis antibody to acetyl choline receptor. *Proc. Natl. Acad. Sci. USA*, **77**, 3635–9.

Buckingham J.M., Howard F.M., Bernatz P.E. *et al.* (1976) The value of thymectomy in myasthenia gravis. A computer matched study. *Ann. Surg.*, **184**, 453–8.

Budman D.R. & Steinberg A.D. (1977) Hematologic aspects of systemic lupus erythematosus. *Ann. Intern. Med.*, **86**, 220–9.

Burrow G., Klatskin E. & Genel M. (1978) Intellectual development in children whose mothers took propylthiouracil during pregnancy. *Yale J. Biol. Med.*, **51**, 151–6.

Cariou R., Tobelem G., Soria C. & Caen J. (1986) Inhibition of protein C activation by endothelial cells in the presence of lupus anticoagulant. *N. Engl. J. Med.*, **314**, 1193–4.

Carloss H.W., McMillan R. & Crosby W.H. (1980) Management of pregnancy in women with immune thrombocytopenic purpura. *JAMA*, **244**, 2756–8.

Carreras L.O., Vermylen J., Spitz B. & Assche A.V. (1981a) 'Lupus' anticoagulant and inhibition of prostacyclin formation in patients with repeated abortion, intrauterine growth retardation and intrauterine death. *Br. J. Obstet. Gynaecol.*, **88**, 890–4.

Carreras L.O., Machin S.J., Defreyn G. *et al.* (1981b) Arterial thrombosis, intrauterine death and 'lupus' anticoagulant: detection of immunoglobulin interfering with prostacyclin formation. *Lancet*, **i**, 244–6.

Carruthers J.A. (1978) Herpes gestationis: clinical features of immunologically proved cases. *Am. J. Obstet. Gynecol.*, **131**, 865–7.

Catterall R.D. (1973) Biological false positive reactions and systemic disease. In *Ninth Symposium on Advanced Medicine* (Ed. by G. Walker), pp. 97–111. Pitman Medical, London.

Chameides L., Truex R.C., Vetter V., Rashkind W.J., Galioto F.M. & Noonan J.A. (1977) Association of maternal systemic lupus erythematosus with congenital heart block. *N. Engl. J. Med.*, **297**, 1204–7.

Cheron R.G., Kaplan M.M., Larsen P.R., Selenkow H.A. & Crigler J.F. (1981) Neonatal thyroid function after propylthiouracil therapy for maternal Graves' disease. *N. Engl. J. Med.*, **304**, 525–8.

Cines D.B. & Schreiber A.D. (1979) Immune thrombocytopenia: the use of a Coombs' antiglobulin test to detect IgG and C3 on platelets. *N. Engl. J. Med.*, **300**, 106–11.

Cines D.B., Dusak B., Tomaski A., Mennuti M. & Schreiber A.D. (1982) Immune thrombocytopenic purpura and pregnancy. *N. Engl. J. Med.*, **306**, 826–31.

Conley C.L. & Hartman R.C. (1952) A hemorrhagic disorder caused by circulating anticoagulant in patients with disseminated erythematosus. *J. Clin. Invest.*, **31**, 621–2.

Cove D.H. & Johnson P. (1985) Fetal hyperthyroidism: experience of treatment in four siblings. *Lancet*, **i**, 430–2.

Daffos F., Forestier F., Muller J.Y. *et al.* (1984) Prenatal treatment of alloimmune thrombocytopenic purpura. *Lancet*, **ii**, 632.

Davies S.V., Murray J.A., Gee H. & Giles H. (1986) Transplacental effect of high-dose immunoglobin in idiopathic thrombocytopenia (ITP). *Lancet*, **i**, 1098–9.

De Castellarnau C., Vila L., Sancho M.J. *et al.* (1983) Lupus anticoagulant, recurrent abortion, and prostacyclin production by cultured smooth muscle cells. *Lancet*, **ii**, 1137–8.

Derue G.J., Englert H.J., Harris E.N. *et al.* (1985) Fetal loss in systemic lupus: association with anticardiolipin antibodies. *J. Obstet. Gynaecol.*, **5**, 207–9.

DeVoe L. & Taylor R.L. (1979) Systemic lupus erythematosus in pregnancy. *Am. J. Obstet. Gynecol.*, **135**, 473–9.

Donaldson J.O., Penn A.S., Lisak R.P. *et al.* (1981) Antiacetylcholine receptor antibody in myasthenia gravis. *Am. J. Dis. Child.*, **135**, 222–6.

Doniach D., Bottazzo G.F.R. & Drexange H.A. (1982) The autoimmune endocrinopathies. In *Clinical Aspects of Immunology*, 4th edn (Ed. by P.J. Lachman & D.K. Peters), pp. 903–37. Blackwell Scientific Publications, Oxford.

Donoldson L.B. & DeAlvarez R.R. (1962) Further observations on lupus erythematosus associated with pregnancy. *Am. J. Obstet. Gynecol.*, **83**, 1461–73.

Drachman D.B., Adams R.N. & Josifek L.F. (1982) Functional activities of autoantibodies to acetylcholine receptors and the clinical activity of myasthenia gravis. *N. Engl. J. Med.*, **307**, 769–75.

Eberst E., Tongio M.M., Eberst B., Mayer S. & Basset A. (1981) Herpes gestationis and anti-HLA immunization. *Br. J. Dermatol.*, **104**, 553–9.

Eden R.D. & Gall S.A. (1983) Myasthenia gravis and pregnancy: a reappraisal of thymectomy. *Obstet. Gynecol.*, **62**, 328–33.

Elias M. & Eldor A. (1984) Thromboembolism in patients with the 'lupus'-type circulating anticoagulant. *Arch. Intern. Med.*, **144**, 510–15.

Endo K., Kasagi K., Konishi J. *et al.* (1978) Detection and properties of TSH-inhibitor immunoglobulins in patients with Graves' disease and Hashimoto's thyroiditis. *J. Clin. Endocrinol. Metab.*, **46**, 734–9.

Engle A.G. (1980) Morphologic and immunologic findings in myasthenia gravis and EMG syndromes. *J. Neurol. Neurosurg. Psychiatry*, **43**, 577–89.

Estes D. & Larson D.L. (1965) Systemic lupus erythematosus and pregnancy. *Clin. Obstet. Gynecol.*, **8**, 307–20.

Exner T., Rickard K.A. & Kronenberg H. (1978) A sensitive test demonstrating lupus anticoagulant and its behavioural patterns. *Br. J. Haematol.*, **40**, 143–51.

Fallon W.W., Greene R.W. & Losner E.L. (1952) The hemostatic defect in thrombocytopenia as studied by the use of ACTH and cortisone. *Am. J. Med.*, **13**, 12–20.

Farquharson R.G., Pearson J.F. & John L. (1984) Lupus anticoagulant and pregnancy management. *Lancet*, **ii**, 228–9.

Fehr J., Hofmann V. & Kappeler U. (1982) Transient reversal of thrombocytopenia in idiopathic thrombocytopenic purpura by high-dose intravenous gammaglobulin. *N. Engl. J. Med.*, **306**, 1254–8.

Fine L.G., Barnett E.V., Danovitch G.M. *et al.* (1981) Systemic lupus erythematosus in pregnancy. *Ann. Intern. Med.*, **94**, 667–77.

Fisher D.A. & Klein A.H. (1981) Thyroid development and disorders of thyroid function in the newborn. *N. Engl. J. Med.*, **304**, 702–12.

Fiumara N.J. (1963) Biological false positive test for syphilis. *N. Engl. J. Med.*, **268**, 401–5.

Foidart J.M., Yaar M., Hall R., Gaspard U. & Katz S.I. (1981) Immunopathological and clinical studies in herpes gestationis. *Br. J. Obstet. Gynaecol.*, **88**, 153–9.

Franco H.L., Weston W.L., Peebles C., Forstot S.L. & Phanuphak P. (1981) Autoantibodies directed against sicca syndrome antigens in the neonatal lupus syndrome. *J. Am. Acad. Dermatol.*, **4**, 67–72.

Gardner D.F., Druikshank D.P., Hays P.M. & Cooper D.S. (1986) Pharmacology of propylthiouracil (PTU) in pregnant hyperthyroid women: correlation of maternal PTU concentrations with cord serum thyroid tests. *J. Clin. Endocrinol. Metab.*, **62**, 217–20.

Goldsmith R.E., McAdams A.J., Larsen P.R., McKensie M. & Hess E.V. (1973) Familial autoimmune thyroiditis: maternal–foetal relationship and the role of generalized autoimmunity. *J. Clin. Endocrinol. Metab.*, **37**, 265–75.

Gordon B. (1967) Herpes gestationis and the 'pill'. *Br. Med. J.*, **1**, 51.

Grob D., Brenner N.G. & Namba T. (1981) The natural course of myasthenia gravis and effect of therapeutic measures. *Ann. N. Y. Acad. Sci.*, **377**, 652–69.

Handin R. (1981) Neonatal thrombocytopenia: the doctor's dilemma. *N. Engl. J. Med.*, **305**, 951–3.

Handin R.I. & Stossel T.P. (1975) Effect of corticosteroid therapy on the phagocytosis of antibody-coated platelets. *Blood*, **46**, 1016.

Harker L.A. & Finch C.A. (1969) Thrombokinetics in man. *J. Clin. Lab. Invest.*, **48**, 963−74.

Harrington C.I. & Bleehen S.S. (1979) Herpes gestationis: immunopathological and ultra-structure studies. *Br. J. Dermatol.*, **100**, 389−99.

Harris E.N., Gharavi A.E., Boey M.L. *et al.* (1983) Anticardiolipin antibodies: detection by radioimmunoassay and association with thrombosis in systemic lupus erythematosus. *Lancet*, **ii**, 1211−14.

Harris E.N., Loizou S., Englert H. *et al.* (1984) Anticardiolipin antibodies and lupus anticoagulant. *Lancet*, **ii**, 1099.

Harris E.N., Gharavi A.E., Loizou S. *et al.* (1985) Crossreactivity of antiphospholipid antibodies. *J. Clin. Lab. Immunol.*, **16**, 1−6.

Hauch T.W. & Rosse W.F. (1977) Platelet-bound complement (C3) in immune thrombocytopenia. *Blood*, **50**, 1129−36.

Hayslett J.P. & Lynn R.I. (1980) Effect of pregnancy in patients with lupus nephropathy. *Kidney Int.*, **18**, 207−20.

Hertz K.C., Katz S.I., Maize J. & Ackerman A.B. (1976) Herpes gestationis. *Arch. Dermatol.*, **112**, 1543−8.

Hokkanen E. (1969) Myasthenia gravis. *Ann. Clin. Res.*, **1**, 94−108.

Hollingsworth D.R. & Alexander N.M. (1983) Amniotic fluid concentrations of iodothyronines and TSH do not reliably predict fetal thyroid status in pregnancies complicated by maternal thyroid disorders or anencephaly. *J. Clin. Endocrinol. Metab.*, **57**, 349−55.

Hollingsworth D.R., Mabry C.C. & Reid M.C.(1980) New observations in congenital Graves' disease. In *Thyroid Research VIII. Proceedings of the Eighth International Thyroid Congress, Sydney, Australia, Feb. 3−8 1980* (Ed. by J.R. Stockigt & S. Nagataki), pp. 587−90. Australian Academy of Science, Canberra.

Holmes L.B., Driscoll S.G. & Bradley W.G. (1980) Contractures in a newborn infant in a mother with myasthenia gravis. *J. Pediatr.*, **96**, 1067−9.

Holmes R.C. & Black M.M. (1980) Herpes gestationis. A possible association with autoimmune thyrotoxicosis (Graves' disease). *J. Am. Acad. Dermatol.*, **3**, 474−7.

Holmes R.C. & Black M.M. (1984) The fetal prognosis in pemphigoid gestationis (herpes gestationis). *Br. J. Dermatol.*, **110**, 67−72.

Holmes R.C., Black M.M., Dann J., James D.C.O. & Bhogal B. (1982) A comparative study of toxic erythema of pregnancy and herpes gestationis. *Br. J. Dermatol.*, **106**, 499−510.

Holmes R.C., Black M.M., Jureca W. *et al.* (1983) Clues to the aetiology and pathogenesis of herpes gestationis. *Br. J. Dermatol.*, **109**, 131−9.

Hougie C. (1985) Circulating anticoagulants. *Recent Adv. Blood Coag.*, **4**, 63−90.

Houser M.T., Fish A.J., Tagatz G.E., Williams P.P. & Michael A. (1980) Pregnancy and systemic lupus erythematosus. *Am. J. Obstet. Gynecol.*, **138**, 409−13.

Hughes G.R.V., Harris E.N. & Gharavi A.E. (1984) The syndrome of thrombosis, abortion, and neurologic disease. *Contrib. Nephrol.*, **43**, 9−11.

Imbach P., d'Apuzzo V., Hirt A. *et al.* (1981) High dose intravenous gamma globulin for idiopathic thrombocytopenic purpura in childhood. *Lancet*, **i**, 1228−31.

Johansson E.A. & Lassus A. (1974) The occurrence of circulating anticoagulants in patients with syphilitic and biologically false positive antilipoidal antibodies. *Ann. Clin. Res.*, **6**, 105−8.

Karpatkin M., Porges R.F. & Karpatkin S. (1981) Platelet counts in infants of women with autoimmune thrombocytopenia. Effect of steroid administration to the mother. *N. Engl. J. Med.*, **305**, 936−9.

Karpatkin S. (1980) Autoimmune thrombocytopenic purpura. *Blood*, **56**, 329−43.

Karpatkin S., Strick N. & Siskind G.W. (1972) Detection of splenic antiplatelet antibody synthesis in idiopathic autoimmune thrombocytopenic purpura. *Br. J. Haematol.*, **23**, 167−76.

Kasinath B.S. & Katz A.I. (1982) Delayed maternal lupus after delivery of offspring with congenital heart block. *Arch. Intern. Med.*, **142**, 2317.

Katz S.I., Hertz K.C. & Yaoita H. (1976) Herpes gestationis. Immunopathology and characterization of the HG factor. *J. Clin. Invest.*, **57**, 1434−41.

Kelton J.G. (1983) Management of the pregnant patient with idiopathic thrombocytopenic purpura. *Ann. Intern. Med.*, **99**, 796−800.

Kelton J.G., Inwood M.J., Barr R.M. *et al.* (1982) The prenatal prediction of thrombocytopenia in infants of mothers with clinically diagnosed immune thrombocytopenia. *Am. J. Obstet. Gynecol.*, **144**, 449−54.

Kephart D.C., Hood A.F. & Provost T.T. (1981) Neonatal lupus erythematosus: new serological findings. *J. Invest. Dermatol.*, **77**, 331−3.

Kolodny R.C. (1969) Herpes gestationis: a new assessment of incidence, diagnosis, and fetal prognosis. *Am. J. Obstet. Gynecol.*, **104**, 39−44.

Lahita R.G., Bradlow L., Fishman J. *et al.* (1982) Estrogen metabolism in systemic lupus erythematosus patients and family members. *Arthritis Rheum.*, **25**, 843−6.

Laros R.K. & Sweet R.L. (1975) Management of idiopathic thrombocytopenic purpura during pregnancy. *Am. J. Obstet. Gynecol.*, **122**, 182−91.

Laster A.J., Conley C.L., Kickler T.S., Dorsch C.A. & Bias W.B. (1982) Chronic immune thrombocytopenic purpura in monozygotic twins. *N. Engl. J. Med.*, **307**, 1495−8.

Lavery J.P., Koontz W.L., Liu Y.K. & Howell R. (1985) Immunologic thrombocytopenia in pregnancy; use of antenatal immunoglobulin therapy: case report and review. *Obstet. Gynecol.*, **66** (suppl.), 41S−43S.

Lawley T.J., Stingl G. & Katz S.I. (1978) Fetal and maternal risk factors in herpes gestationis. *Arch. Dermatol.*, **114**, 552−5.

Lee L.A. & Watson W.L. (1984) New findings in the neonatal lupus syndrome. *Am. J. Dis. Child.*, **138**, 233−6.

Levy D.L. (1985) The effect of maternal autoimmune disease on the fetus and neonate. In *Recent Advances in Perinatal Medicine* (Ed. by M.L. Chiswick), pp. 59−78. Churchill Livingstone, Edinburgh.

Lindstrom J. (1977) An assay for antibodies to human AChR in serum from patients with myasthenia gravis. *Clin. Immunol. Immunopathol.*, **7**, 36−43.

Litsey S.E., Noonan J.A., O'Connor W.N., Cottrill C.M. & Mitchell B. (1985) Maternal connective tissue disease and congenital heart block: demonstration of immunoglobulin in cardiac tissue. *N. Engl. J. Med.*, **312**, 98−100.

Lockshin M.D., Druzin M.L., Goei S. *et al.* (1985) Antibody to cardiolipin as a predictor of fetal distress or death in pregnant patients with systemic lupus erythematosus. *N. Engl. J. Med.*, **313**, 152−6.

Logaridis T.E., Doran T.A., Scott J.G., Gare D.G. & Thomas H.C. (1983) The effect of maternal steroid administration on fetal platelet count in immunologic thrombocytopenic purpura. *Am. J. Obstet. Gynecol.*, **145**, 147−51.

Lubbe W.F. & Walker E.B. (1983) Chorea gravidarum associated with circulating lupus anticoagulant: successful outcome of pregnancy with prednisone and aspirin therapy. Case report. *Br. J. Obstet. Gynaecol.*, **90**, 487−90.

Lubbe W.F., Palmer S.J., Butler W.S. & Liggins G.C. (1983) Fetal survival after prednisone suppression of maternal lupus-anticoagulant. *Lancet*, **i**, 1361−3.

Lurhuma A.Z., Riccomi H. & Masson P.L. (1977) The occurrence of circulating immune complexes and viral antigens in idiopathic thrombocytopenic purpura. *Clin. Exp Immunol.*, **28**, 49−55.

McCue C.M., Mantakas M.E., Tingelstad J.B. & Ruddy S. (1977) Congenital heart block in newborns of mothers with connective tissue disease. *Circulation*, **56**, 82−90.

McMillan C., Longmire R.L., Tavassoli M. *et al.* (1974) In vitro platelet phagocytosis by splenic leukocytes in idiopathic thrombocytopenic purpura. *N. Engl. J. Med.*, **290**, 249−51.

McMillan R. (1981) Chronic idiopathic thrombocytopenic purpura. *N. Engl. J. Med.*, **304**, 1135−47.

McMillan R., Yelenosky R.J., & Longmire R.L. (1976) Antiplatelet antibody production by the spleen and bone marrow in immune thrombocytopenic purpura. In *Immunological Aspects of the Spleen* (Ed. by J.R. Battias & J.W. Streilein), p. 227. North-Holland, Amsterdam.

Maddison P., Mogavero H., Provost T.T. & Reichlin M. (1979) The clinical significance of autoantibodies to a soluble cytoplasmic antigen in systemic lupus erythematosus and other connective tissue disease. *J. Rheumatol.*, **6**, 189–95.

Maxwell K.D., Kearney K.K., Johnson J.W.C., Eagan J.W. & Tyson J.E. (1980) Fetal tachycardia associated with intrauterine fetal thyrotoxicosis. *Obstet. Gynecol.*, **55** (suppl.), 18S–22S.

Mizunuma H., Takahashi Y., Taguchi H. *et al.* (1984) A new approach to idiopathic thrombocytopenic purpura during pregnancy by high-dose immunoglobulin G infusion. *Am. J. Obstet. Gynecol.*, **148**, 218–19.

Momotani N., Noh J., Oyanagi H., Ishikawa N. & Ito K. (1986) Antithyroid drug therapy for Graves' disease during pregnancy optimal regimen for fetal thyroid status. *N. Engl. J. Med.*, **315**, 24–8.

Moncada S. & Vane J.R. (1978) Pharmacology and endogenous roles of prostaglandin endoperoxides, thromboxane A2, and prostacyclin. *Pharmacol. Rev.*, **30**, 293–331.

Moncada S., Higgs E.A. & Vane J.R. (1977) Human arterial and venous tissues generate prostacyclin (prostaglandin X), a potent inhibitor of platelet aggregation. *Lancet*, **i**, 18–21.

Montoro M. & Mestman J.H. (1981) Graves' disease and pregnancy. *N. Engl. J. Med.*, **305**, 48.

Mujtaba Q. and Burrow G.N. (1975) Treatment of hyperthyroidism in pregnancy with propylthiouracil and methimazole. *Obstet. Gynecol.*, **46**, 282–6.

Mund A., Simson J. & Rothfield N. (1963) Effect of pregnancy on the course of systemic lupus erythematosus. *JAMA*, **183**, 917–20.

Myers T.J., Kim R., Steiner M. & Baldini M. (1982) Platelet associated complement C3 in immune thrombocytopenic purpura. *Blood*, **59**, 1023–8.

Namba T., Brown S.B. & Grob D. (1970) Neonatal myasthenia gravis: report of two cases and review of the literature. *Pediatrics*, **45**, 488–504.

Newland A.C., Treleavan J.G., Minchinton R.M. & Waters A.H. (1983) High dose intravenous IgG in adults with autoimmune thrombocytopenia. *Lancet*, **i**, 84–7.

Newsom-Davis J. & Vincent A. (1982) Myasthenia gravis. In *Clinical Aspects of Immunology*, 4th edn (Ed. by P.J. Lachman & D.K. Peters), pp. 1032–43. Blackwell Scientific Publications, Boston.

Olanow C.W., Wechsler A.S. & Roses A.D. (1982) A prospective study of thymectomy and serum acetylcholine receptor antibodies in myasthenia gravis. *Ann. Surg.*, **196**, 113–21.

O'Reilly R. & Taber B. (1978) Immunological thrombocytopenic purpura and pregnancy. *Obstet. Gynecol.*, **51**, 590–7.

Osserman K.E. & Genkins G. (1971) Studies in myasthenia gravis: review of a twenty year experience in over 1200 patients. *Mt Sinai. J. Med. (NY)*, **38**, 497–537.

Pappas C. (1986) Placental transfer of immunoglobulins in immune thrombocytopenic purpura. *Lancet*, **i**, 389.

Pekonen F., Teramo K., Makinen T., Ikonen E., Osterlund K. & Lamberg B. (1984) Prenatal diagnosis and treatment of fetal thyrotoxicosis. *Am. J. Obstet. Gynecol.*, **150**, 893–5.

Peterson O.H. & Larson D. (1954) Thrombocytopenic purpura in pregnancy. *Obstet. Gynecol.*, **4**, 454–69.

Plauche W.C. (1983) Myasthenia gravis. *Clin. Obstet. Gynecol.*, **26**, 592–604.

Provost T.T. & Tomasi T.R. Jr (1973) Complement activation via the alternate pathway in skin diseases. I. Herpes gestationis, systemic lupus erythematosus, and bullous pemphigoid. *J. Clin. Invest.*, **52**, 1779.

Remuzzi G., Marchesi D., Zoja C. *et al.* (1980) Reduced umbilical and placental vascular prostacyclin in severe preeclampsia. *Prostaglandins*, **20**, 105−10.

Reunala T., Karvonen J., Tiilikainen A. & Salo O.P. (1977) Herpes gestationis: a high titre of anti-HLA-B8 antibody in the mother and pemphigoid-like immunohistological findings in the mother and the child. *Br. J. Dermatol.*, **96**, 563−8.

Roses A.D., Olanow C.W. & McAdams M.W. (1981) No direct correlation between serum antiacetylcholine receptor antibody levels and clinical state of individual patients with myasthenia gravis. *Neurology*, **31**, 220−4.

Rote N.S. (1985) The immune response. In *Immunology in Obstetrics and Gynecology* (Ed. by J.R. Scott & N.S. Rote), pp. 27−54. Appleton-Century-Crofts, Norwalk, Conn.

Rote N.S., Nielsen K.G., Nielsen V.D. *et al.* (1983) Studies by enzyme-linked immuno-sorbent assay (ELISA) of antiplatelet antibody and transient neonatal thrombo-cytopenic purpura. *Am. J. Reprod. Immunol.*, **3**, 178−82.

Sanfelippo M.J. & Drayna C.J. (1982) Prekallikrein inhibition associated with the lupus anticoagulant. *Am. J. Clin. Pathol.*, **77**, 275−9.

Schleider M.A., Nachman R.L., Jaffe E.A. & Coleman N. (1976) A clinical study of the lupus anticoagulant. *Blood*, **48**, 499−509.

Scott J.R., Cruikshank D.P., Kochenour N.K., Pitkin R.M. & Warenski J.C. (1980) Fetal platelet counts in the obstetric management of immunologic thrombocytopenic purpura. *Am. J. Obstet. Gynecol.*, **136**, 495−9.

Scott J.R., Rote N.S. & Cruikshank D.P. (1983) Antiplatelet antibodies and platelet counts in pregnancies complicated by autoimmune thrombocytopenic purpura. *Am. J. Obstet. Gynecol.*, **145**, 932−9.

Scott J.S. (1977) Immunologic diseases in pregnancy. *Prog. Allergy*, **23**, 321−66.

Scott J.S. (1984) Connective tissue disease antibodies and pregnancy. *Am. J. Reprod. Immunol.*, **6**, 19−24.

Scott J.S., Maddison P.J., Taylor P.V., Esscher E., Scott O. & Skinner R.P. (1983) Connective-tissue disease, antibodies to ribonucleoprotein, and congenital heart block. *N. Engl. J. Med.*, **309**, 209−12.

Shenker J.G. & Polishuk W.F. (1968) Idiopathic thrombocytopenic purpura in pregnancy. *Gynaecologia (Basel)*, **165**, 271.

Shornick J.K., Stastny P. & Gilliam J.N. (1981) High frequency of histocompatibility antigens HLA-DR3 and DR4 in herpes gestationis. *J. Clin. Invest.*, **68**, 553−5.

Shornick J.K., Stastny P. & Gilliam J.N. (1982) Anti-HLA antibodies and paternal HLA typing in herpes gestationis. *J. Invest. Dermatol.*, **78**, 340.

Shornick J.K., Bangert J.L., Freeman R.G. & Gilliam J.N. (1983) Herpes gestationis: clinical and histologic features of twenty-eight cases. *J. Am. Acad. Dermatol.*, **8**, 214−24.

Shulman N.R. & Jordan J.V. (1982) Platelet immunology. In *Textbook of Hemostasis and Thrombosis* (Ed. by R. Coleman, V. Marder & E. Salzmann), p. 274. J.B. Lippincott, Philadelphia.

Stephensen O., Cleland W.P. & Hallidie-Smith K. (1981) Congenital complete heart block and persistent ductus arteriosus associated with maternal lupus erythematosus. *Br. Heart J.*, **46**, 104−6.

Syrop C.H. & Varner M.W. (1983) Systemic lupus erythematosus and pregnancy. *Clin. Obstet. Gynecol.*, **26**, 547−57.

Tan E.M., Cohen A.S., Fries J. *et al.* (1982) Criteria for the classification of systemic lupus erythematosus. *Arthritis Rheum.*, **25**, 735−6.

Tancer M.L. (1960) Idiopathic thrombocytopenic purpura and pregnancy. *Am. J. Obstet. Gynecol.*, **79**, 148−53.

Taylor P.V., Scott J.S., Gerlis L.M., Esscher E. & Scott O. (1986) Maternal antibodies against fetal cardiac antigens in congenital complete heart block. *N. Engl. J. Med.*, **315**, 667−72.

Tchernia G., Dreyfus M., Laurian Y., Derycke M., Mirica C. & Kerbrat G. (1984) Management of immune thrombocytopenia in pregnancy: response to infusions of immuno-globulins. *Am. J. Obstet. Gynecol.*, **148**, 225−6.

Territo M., Finklestein J., Oh W., Hobel C. & Kottlove H. (1973) Management of auto-immune thrombocytopenia in pregnancy and in the neonate. *Obstet. Gynecol.,* **41,** 579–84.

Thiagarajan P., Shapiro S.S. & DaMarco L. (1980) Monoclonal immunoglobin M lambda coagulation inhibitor with phospholipid specificity: mechanisms of a lupus anti-coagulant. *J. Clin. Invest.,* **66,** 397–405.

Varner M.W., Meehan R.T., Syrop C.H., Strottmann M.P. & Goplerud C.P. (1983) Pregnancy in patients with systemic lupus erythematosus. *Am. J. Obstet. Gynecol.,* **145,** 1025–40.

Wallgren G. & Agoria E. (1960) Congenital complete A–V block in three sibs. *Acta Paediatr. Scand.,* **49,** 49–56.

Weksler B.B., Pett S.B., Alonso D., Richter R.C., Stelzer P. & Subramanian V. (1983) Differential inhibition by aspirin of vascular and platelet prostaglandin synthesis in atherosclerotic patients. *N. Engl. J. Med.,* **308,** 800–5.

Wilroy R.S. & Etteldorf J.N. (1971) Familial hyperthyroidism including two siblings with neonatal Graves' disease. *J. Pediatr.,* **78,** 625–32.

Zilliacus H. (1964) Thrombocytopenia in pregnancy. *Clin. Obstet. Gynecol.,* **2,** 404–25.

10

Fetal Influence on Human Parturition

J.E. BLEASDALE & G.C. DI RENZO

Introduction

It is unquestioned that the potential consequences of an untimely birth are serious and extend far beyond the neonatal period. Despite major advances in reducing perinatal mortality and morbidity from other causes, preterm birth complicates about 5–10% of all pregnancies and is associated with numerous morbid sequelae and neonatal deaths. Since reliable biochemical indices that may be useful in identifying pregnant women destined to experience preterm labour are not known, inhibition of preterm labour rather than prevention of preterm labour has been the basis of treatment. The limited success of tocolytic therapy (Creasy 1983), however, may be due, in part, to the relatively few tocolytic agents available and to the unproven assumption of a common mechanism underlying preterm labour, i.e. that preterm labour is precocious normal labour. Some cases of preterm labour may result from a normal fetal response to an intrauterine environment that has become hostile, while other cases may result from an abnormal activation of a normal system primed for labour. Several factors that appear to predispose pregnant women to preterm labour have been identified (reviewed by Fuchs 1983). Most of these factors induce responses in the fetus that are symptomatic of fetal stress. These clinical findings constitute indirect evidence that the fetus may influence the timing of parturition.

The concept that the fetus initiates parturition is old (reviewed by Thorburn 1983). Hippocrates (460–370 BC) suggested that the fetus 'becomes agitated and breaks through the membranes'; and William Harvey in the 17th century wrote that 'The assistance of the foetus is chiefly required in the birth, is evident, not in Birds only, which do by their own industry without help of their Parents break up the shell, but also in other Animals; ...' (*De Generatione Animalium*, London, 1651). Van Deventer (18th century) envisioned a prominent role for the fetus in the initiation of parturition. In 1882, Spiegelberg recognized the importance of the uterus in parturition, but concluded still that the fetus provided the signal for uterine activity. Malpas, in 1933, observed that when the fetus is anencephalic pregnancy is sometimes prolonged markedly and this observation was the basis for the subsequent proposition that the hypothalamus−pituitary−adrenal axis is involved in stimulation of uterine contractions. This conclusion was supported by the findings of delayed parturition in cattle whose fetuses suffered a genetic malformation of the pituitary−adrenal axis (Kennedy *et al.* 1957; Holm 1967) and in sheep whose fetuses had defective pituitaries because of either maternal ingestion of a teratogenic toxin (Binns *et al.* 1963) or surgical ablation (Liggins *et al.* 1967). These latter investigations heralded the modern era of investigation of the initiation of parturition.

Experimental models of human parturition

Parturition has been investigated more extensively in sheep than in any other species and the pioneering work of Liggins and colleagues (Liggins *et al.* 1967; Liggins 1969a,b) has contributed greatly to an understanding of the critical function of the fetal pituitary−adrenal axis in the initiation of ovine parturition (Fig. 10.1). Progesterone secretion by the corpus luteum is essential for the maintenance of early pregnancy in all mammals, but in many species (including sheep and human) the placenta adopts the role of maintaining progesterone status at some stage of pregnancy. In all 'corpus luteum-dependent' species, and some 'placenta-dependent' species (including sheep but not human), parturition is signalled by a withdrawal of progesterone. Liggins (1983) noted that the placenta-dependent species that exhibit progesterone withdrawal at term are those that possess a placental progesterone 17α-hydroxylase and are capable of metabolizing progesterone or pregnenolone to oestrogen. The ovine placenta at term, given a supply of cholesterol (from *de novo* synthesis *in situ* and from uptake of serum lipoproteins), is self-sufficient in its production of oestrogen and progesterone. The rate of conversion of progesterone to oestrogen, however, is low in the placenta before term because of low activities of progesterone 17α-hydroxylase and 17α-hydroxyprogesterone 17,20-lyase. Instead, progesterone is secreted by the placenta, which is responsible for the high concentration of progesterone in maternal blood during the second and third trimesters of gestation. The fetal sheep adrenal gland, following a period of responsiveness to ACTH, becomes relatively refractory (by day 100 of gestation)

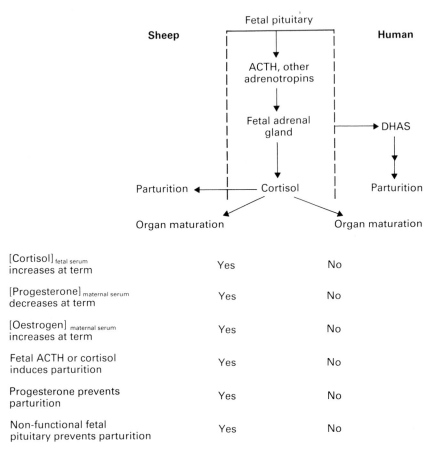

Fig. 10.1. Fetal endocrine relationships and their proposed involvement in parturition and organ maturation in sheep and humans. (Adapted from Challis *et al.* 1983a and Liggins 1983.)

before regaining responsiveness to ACTH (and probably other trophic factors) by day 130 of gestation (Wintour *et al.* 1975; Glickman & Challis 1980). Induction of 17α-hydroxylase activity in the fetal adrenal by ACTH results in a greatly increased concentration of cortisol in fetal serum (Challis *et al.* 1983a,b). Fetal cortisol promotes the initiation of surfactant production by the fetal lungs (reviewed by Ballard 1982), and the maturation of other fetal organs (reviewed by Buster 1980). In addition, fetal cortisol induces increased activities of 17α-hydroxylase and 17,20-lyase in the placenta and thus promotes the conversion of progesterone to oestrogen (Anderson *et al.* 1975; Steele *et al.* 1976). The consequences of the resultant fall in the ratio of progesterone to oestrogen are many and include heightened excitability and increased electrical coupling of cells of the myometrium (Fuchs 1978; Verhoeff & Garfield 1986), an increase in myometrial sensitivity to oxytocin (Soloff 1975; Fuchs *et al.* 1983b) and increased synthesis of prostaglandins by several intrauterine tissues (Castracane & Jordan 1975), which together promote parturition.

In spite of the clinical evidence that a malfunctioning fetal pituitary—adrenal axis affects the timing of human parturition (reviewed by Casey *et al.* 1983c), the role of the fetal adrenal in human parturition has not been defined clearly. In primates, the fetal adrenal cortex consists of a definitive zone which secretes predominantly cortisol and a fetal zone which secretes dehydroepiandrosterone sulphate (DHAS). Fetal cortisol is apparently involved in fetal lung maturation in the human as well as the sheep (Ballard 1982). In contrast to the sheep, however, there is no abrupt rise in the concentration of cortisol in human fetal serum at term, and neither ACTH nor cortisol when administered at term will induce labour (Liggins *et al.* 1977a,b). Furthermore, the human placenta, unlike the ovine placenta, lacks 17α-hydroxylase and is essentially unable to convert progesterone to oestrogen. The relative rates of secretion of progesterone and oestrogen are, therefore, not sensitive directly to changes in the concentration of cortisol in fetal serum. The human placenta instead is dependent upon a source of exogenous androgen to support oestrogen synthesis and the fetal adrenal satisfies this demand by providing DHAS. The human fetal adrenal (unlike the ovine fetal adrenal) has high DHA sulphokinase activity and the placenta has high activity of the corresponding sulphatase. Therefore, control by the human fetal adrenal of the relative rates of production of progesterone and oestrogen by the placenta is exerted not through cortisol but through DHAS (Fig. 10.1). This endocrine relationship accounts for the increased incidence of delayed parturition in pregnancies that are complicated by anencephaly (Honnebier & Swaab 1973), fetal adrenal hypoplasia (O'Donohoe & Holland 1968) or placental sulphatase deficiency (France *et al.* 1973). Each of these complications results in diminished production of non-esterified oestrogen. Therefore, in contrast to ovine parturition, which is integrated with maturation of the fetal lungs and is dependent upon increased fetal production of cortisol, human parturition does not appear to be integrated closely with maturation of the fetal lungs, and regulation of the initiation of parturition appears to be multifactorial.

The evolutionary advantages, if any, of multifactorial control of parturition might be expected to include a reduced risk of preterm labour. It has been noted, however, that, whereas preterm parturition in sheep is relatively rare (less than 1% of pregnancies), it is relatively common in humans (approx. 5–10% of pregnancies) (Challis & Thorburn 1975). Importantly, with respect to a definition of the functions of the fetus in the initiation of parturition, the distinct and well-characterized changes in concentrations of various hormones in the plasma of fetal sheep near term are absent in the human (Fig. 10.1).

Contributions of the human fetus to endocrine changes at term

Steroid hormones

There is an approximately linear increase in the concentration of oestrogens in the maternal circulation throughout gestation such that, at term, the concentrations of oestradiol-17β, oestrone, oestriol, oestetrol and their corresponding conjugates are all more than ten times greater than in normal ovulatory women (Adlercreutz 1974). It has been estimated that, in pregnant women at term, daily oestrogen production may exceed that produced by normal ovulatory women in three years (MacDonald & Porter 1983). This hyperoestrogenic state of human pregnancy is unique among animals and is even more remarkable when one considers that, near term, most of the oestrogen originates from the placenta, which is dependent totally upon an extraplacental supply of androgens to support oestrogen biosynthesis. The fetal adrenals are the principal source of this androgen in the form of DHAS. The weight of the human fetal adrenal increases progressively after the 20th week of gestation, largely as a result of a massive enlargement of the fetal zone of the adrenal cortex, which is the source of secreted DHAS (and other C_{19}-steroids) (Carr & Simpson 1981). Steroid secretion by the fetal adrenals at term may be more than ten times that of adult adrenals (Siiteri & MacDonald 1966; MacDonald & Porter 1983). Paradoxically, the fastest rate of growth of the fetal adrenal occurs in the last 4–6 weeks of gestation, when ACTH concentration in the fetal circulation is declining (Carr & Simpson 1981). This has led to the suggestion that there is increased responsiveness of the human fetal adrenal to ACTH near term (Casey *et al.* 1983c). In addition, it is likely that the fetal adrenal responds to other trophic stimuli. The human fetal adrenal has prolactin receptors

(Posner *et al.* 1974) and changes in prolactin concentration in fetal serum in late gestation parallel the growth of the fetal adrenal (Winters *et al.* 1975). If prolactin is a second trophic stimulus for the human fetal adrenal, its effect appears to be on adrenal growth rather than a direct effect on steroidogenesis (Casey *et al.* 1983c).

Changes in the concentrations of various steroid hormones in the plasma of the chronically catheterized fetus of the rhesus monkey have been monitored (Fig. 10.2) (Walsh *et al.* 1984). During the last 4 days of gestation, the concentrations of DHAS and oestrone in fetal plasma increase. Similarly, a 2·5-fold increase in concentration of DHAS in the human fetal circulation during the final week of gestation has been measured (Parker *et al.* 1982). Some of the fetal DHAS is transferred to the maternal circulation, and most of the remainder is converted to oestrogen by the placenta (Tulchinsky 1973; Parker *et al.* 1982). In the final 6 weeks of gestation, placental synthesis of oestriol relative to that of other oestrogens increases (Tulchinsky *et al.* 1972). The gradual increase in oestrogen in the maternal circulation during gestation is paralleled by an increase in oestrogen (principally oestrone sulphate) in the amniotic fluid (Jolivet & Gautray 1978). Whereas there is no dramatic increase in maternal circulating oestrogen immediately prior to parturition, the concentration of oestrone sulphate in amniotic fluid doubles during the last 2−3 weeks of gestation (Challis & Mitchell 1981). Furthermore, oestrone sulphate in amniotic fluid may be converted to a biologically active form since human fetal membranes appear to have high oestrogen sulphatase activity (Diczfalusy *et al.* 1963).

The human placenta is also the major site of progesterone production in the second half of gestation. The marked fall in progesterone concentration in maternal plasma and the reciprocal increase in oestrogen concentration that herald parturition in sheep are absent in the human. Furthermore, progestogens may have some prophylactic benefit when administered, before preterm labour, to women at high risk of experiencing preterm labour, but do not inhibit preterm labour that is in progress (Fuchs & Stakemann 1960; Ovlisen & Iversen 1963). Not until after labour has commenced are there abrupt changes (decreases) in the concentrations of oestrogen and progesterone in maternal plasma (Willcox *et al.* 1985). More than 97% of oestrogen and progesterone in the circulation of pregnant women is bound to plasma proteins and the proportion of total hormone that is free does not change during the final two weeks of gestation (Willcox *et al.* 1985). Nevertheless, the ratio of plasma concentrations of oestrogen to progesterone at term is higher

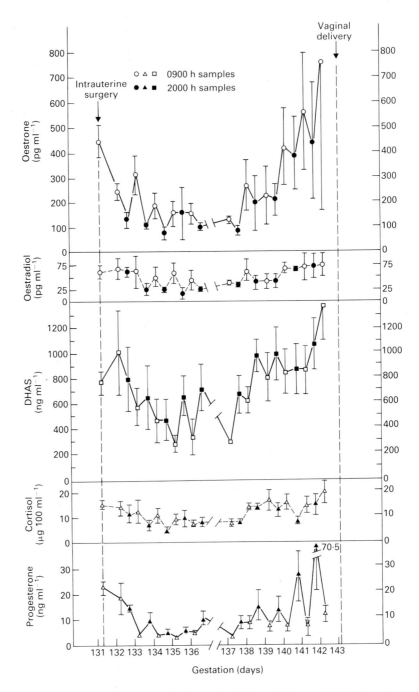

Fig. 10.2. Steroid concentrations in fetal peripheral plasma before vaginal delivery in chronically catheterized rhesus monkeys. Data are normalized to the mean gestational age at intrauterine surgery (range, 129–132 days) and the mean gestational age at vaginal delivery (range, 141–145 days) and are mean values ± SEM ($n = 4$ for DHAS, $n = 3$ for other hormones). (From Walsh *et al.* 1984 with permission of the Endocrine Society.)

than at mid-gestation and the possibility that the slowly rising oestrogen: progesterone ratio reaches a threshold at which parturition is triggered cannot be discounted. Cells isolated from human chorion convert exogenous pregnenolone to progesterone (Gibb *et al.* 1978) and, while some investigators have observed that this process is stimulated by gonadotrophin-releasing hormone (Challis & Mitchell 1981), others have not (Das *et al.* 1985). The quantitative importance of this production of progesterone is unclear, but the synthesis of progesterone by chorion may constitute a mechanism, additional to the provision of fetal DHAS, by which the fetus contributes to the maintenance of progesterone status. Furthermore, it has been proposed that the increased production of DHAS by the fetal adrenal (which results in increased oestrogen synthesis by the placenta) is accompanied by inhibition of the conversion of pregnenolone to progesterone in fetal membranes and there is consequently an increase in the 'local' oestrogen: progesterone ratio (Siiteri & Séron-Ferré 1981). It also has been proposed that the synthesis of a progesterone-binding protein in fetal membranes at term reduces the local concentration of biologically active progesterone (Schwarz *et al.* 1977), but this has not been proved experimentally. A major role of the fetal membranes in regulation of the oestrogen: progesterone ratio seems unlikely, however, not only because progesterone synthesis by human fetal membranes is greater after labour than before (Shaughnessy *et al.* 1983), but also because progesterone degradation by fetal membranes, which is substantial in midgestation, is greatly reduced at term (MacDonald *et al.* 1978).

These various mechanisms by which the fetus may influence oestrogen and progesterone status are pertinent to a consideration of the functions of the fetus in the initiation of parturition because oestrogens and progesterone are involved intimately in the mechanism of parturition. Cervical maturation is influenced by oestrogen and progesterone. The transformation of the cervix from a hard, inflexible structure to one that is soft, oedematous and flexible is accompanied by marked ultrastructural and biochemical changes (reviewed by Golichowski 1986). Smooth muscle, collagen and connective tissue extracellular matrix comprise the three principal structural components of the cervix. Before cervical maturation, collagen fibres form a dense framework by binding to dermatan sulphate and chondroitin sulphate of the extracellular matrix and provide resistance to cervical distension. During cervical maturation, the content of dermatan sulphate and chondroitin sulphate falls while the content of hyaluronic acid and water increases. As a result, the collagen framework is disrupted and the cervix becomes soft and distensible. Accumulation of hyaluronic acid correlates with the major structural changes of the cervix. Although the hormonal control of hyaluronic acid synthesis in the human cervix has not been defined, oestrogens stimulate the accumulation of hyaluronic acid in rabbit uterine horns (Endo & Yosizawa 1973). Associated with the disruption of the collagen framework is an increase in collagen degradation, which is catalysed by an endogenous collagenase that exists as a zymogen (procollagenase) before the onset of cervical maturation. Regulation of collagenolysis is complex and includes control of procollagenase synthesis, regulation of procollagenase conversion to collagenase and modulation of active collagenase (Golichowski 1986). Oestrogens appear to stimulate collagenolysis both directly and indirectly, as a result of their promotion of prostaglandin synthesis. Human cervical stroma possesses oestrogen receptors (Sanborn *et al.* 1980), and in the rat the number of cervical oestrogen receptors increases at term (Huszar & Naftolin 1984). Treatment of experimental animals with oestrogen stimulates collagenolysis (Huszar & Naftolin 1984), and parenteral administration of DHAS to pregnant women between the 38th and 42nd weeks of gestation accelerates cervical maturation (Mochizuki & Tojo 1980). In contrast, collagenolysis in explants of cervical tissue from non-pregnant women is inhibited by progesterone (Hillier & Wallis 1981).

The influences of oestrogen and progesterone on the cervix are paralleled by effects of these hormones on the myometrium. Cholinergic and adrenergic nerve terminals, which are abundant in myometrium in early gestation, are essentially absent at term (Morizaki *et al.* 1987). Consequently, regulation of myometrial contractions is believed to be mainly hormonal rather than neural. Oestrogens have several actions in myometrium that are consistent with oestrogenic preparation of the uterus for parturition. Oestrogens promote the synthesis of the contractile proteins actin and myosin and are required for the maintenace of high intracellular concentrations of ATP that are necessary for muscle activity (Clark & Peck 1979). Oestrogens promote the maintenance of a large potential difference across the muscle plasma membrane, which serves to suppress random asynchronous contractions (Jung 1963). Oestrogens are further involved in the synchronization of myometrial contractions by promoting the formation of gap junctions, the intercellular organelles that permit electrical coupling of contiguous muscle cells. Oestrogens appear to stimulate gap junction formation by increasing the synthesis of gap junction proteins (connexins), while progesterone decreases the synthesis of connexins (Verhoeff & Garfield 1986). Consistent with a progestogenic (inhibitory) effect on gap junctions is the observation that the antiprogesterone, RU-486, initiates gap junction formation and pre-term labour in rats. RU-486-induced labour, but not RU-486-induced gap junction formation, was blocked by oestradiol (Garfield *et al.* 1987). Oestrogens increase the expression of myometrial receptors for some hormones, e.g. oxytocin (Soloff 1975; Nissenson *et al.* 1978) and α-adrenergic agonists (Roberts *et al.* 1981), but decrease the expression of receptors for other hormones, e.g. β-adrenergic agonists (Roberts *et al.* 1981). The expression of myometrial receptors for some other hormones, e.g. prostaglandin E_2 and prostaglandin $F_2α$ is unaffected by oestrogens (Wakeling & Wyngarden 1974). In contrast, progesterone appears to increase the expression of receptors for prostaglandins (Wakeling & Wyngarden 1974) and for β-agonists (Roberts *et al.* 1981), but decreases the expression of oxytocin receptors (Nissenson *et al.* 1978). It should be noted, however, that some of the hormonally induced changes in receptor density summarized above were observed in experimental animals and the relevance of these observations to human myometrial receptors has not been established in every case. Dominance of the influence of progesterone until term is exerted at three levels or more: through the inhibition by progesterone of oestrogen receptor synthesis (Clark *et al.* 1977), by induction of the synthesis of certain proteins, e.g. β-receptors, and by effects independent of protein synthesis, e.g. promotion of sequestration by the sarcoplasmic reticulum of Ca^{2+} required for muscle activity (Carsten 1979). At term, an increase in the oestrogen : progesterone ratio above a critical threshold or a larger local increase in oestrogen : progesterone would, therefore, not only promote cervical maturation but also prepare the myometrium for synchronous contractions in response to a variety of stimuli.

Although it has been noted that an increase in the concentration of plasma cortisol is universal at or near term in mammalian fetuses (Liggins 1976), the surge in the concentration of cortisol in fetal plasma that is associated intimately with the initiation of parturition in sheep is absent in women (Liggins 1983). Indeed, much of the cortisol in human fetal plasma at term may be of maternal origin (Murphy *et al.* 1974). The increase in cortisol in fetal plasma observed after labour is apparently due to fetal stress associated with vaginal delivery rather than a direct cause or effect of labour itself (reviewed by Casey *et al.* 1983c). Administration of glucocorticosteroids to pregnant women does not induce labour except when the pregnancy is post-term (Mati *et al.* 1973). Furthermore, the length of gestation is normal in pregnancies complicated by congenital adrenal hyperplasia (Price *et al.* 1971). Human fetal adrenals produce also non-glucocortico-11β-hydroxysteroids in amounts that increase in late gestation and it has been proposed that these steroids enter the amniotic fluid and influence prostaglandin production by the fetal membranes (Murphy 1980). Glucocorticosteroids inhibit prostaglandin production in some tissues, but in human amnion prostaglandin synthesis is stimulated by dexamethasone (Casey *et al.* 1985; Mitchell *et al.* 1988). A direct effect of cortisol on myometrial activity has not been demonstrated and the proposition that cortisol at term may act to promote parturition by competing with progesterone for occupancy of progesterone receptors has not been proved experimentally (Elsner *et al.* 1979).

Peptide hormones

Oxytocin, at picomolar concentrations, stimulates uterine activity and has been used extensively to induce labour in women. The concept that oxytocin fulfils this function in spontaneous labour, however, is controversial. Confusion regarding reported changes in plasma concentrations of oxytocin at the onset of parturition may be attributable to differences in radioimmunoassays, to the low concentration of oxytocin in plasma and to the pulsatile nature of oxytocin secretion (Chard 1983). At term, the concentration of oxytocin in umbilical arterial plasma is higher than that in either umbilical venous plasma or maternal peripheral venous plasma (Chard 1983), suggesting that the fetus actively produces oxytocin at this stage of gestation. The umbilical arterial–venous difference in oxytocin concentration is reversed when oxytocin is administered to induce labour and this is suggestive that, in the human, oxytocin is transferred across the placenta in spite of high activity *in vitro* of placental oxytocinase that destroys biological activity (Dawood 1983; Fields *et al.* 1983). It is generally accepted that oxytocin concentrations in maternal and fetal plasma do not increase abruptly before the onset of labour. After labour has commenced, oxytocin concentrations in maternal and fetal plasma increase, so that during active labour oxytocin concentrations are 2–4 times greater than those before labour (Fig. 10.3) (Fuchs *et al.* 1983a).

A stimulus for maternal secretion of oxytocin in the sheep (but not in the human) is the Ferguson reflex, a neural response to stretching of the cervix. The stimulus for oxytocin secretion by the fetus is not known

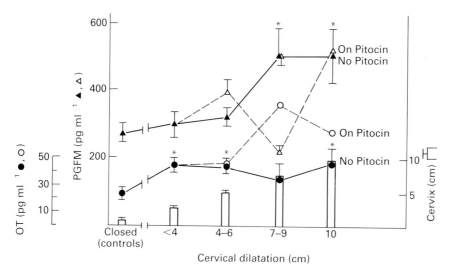

Fig. 10.3. Concentrations of oxytocin and 13,14-dehydro-15-keto-PGF$_2\alpha$ in peripheral plasma of pregnant women during the first stage of spontaneous labour. Oxytocin (OT, circles) and PGFM (triangles) in the peripheral plasma of 15 pregnant women were quantitated during spontaneous labour. Three to four serial samples were collected from each patient and the extent of cervical dilatation at time of sampling was noted. Control values are the mean concentrations of oxytocin and PGFM in plasma of 15 women in late pregnancy before the onset of labour. Asterisks indicate significant differences from the controls. (From Fuchs & Fuchs 1984b with permission of the MacMillan Publishing Company.)

but has been attributed to the 'stress' of delivery (Chard 1983; Fuchs & Fuchs 1984a). It has been proposed that oxytocin may induce increased uterine activity even in the absence of a marked increase in the plasma concentration of oxytocin at term because there is an increase in oxytocin receptor density at this time, which may result in increased sensitivity of the myometrium to oxytocin. Oxytocin receptor density in human myometrium increases 30–200-fold during the course of gestation, and the asymmetric distribution of receptors over the uterus changes in late gestation so that the highest density is no longer in the fundus but in the lower segment of the uterus (Fuchs *et al.* 1983b; Bottari *et al.* 1987). As discussed earlier, these changes in receptor density are influenced by oestrogen and progesterone.

It has been proposed that oxytocin has at least two actions that promote labour (Fuchs *et al.* 1982). First, oxytocin stimulates myometrial contractions by promoting an increase in cytosolic free Ca^{2+} that is required for contractile activity (a hormonal response that apparently involves inositol trisphosphate as a second messenger; Tomasi *et al.*

1987). Second, oxytocin (10 mU ml^{-1}) appears to increase prostaglandin synthesis in decidua, which, like myometrium, possesses oxytocin receptors (Fuchs *et al.* 1982). Strickland *et al.* (1982), however, were unable to detect an effect of oxytocin (at concentrations up to 500 μU ml^{-1}) on prostaglandin production by superfused human decidua vera tissue. The synthesis of prostaglandins by myometrium is unaffected by oxytocin (Fuchs *et al.* 1982). Indirect evidence that oxytocin-dependent production of prostaglandins by decidua may be required for successful parturition includes the finding that treatment with indomethacin (an inhibitor of prostaglandin synthesis) reduces the efficacy of oxytocin in inducing labour even though the effect of oxytocin on uterine contractions is unaltered (Husslein *et al.* 1981). This requirement for oxytocin-induced synthesis of prostaglandins, however, may be an artefact of induction of labour and may reflect the importance of prostaglandins in cervical maturation, a process that in spontaneous labour is already well under way before plasma concentrations of oxytocin increase.

Oxytocin enters the amniotic sac with the fetal urine and reaches its greatest concentration in amniotic fluid at term (Dawood *et al.* 1979). In spite of the presence of oxytocinase in amniotic fluid, oxytocin could potentially alter prostaglandin synthesis by the fetal membranes (Fuchs & Fuchs 1984a) and this action, if significant, would afford another mechanism by which fetal oxytocin influences myometrial activity. The influence of oxytocin on prostaglandin synthesis by the fetal membranes, however, has not been evaluated fully. Thus, although an initiator function of oxytocin in parturition has been argued (Fuchs & Fuchs 1984a), others have suggested that the functions of oxytocin are in the late stages of labour (including delivery of the placenta and uterine contractions to reduce blood loss), and in the maternal response to suckling (Chard 1983; MacDonald 1984). The recent availability of oxytocin analogues that act as antagonists (e.g. ORF 22164; Demarest *et al.* 1987) will facilitate investigations of the function of oxytocin in the initiation of labour and may be prototypes of a new class of tocolytic agents.

Vasopressin is present in maternal plasma at concentrations that remain low throughout pregnancy and labour (Hoppenstein *et al.* 1968). In contrast, the vasopressin concentration in umbilical arterial plasma is 10 to 20 times greater than that of oxytocin (Chard 1983). The high ratio of vasopressin concentration in the umbilical artery to that in the vein is suggestive of active fetal production of vasopressin and is consistent with the presence of vasopressin in human fetal pituitary. The human uterus possesses specific receptors for vasopressin (Bottari *et al.* 1987) and, before pregnancy, the uterus is more sensitive to vasopressin than to oxytocin (Embrey & Moir 1967). During pregnancy, the large increase (30- to 200-fold) in oxytocin receptor density is accompanied by a more modest increase (approx. 5-fold) in vasopressin receptor density and, consequently, the uterus at term is approximately ten times more sensitive to oxytocin than to vasopressin (Fuchs 1983; Bottari *et al.* 1987). Nevertheless, because the concentration of vasopressin in fetal plasma is much greater than that of oxytocin, vasopressin may have a significant effect on the myometrium. Such an effect could be direct or indirect by modulation of prostaglandin production by the fetal membranes since biologically active vasopressin is present in amniotic fluid (Fuchs & Fuchs 1984a). An apparently stress-induced release of vasopressin into the fetal circulation at term has been observed (DeVane & Porter 1980), and, because several of the factors that predispose pregnant women to preterm labour also cause fetal stress (Fuchs 1983), it is possible that vasopressin could be involved in the initiation of preterm labour. Pre-eclampsia may result in a stress-induced increase in fetal plasma concentration of vasopressin, but this is not manifest as an increase in vasopressin concentration in maternal peripheral plasma (DeVane 1985). Thus, if fetal vasopressin functions in the initiation of preterm labour, its mechanism of action presumably involves entry into the amniotic fluid and stimulation of prostaglandin production by the fetal membranes. The increased incidence of preterm deliveries in pregnancies complicated by pre-eclampsia, however, is largely iatrogenic (i.e. elective delivery before term).

The properties of relaxin as a smooth muscle relaxant have been known for more than 50 years, but the functions of this hormone in human pregnancy and parturition remain undefined (reviewed by Sanborn 1986). Relaxin may be synthesized by uterine decidua (Bigazzi *et al.* 1980), but the corpus luteum is by far the principal site of synthesis (Weiss *et al.* 1977). Changes in the concentration of relaxin in peripheral plasma during pregnancy vary between species, but in the human the concentration of relaxin increases during the first trimester, then remains low for the rest of gestation (Szlachter *et al.* 1982). Relaxin receptors are found in myometrium and cervix in several species, and in the rat and pig relaxin receptor density is increased after treatment with oestrogens (Mercado-Simmen *et al.* 1982). A developmental decline in relaxin receptor density in rat myometrium occurs in late gestation (Mercado-Simmen *et al.* 1982). In non-pregnant animals, relaxin inhibits uterine contractions induced by either oxytocin or prostaglandins only when the concentrations of these stimulants are low (Sanborn 1986). Effects of relaxin on myometrial activity during pregnancy, however, have been difficult to demonstrate, perhaps because of the development of refractoriness to relaxin, or because of modulation of relaxin responses by other hormones. In addition to altering myometrial contractility, relaxin decreases uterine degradation of glycogen and collagen, and alters the physical properties of the uterus (Sanborn 1986). At least some of the actions of relaxin are mediated by cyclic AMP (Sanborn *et al.* 1980). Since, in pregnant women, the most dramatic changes in plasma relaxin concentration occur in the first trimester, it has been proposed that the function of relaxin is to maintain uterine quiescence until that role is assumed by progesterone. The function of relaxin, if any, in the initiation of parturition is unknown but, given the ovarian origin of this hormone, fetal involvement in any function of relaxin in initiation of parturition is likely to be only indirect (e.g. via oestrogenic regulation of relaxin receptors).

Prolactin is present in fetal plasma in amounts that increase in late gestation in parallel with the growth of the fetal adrenals (Winters *et al.* 1975) and, as discussed earlier, a trophic action of prolactin on the fetal adrenals has been proposed. Prolactin is also found in amniotic fluid and the source of this prolactin appears to be, not the fetal pituitary, but the uterine decidua (Golander *et al.* 1979; Tomita *et al.* 1982). It has been proposed that the decrease in the concentration of prolactin in amniotic fluid that occurs in late gestation is due not to decreased decidual synthesis but rather to impaired transfer of prolactin from the decidua to the amniotic fluid when cellular contact between chorion and amnion is disrupted (McCoshen *et al.* 1982). Tyson *et al.* (1985) found that prostaglandin E_2 (PGE_2) production by human amnion *in vitro* is inhibited by prolactin. They proposed that decidual prolactin attenuates PGE_2 production in amnion until term, when structural changes in the fetal membranes impair prolactin transfer and result in accelerated PGE_2 production by the amnion. The concentration of prolactin in amniotic fluid is also influenced, however, by maternal diabetes and by fetal gender, without any consistent effect on the initiation of parturition (McCoshen 1987). Thus, elucidation of the function of prolactin (from decidua or fetal pituitary) in the initiation of parturition awaits further investigation.

Other peptide hormones (e.g. bradykinin, angiotensin) have uterotonic actions but their involvement in the initiation of parturition remains to be defined. In addition, a variety of peptide growth factors are present in amniotic fluid in amounts that, in some cases, increase in late gestation and, as discussed later, are sufficient to influence prostaglandin production by the fetal membranes.

It is apparent that the influence of the human fetus on endocrine changes at term of gestation is multiple, and that any fetal contribution to the initiation of parturition cannot be attributed to a single hormone. Furthermore, several of the endocrine changes in which the fetus participates result in stimulation of prostaglandin production by intrauterine tissues at term. Prostaglandin action, therefore, may afford a mechanism of complementation or synergism between the various fetal stimuli that promote parturition.

Prostaglandins and the initiation of parturition

Prostaglandin production and action during parturition

The prostaglandins are members of a diverse family of biologically active compounds that are derived by oxidation of polyunsaturated fatty acids. The most abundant prostaglandins are those of the '2-series' (e.g. PGE_2 and $PGF_2\alpha$), which are derived from arachidonic acid. Prostaglandins are involved in numerous fetoplacental processes, which include regulation of umbilical haemodynamics (Tuvemo *et al.* 1976), maintenance of patency of the ductus arteriosus (Coceani *et al.* 1976), control of fetal breathing (Kitterman *et al.* 1983), regulation of steroid aromatization by the placenta (Lehmann 1974) and regulation of fetal urine flow (Kirshon *et al.* 1987). The first evidence of a possible involvement of prostaglandins in parturition was obtained by Kurzrok & Lieb (1930), who observed that an extract of human semen induced strips of human myometrium to contract and relax. Shortly thereafter, Von Euler (1935) introduced the name prostaglandin to describe biologically active material that was purified partially from prostate and seminal vesicles. Luukkainen and Csapo (1963) found that responsiveness of the rabbit uterus to oxytocin was increased when a lipid emulsion was infused intravenously. The active compound in the lipid emulsion was found subsequently to be linoleic acid, a precursor of arachidonic acid (Lanman *et al.* 1974), and it was confirmed that arachidonic acid administered intravenously to pregnant rabbits induced parturition (Nathanielsz *et al.* 1973). Arachidonic acid is metabolized to prostaglandins and to a variety of other biologically active derivatives (Fig. 10.4). Since the biologically active products of arachidonic acid metabolism are in most cases short-lived, the prostaglandins that influence uterine activity are local hormones produced by

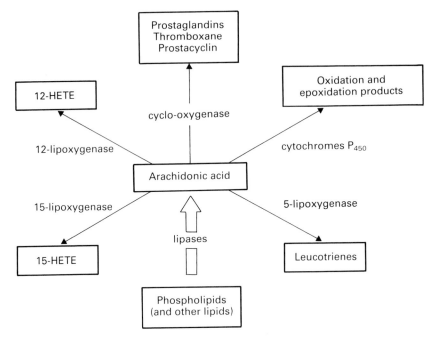

Fig. 10.4. Summary of the metabolism of arachidonic acid to biologically active derivatives. 12-HETE = 12-hydroxy-5,8,10,14-eicosatetraenoic acid, 15-HETE = 15-hydroxy-5,8,11,13-eicosatetraenoic acid.

intrauterine tissues. Each of the metabolic pathways indicated (Fig. 10.4) is functional in one or more of the intrauterine tissues (reviewed by Mitchell 1986).

The presence of prostaglandins in amniotic fluid was first reported by Karim and coworkers (Karim 1966; Karim & Devlin 1967), who observed that in amniotic fluid obtained during labour the concentration of prostaglandins of both the E and F series were greater than those in amniotic fluid obtained before labour. Prostaglandins were found to increase the intensity of spontaneous uterine contractions (Karim & Devlin 1967) and, when administered intravenously to pregnant women, prostaglandins induced labour at or near term (Bygdeman *et al.* 1968; Karim *et al.* 1968) and abortion in the first and second trimesters (Karim & Filshie 1970). Instillation of arachidonic acid (but not oleic acid) into the human amniotic sac induced second-trimester abortion and delivery at term (MacDonald *et al.* 1974). Conversely, administration of inhibitors of cyclo-oxygenase (Fig. 10.4), such as aspirin and indomethacin, was found to prolong gestation (Lewis & Schulman 1973) and to delay

second-trimester abortion induced by hypertonic saline (Waltman *et al.*
1972). Indomethacin has the advantage of being a reversible inhibitor of
cyclo-oxygenase and has been used successfully to halt preterm labour,
even though it has the disadvantage of being transferred to the fetal
circulation and so has potential for causing fetal complications (reviewed
by Witter & Niebyl 1986).

Whereas the clinical efficacy of prostaglandins and inhibitors of
prostaglandin synthesis has been proved, documentation of changes in
concentrations of circulating prostaglandins at or near the onset of
spontaneous labour has been difficult (reviewed by Mitchell 1986). In
sheep, the concentration of $PGF_2\alpha$ in the utero-ovarian venous blood
increases significantly during the last day of gestation, before the onset
of labour (Liggins & Grieves 1971). Corresponding measurements cannot
be made in women, but no significant changes in concentration of either
PGE_2 or $PGF_2\alpha$ in peripheral plasma were detected during labour (Mitchell
et al. 1978b). PGE_2 and $PGF_2\alpha$, however, are essentially metabolized
completely during a single passage through the lungs and so an increased
production of prostaglandins during labour may not be reflected in a
single measurement of prostaglandin concentration in plasma. When
the concentrations of the major metabolites of $PGF_2\alpha$ (PGFM, 13,14-
dihydro-15-keto-$PGF_2\alpha$) and PGE_2 (PGEMII, 11-deoxy-13,14-dihydro-
15-keto-11,l6-cyclo-PGE_2) in peripheral plasma were measured, an
increase in the concentration of PGFM but not PGEMII occurred during
labour (Fig. 10.3) (Mitchell *et al.* 1978b, 1982; Fuchs *et al.* 1983a). The
concentration of thromboxane B_2 (TXB_2, a biologically inactive metabolite of thromboxane A_2) in maternal peripheral plasma remained unchanged before and during labour (Ylikorkala & Viinikka 1980). The
concentration of 6-keto-$PGF_1\alpha$ (an inactive metabolite of prostacyclin)
was increased during late pregnancy and again during labour (Barrow *et
al.* 1983).

Concentrations of prostaglandins in plasma obtained from umbilical
artery and vein before and during labour have also been measured. The
concentrations of PGE_2 and $PGF_2\alpha$ in fetal plasma are much greater than
those in maternal plasma, reflecting, in part, the low metabolism of
prostaglandins by the fetal lungs (MacKenzie *et al.* 1980). The arteriovenous difference in concentration of PGE_2 in the umbilical cord is
suggestive that the placenta is a major source of PGE_2 in the fetal
circulation. It has been proposed that, in the fetus, PGE_2 is a circulating
hormone which functions in the maintenance of patency of the ductus
arteriosus (Mitchell 1986). The concentrations of PGE_2, $PGF_2\alpha$ and 6-

keto-PGF$_1\alpha$ are increased in the plasma of fetal sheep during labour and the concentrations of PGE$_2$, PGF$_2\alpha$ and PGFM (but not TXB$_2$ or 6-keto-PGF$_1\alpha$) are greater in human fetal plasma obtained after spontaneous labour and delivery than after delivery by caesarean section without labour (Mitchell 1986). Changes in concentrations of lipoxygenase products (Fig. 10.4) in maternal or fetal plasma in association with labour have not been well defined.

The concentrations of prostaglandins and their metabolites in maternal urine have been measured as an approximate index of total prostaglandin production by uterine tissues. Concentrations of the urinary metabolites of PGE$_2$ and PGF$_2\alpha$ increased throughout gestation and the urinary excretion rate of the major metabolite of PGF$_2\alpha$ doubled at the onset of parturition (Hamberg 1974). PGE$_2$, PGF$_2\alpha$, PGFM and 6-keto-PGF$_1\alpha$ were all found in the first-voided urine of human newborn infants in amounts that were greater if delivery by caesarean section occurred after labour had commenced (Casey *et al.* 1983a). Although fetal urine is the major contributor to amniotic fluid volume at term, the amounts of prostaglandins in fetal urine are insufficient to account for the large increase in concentrations of prostaglandins found in amniotic fluid during labour. Concentrations of PGE$_2$ and PGF$_2\alpha$ in amniotic fluid increase slowly during the latter half of gestation, and then increase abruptly at the onset of labour and as labour progresses (Keirse *et al.* 1977b; Keirse 1979). Concentrations of TXB$_2$ and 6-keto-PGF$_1\alpha$ in human amniotic fluid are greater during labour, but do not increase progressively with labour (Mitchell 1986). During labour, the concentrations of leucotriene B$_4$ (LTB$_4$) and 12-hydroxy-5,8,10,14-eicosatetraenoic acid (12-HETE) in human amniotic fluid are approximately doubled and the concentration of 15-hydroxy-5,8,11,13-eicosatetraenoic acid (15-HETE) increases approx. sevenfold (Romero *et al.* 1987a). Since these latter changes in concentrations of lipoxygenase products are less than those for cyclo-oxygenase products, the onset of parturition is characterized not only by quantitive changes but also by qualitative changes in biologically active metabolites of arachidonic acid.

Sources of prostaglandins during labour

Because the major source of arachidonic acid metabolites in amniotic fluid is apparently not fetal urine, and since neither biosynthesis nor degradation of prostaglandins occurs in amniotic fluid itself, other sources must be evaluated. Placenta, myometrium, cervix, decidua vera, chorion laeve and amnion tissues all metabolize arachidonic acid and produce characteristic spectra of biologically active products (Mitchell 1986). When prostaglandin production rates are measured in superfused tissue minces, amnion is the most active uterine tissue and PGE_2 (then 6-keto-$PGF_1\alpha$ and TXB_2) is the most abundant product (Mitchell *et al.* 1978a; Okazaki *et al.* 1981a). Amnion tissue obtained after spontaneous vaginal delivery exhibits greater rates of production of PGE_2 and 6-keto-$PGF_1\alpha$ (but not TXB_2) than does amnion tissue obtained at term before labour (Skinner & Challis 1985). When amnion tissue is incubated *in vitro* in the presence of $[^{14}C]$arachidonic acid, the principal radio-labelled lipoxygenase product is 12-HETE, but 15-HETE is the most abundant lipoxygenase product of chorion laeve and decidua vera (Mitchell 1986).

The concentrations of prostaglandin metabolites in amniotic fluid increase in parallel with the concentrations of their parent prostaglandins (Keirse *et al.* 1977a). This finding, together with the observation that activities of enzymes involved in prostaglandin degradation do not change in association with labour (Keirse 1979) is suggestive that increased prostaglandin concentrations do not result from decreased prostaglandin degradation. Furthermore, there is evidence that increased synthesis of prostaglandins in human amnion and myometrium is due, at least in part, to increased amounts of biosynthetic enzymes (cyclo-oxygenase and prostacyclin synthase) (Okazaki *et al.* 1981a; Moonen *et al.* 1984).

This increased capacity for prostaglandin synthesis by some intra-uterine tissues during labour, however, can result in increased prosta-glandin production only if there is an adequate supply of substrate, i.e. non-esterified arachidonic acid. Intracellular concentrations of non-esterified fatty acids, however, are maintained at low levels by acyltrans-ferases involved in the oxidation and esterification of fatty acids. Liberation of non-esterified fatty acids is catalysed by lipases and is a prerequisite of the acute stimulation of prostaglandin synthesis (Lands & Samuelsson 1968; Vonkeman & van Dorp 1968). Indeed, the increase in concen-trations of prostaglandins in amniotic fluid at the onset of labour is accompanied by a six- to tenfold increase in the concentration of non-esterified arachidonic acid (MacDonald *et al.* 1974), and the concentration of arachidonic acid in amniotic fluid increases further as labour pro-gresses (Keirse *et al.* 1977a). The significance of arachidonic acid in amniotic fluid is illustrated by the finding that either delivery at term (after fetal demise) or second-trimester abortion was induced when arachidonic acid was instilled into the amniotic fluid (MacDonald *et al.* 1974). The source of the arachidonic acid that appears in amniotic fluid during early labour (cervical dilatation 4 cm or less) has been investigated (Okita *et al.* 1982a). Several lipids in amnion and chorion are rich in arachidonic acid, and during early labour the amount of arachidonic acid that remains esterified in lipids of fetal membranes declines. It has been computed that the amount of arachidonic acid mobilized from fetal membranes during early labour (approx. 1 μmol) is sufficient to account for the increased amounts of non-esterified arachidonic acid, prostaglandins and prostaglandin metabolites in amniotic fluid, maternal plasma and maternal urine during this period (Okita *et al.* 1982a). Thus, it is evident that arachidonic acid mobilization and prostaglandin production by fetal membranes, and amnion in particular, may be important components of the initiation of spontaneous labour.

Several characteristics of human amnion are consistent with an active role of this tissue in the initiation of parturition. First, amnion is a metabolically active tissue with an estimated O_2 consumption per g tissue greater than that of either fetal brain or fetal muscle (Liggins *et al.* 1977b). Second, among intrauterine tissues, amnion is the most active producer of prostaglandins (Okazaki *et al.* 1981a; Mitchell 1986). Third, amnion is essentially devoid of 15-hydroxyprostaglandin dehydrogenase, an important enzyme in the inactivation of prostaglandins (Okazaki *et al.* 1981a). Consequently, prostaglandins produced in amnion are not metabolized *in situ* but are free to diffuse into the amniotic fluid and to neighbouring tissues. Fourth, the amnion has a large surface area (approx. $0.6m^2$, not including the increased surface area afforded by numerous microvilli) that is ideally suited for absorptive processes and for responding to hormones and other substances in amniotic fluid. A close metabolic relationship between human amnion and amniotic fluid is likely because the amnion is avascular and non-innervated. Fifth, the amnion is contiguous with the chorion and in close proximity to decidua vera which are active producers of prostaglandins that can stimulate contractions in the underlying myometrium.

Mobilization of arachidonic acid to support prostaglandin biosynthesis

Sources of arachidonic acid

During early labour, the decrease in amount of arachidonic acid esterified in amnion lipids (approx. 27%) is more than sufficient to account for the increase in arachidonic acid and prostaglandins in amniotic fluid during this period (Okita *et al.* 1982a). This arachidonic acid was found to be mobilized selectively from two phospholipids in amnion, phosphatidylinositol and phosphatidylethanolamine (Okita *et al.* 1982a). Subsequently, enzymatic mechanisms that can account for the selective mobilization of arachidonic acid from phosphatidylinositol and phosphatidylethanolamine were defined (Fig. 10.5) (Bleasdale & Johnston 1984). Mobilization of arachidonic acid from phosphatidylethanolamine appears to occur in a single reaction catalysed by a phospholipase A_2 that exhibits substrate preference for phosphatidylethanolamine molecules that contain arachidonic acid, and this phospholipase A_2 has optimal activity *in vitro* at pH 7 to 8 in the presence of calcium (Okazaki *et al.* 1978). The pH dependence and calcium requirement are indicative that this phospholipase A_2 is not lysosomal and so it is unlikely that lysosomes are involved in arachidonic acid mobilization in amnion, as was proposed for decidua (Gustavii 1972). Three enzymes appear to act concertedly to catalyse the mobilization of arachidonic acid from phosphatidylinositol in amnion (Fig. 10.5), and none of these enzymes is lysosomal (Di Renzo *et al.* 1981; Okazaki *et al.* 1981a,b,c,). A calcium-dependent phospholipase C catalyses the hydrolysis of phosphatidylinositol to produce a diacylglycerol that has at least two potential metabolic fates: phosphorylation to phosphatidic acid in a reaction catalysed by diacylglycerol kinase, and hydrolysis to monoacylglycerol in a reaction catalysed by diacylglycerol lipase. Diacylglycerol kinase is part of a mechanism by which diacylglycerol may be recycled to phosphatidylinositol and is inhibited by calcium (Fig. 10.5). In contrast, activity of diacylglycerol lipase, which catalyses the next reaction in the sequence that results in liberation of non-esterified arachidonic acid (Fig. 10.5), is not affected directly by calcium. Calcium, therefore, may have an important function in the mobilization of arachidonic acid from amnion lipids during early labour. It was proposed (Bleasdale & Johnston 1984) that in resting amnion cells the concentration of cytosolic free Ca^{2+} is low and consequently phospholipase A_2 activity is suppressed and any diacylglycerol formed by the action of phospholipase C is recycled to phosphatidylinositol. In response to a variety of stimuli, the cytosolic free Ca^{2+} concentration increases, activities of phospholipases A_2 and C increase, recycling of diacylglycerol is inhibited and arachidonic acid mobilization is stimulated (Fig. 10.5). Consistent with a role for calcium in the regulation of prostaglandin production are the observations that either removal of extracellular Ca^{2+} or blocking calcium entry into amnion cells by use of methoxyverapamil greatly reduced PGE_2 produc-

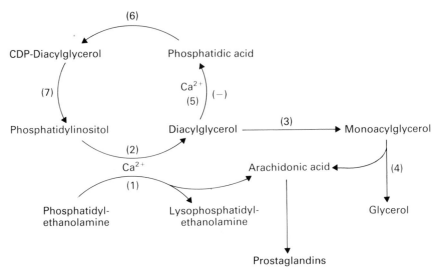

Fig. 10.5. Proposed pathways for the mobilization of arachidonic acid from phosphatidylinositol and phosphatidylethanolamine in amnion. The reactions illustrated are catalysed by (1) phospholipase A_2, (2) phospholipase C, (3) diacylglycerol lipase, (4) monoacylglycerol lipase, (5) diacylglycerol kinase, (6) CTP: phosphatidic acid cytidylyltransferase, and (7) phosphatidylinositol synthase. Calcium stimulates the activities of phospholipase A_2 and phospholipase C, but inhibits diacylglycerol kinase activity.

tion, whereas the use of a calcium ionophore, A23187, to promote calcium entry into amnion cells increased PGE_2 production (Olson *et al.* 1983a).

Regulation of arachidonic acid mobilization

In view of the importance of arachidonic acid mobilization to support the synthesis of prostaglandins that are involved in parturition, it is likely that hormones that influence arachidonic acid mobilization may function in the initiation of spontaneous labour at term or in the precipitation of preterm labour. It does not appear that suppression of arachidonic acid mobilization until term is due to a deficiency of one or more of the enzymes involved in mobilization. For instance, the specific activities of diacylglycerol lipase, diacylglycerol kinase and monoacylglycerol lipase in amnion were unchanged throughout gestation and during early labour (Okazaki *et al.* 1981c). Although the specific activities of phospholipases A_2 and C in amnion tissue obtained at term were more than three times greater than the corresponding activities in amnion obtained between the 13th and 17th weeks of gestation, activities of these phospholipases in amnion obtained at term after labour were not different from those in amnion at term before labour (Okazaki *et al.* 1981c). Thus, development of the enzymatic mechanisms for the mobilization of arachidonic acid in amnion is apparently complete before the initiation of parturition, at which time these mechanisms are activated.

Because human amnion is avascular and has no nerve supply, it is reasonable to suspect that humoral modulation of arachidonic acid mobilization and prostaglandin production in amnion may be exerted by substances in amniotic fluid. Indeed, amniotic fluid contains several substances that influence prostaglandin production by amnion. Some of these substances appear to stimulate prostaglandin production by satisfying the Ca^{2+} requirement for arachidonic acid mobilization. Human amniotic fluid obtained at term after labour has commenced contains platelet-activating factor (PAF, 1-0-alkyl-2-acetyl-glycero-3-phosphocholine) at concentrations at which this lipid is biologically active (Billah & Johnston 1983). PAF is undetectable, however, in amniotic fluid obtained at term before labour. Although PAF was described originally as a potent activator of platelets (Demopoulos *et al.* 1979) and as a hypotensive factor (Blank *et al.* 1979), PAF has other biological activities and was found to increase PGE_2 production by amnion tissue *in vitro* (Billah *et al.* 1985). Stimulation of amnion PGE_2 production by PAF was blocked by the calcium chelator, EGTA. This action of PAF is consistent with its actions on a variety of blood cells to increase the concentrations of cytosolic free Ca^{2+}, resulting in activation of phospholipases, mobilization of arachidonic acid and increased prostaglandin production (e.g. Lee *et al.* 1981).

Human amnion is capable not only of responding to PAF but also of synthesizing PAF (Billah *et al.* 1985), and the amounts of PAF in amnion more than double during labour (Ban *et al.* 1986). Secretion of PAF by amnion tissue *in vitro*, however, has not been observed, and other sources of the PAF in amniotic fluid during labour have been considered. There is no synthesis of PAF in amniotic fluid but amniotic fluid does contain high activity of PAF acetylhydrolase, an enzyme that catalyses deacetylation (inactivation) of PAF (Billah & Johnston 1983). 1-0-Alkyl-glycero-3-phosphocholine acetyltransferase, the enzyme that catalyses the final reaction in the predominant pathway for PAF biosynthesis in most tissues, is active not only in amnion but also in chorion, decidua, fetal kidney and fetal lung (Johnston *et al.* 1987). Although PAF was detected in first-voided urine of newborn infants (Billah & Johnston

1983), the fetal kidney is unlikely to be the source of most of the PAF in amniotic fluid. This is because PAF in human amniotic fluid is predominantly 1-octadecyl-2-acetyl-glycero-3-phosphocholine whereas kidney synthesizes largely 1-hexadecyl-2-acetyl-glycero-3-phosphocholine (Nishihira *et al.* 1984).

The possibility that PAF in amniotic fluid originates in the fetal lung was supported by the finding that some of the PAF in amniotic fluid was associated with lamellar bodies (the organelle of lung surfactant storage) (Billah & Johnston 1983). The amount of PAF and the activity of acetyltransferase increase markedly in fetal rabbit lung near the onset of production of lung surfactant (Hoffman *et al.* 1986b); and, in explants of human fetal lung tissue, differentiation of type II pneumonocytes (the cells that synthesize lung surfactant) is accompanied by an increase in acetyltransferase activity (Hoffman *et al.* 1986a; Johnston *et al.* 1987). Precursors for PAF biosynthesis and enzymes for PAF metabolism also are found in type II pneumonocytes (Hoffman *et al.* 1986b). Johnston and co-workers have presented evidence in support of the hypothesis that, in fetal type II pneumonocytes, PAF stimulates utilization of glycogen, which is required to fuel surfactant biosynthesis at this stage of development (Johnston *et al.* 1987). In addition, it was proposed that PAF is secreted from fetal lungs as a component of lung surfactant and enters the amniotic fluid. Near term, PAF accumulates in amniotic fluid, perhaps because the capacity for hydrolysis by PAF acetylhydrolase is either exceeded or compromised, and PAF then stimulates PGE_2 production by the amnion. PAF may increase uterine activity not only by stimulation of prostaglandin production, but also by direct action on the myometrium (Nishihira *et al.* 1984). It is not known, however, whether PAF in human amniotic fluid gains access to the myometrium. Other questions regarding the possible involvement of PAF in surfactant production by fetal lungs and in the initiation of parturition remain unanswered. For instance, the factors that stimulate PAF production by the fetal lungs in late gestation are unknown, and direct evidence that PAF stimulates glycogenolysis is lacking. It is not clear why PAF can be detected in amniotic fluid only *after* labour has commenced or why PAF is not present in all specimens of amniotic fluid obtained during labour (Billah & Johnston 1983). Nevertheless, this hypothesis provides a plausible explanation of how a fetal contribution (i.e. PAF) to the initiation of parturition is coordinated with the functional maturation of a vital organ (the fetal lungs) (Fig. 10.6).

Other substances in amniotic fluid, like PAF, have potential for affecting the calcium requirement for arachidonic acid mobilization in

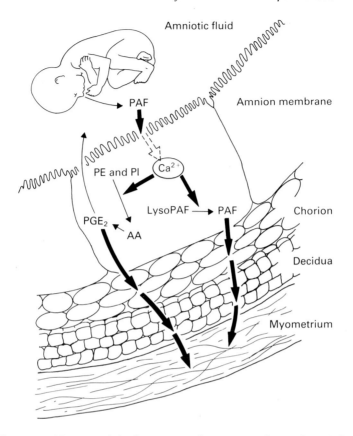

Fig. 10.6. Proposed function of platelet-activating factor in stimulation of prostaglandin production in amnion by the fetal lungs. PAF enters the amniotic fluid as a component of lamellar bodies (the organelles of lung surfactant storage). PAF accumulates in amniotic fluid only at the time of parturition, perhaps as the capacity for PAF hydrolysis by PAF acetylhydrolase is exceeded, and acts on amnion. PAF increases cytosolic free calcium concentration in amnion, perhaps via an increase in inositol trisphosphate, and thus activates the mechanisms of mobilization of arachidonic acid that are illustrated in Fig. 10.5. As a consequence, prostaglandin production is increased. In addition, the increase in cytosolic free calcium may stimulate PAF synthesis in amnion. Prostaglandins and PAF originating in amnion diffuse to neighbouring tissues and elicit responses that include further stimulation of prostaglandin production and induction of myometrial contractions. PE, phosphatidylethanolamine; PI, phosphatidylinositol; AA, arachidonic acid; PAF, platelet-activating factor; PGE_2, prostaglandin E_2. (From Johnston *et al.* 1987 with permission of Plenum Press, New York.)

amnion. For example 1,25-dihydroxyvitamin D_3, which is involved in Ca^{2+} uptake by various cells, is present in amniotic fluid at term (Lazebnik *et al.* 1983) and stimulates PGE_2 efflux from human amnion cells in primary culture (Casey *et al.* 1986). The source of 1,25-dihydroxyvitamin D_3 may be the fetal kidney or decidua vera (Weisman *et al.* 1979; Fraser

1980). It has not been proved, however, that the stimulation of PGE_2 production in amnion by 1,25-dihydroxyvitamin D_3 involves an increase in the concentrations of cytosolic free Ca^{2+}. Polyamines, e.g. spermine, which are also present in amniotic fluid, may stimulate arachidonic acid mobilization in amnion by reducing the Ca^{2+} requirement for phospolipase C activity (Sagawa *et al.* 1983; Bleasdale & Johnston 1984).

Calcium may stimulate arachidonic acid mobilization in amnion by mechanisms other than direct interaction with phospholipases A_2 and C. For instance, Olson *et al.* (1983a) found that production of PGE_2 by amnion cells was inhibited by calmidazolium and trifluoperazine, two antagonists of the calcium-binding protein calmodulin. It is possible, therefore, that some of the functions of Ca^{2+} in the regulation of prostaglandin production by amnion may be mediated by calmodulin. Another mechanism by which Ca^{2+} may stimulate arachidonic acid mobilization involves activation of protein kinase C. This calcium- and diacylglycerol-dependent protein kinase is ubiquitous and has many substrates (Nishizuka 1984), which include lipocortins (Hirata 1981; Khanna *et al.* 1986). Lipocortins 1 and 2 are structurally related proteins of approx. M_r 36 000 that exhibit Ca^{2+}-dependent binding to phospholipids, which, under certain conditions, results in inhibition of phospholipase A_2 activity (Davidson *et al.* 1987). Phosphorylation of lipocortins is catalysed *in vitro* by protein kinase C (and other kinases) and has been reported to reduce the phospholipase A_2 inhibitory activity of lipocortins. Thus, calcium-dependent activation of protein kinase C could stimulate arachidonic acid mobilization in amnion via phosphorylation of lipocortins, which results in disinhibition of phospholipase A_2 activity. This mechanism is attractive because in amnion the concentration of diacylglycerol (another cofactor for protein kinase C activity) increases markedly during early labour (Okita *et al.* 1982b). Although it has been observed that phorbol esters (activators of protein kinase C) stimulate PGE_2 production by human amnion cells in culture (Lytton & Mitchell 1988), it has not been proved that lipocortins are substrates for amnion protein kinase C *in vivo* or that endogenous lipocortins limit arachidonic acid mobilization in amnion. Furthermore, because glucocorticosteroids stimulate lipocortin synthesis in several tissues (Flower *et al.* 1984), glucocorticosteroids might be expected to inhibit prostaglandin production by amnion. Interestingly, however, dexamethasone inhibited prostaglandin production by human myometrial cells in culture (Casey *et al.* 1985) but stimulated PGE_2 production by amnion cells (Mitchell *et al.* 1988).

Some substances in amniotic fluid may alter arachidonic acid mobilization and prostaglandin production in amnion by mechanisms that are apparently Ca^{2+}-independent. Catecholamines perform regulatory functions in a number of processes in the perinatal period, including control of placenta blood flow, neonatal thermogenesis and secretion of lung surfactant (Phillippe 1983). Catecholamines in the maternal circulation are unlikely to influence PGE_2 production by amnion since the placenta is believed to effectively metabolize (inactivate) catecholamines (Saarikoski 1974). Several catecholamines and their metabolites, however, are found in amniotic fluid in amounts that are greater during the third trimester than during the first trimester (Divers *et al.* 1981; Phillippe & Ryan 1981). Some of these catecholamines enter the amniotic sac as components of fetal urine (Dalmaz *et al.* 1980). Human amnion possesses β_2-adrenergic receptors and the density of receptors increases threefold between mid-gestation and term (Fig. 10.7) (Di Renzo *et al.* 1984a). Amnion β-receptors are apparently functional, since exposure of amnion tissue *in vitro* to a β-agonist resulted in an increase in the tissue content of cyclic AMP that was blocked by the prior addition of the β-antagonist, propranolol (Di Renzo *et al.* 1984a). The transitory increase in intracellular cyclic AMP concentration induced by isoproterenol was accompanied by an increased efflux of arachidonic acid and PGE_2 from the tissue (Fig. 10.8) (Di Renzo *et al.* 1984b). The mechanism by which an increase in intracellular cyclic AMP in amnion results in increased PGE_2 is unknown. The effects of other catecholamines and their metabolites that are found in amniotic fluid on PGE_2 production in amnion have not been defined. The acute efflux of prostaglandins from freshly dispersed amnion cells, however, is stimulated by catecholoestrogens (Olson *et al.* 1983b).

A function of catecholamines in the initiation of parturition is attractive also because, at term, the human cervix (in contrast to the corpus uteri) contains numerous adrenergic nerve terminals and there is indirect evidence that activation of these terminals promotes cervical maturation (Huszar & Naftolin 1984). Catecholamines, therefore, have potential for influencing cervical maturation by increasing PGE_2 production in the cervix as well as influencing the initiation of parturition by increasing PGE_2 production in the amnion. Although the proposal that catecholamines are involved in the initiation of parturition is consistent with the observation that norepinephrine instilled into the amniotic sac of women near term stimulated uterine activity (Amy & Karim 1974), it may appear to conflict with the therapeutic use of ritodrine (a β-mimetic)

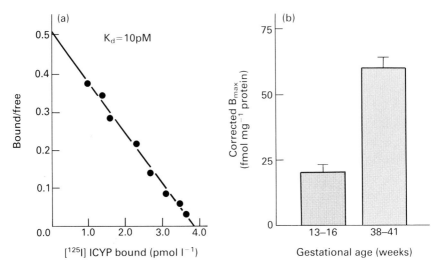

Fig. 10.7. Beta-adrenergic receptors in human amnion tissue. (a) Scatchard analysis of the binding of $[^{125}I]$ iodocyanopindolol (ICYP) to a membrane fraction prepared from human amnion tissue obtained at term. (b) Comparison of maximal binding capacity (B_{max}) for ICYP by membrane fractions prepared from human amnion tissue obtained either at 13–16 weeks of gestation $(n = 5)$ or at 38–41 weeks of gestation $(n = 11)$. The B_{max} value at 38–41 weeks of gestation is significantly greater $(p < 0.01)$ than that at 13–16 weeks of gestation. (Data from Di Renzo *et al.* 1984a.)

to inhibit preterm labour. Maintenance of uterine quiescence by ritodrine appears to involve activation of myometrial β-receptors. Administration of ritodrine to pregnant sheep for 24 h, however, results in a loss of receptors from the myometrium, which is accompanied by increased sensitivity of the myometrium to oxytocin (Ward *et al.* 1987). It was suggested that this desensitization of the myometrium to β-agonists accounts for the increase in the concentrations of PGFM and $PGF_2\alpha$ in the plasma of pregnant sheep treated chronically with ritodrine (Casper & Lye 1987). It has not been proved, however, that functional myometrial β-receptors are necessary for maintenance of human pregnancy. For example, treatment of hypertensive pregnant women with large doses of a β-antagonist, propranolol, does not induce preterm labour (Liggins *et al.* 1977b). Additional mechanisms of the tocolytic action of ritodrine, therefore, cannot be precluded. Ritodrine is transferred from the maternal circulation to the fetus and can be detected in human amniotic fluid (Van Lierde & Thomas 1982) and so may act on the amnion. Ritodrine, at concentrations up to 0·1 mM, did not increase the intracellular concentration of cyclic AMP in amnion tissue *in vitro* and so did

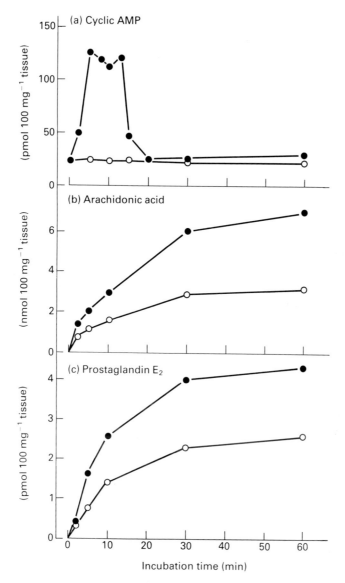

Fig.10.8. Isoproterenol-induced increase in the cyclic AMP content of amnion tissue pieces and the release of arachidonic acid and prostaglandin E_2. Amnion tissue pieces (35−40 mg wet weight) were preincubated for 2 h in pseudoamniotic fluid, rinsed briefly, blotted and transferred to fresh pseudoamniotic fluid with (●) or without (○) isoproterenol (10^{-5}M). After various periods of further incubation, amounts of cyclic AMP in the pieces of amnion (a) and amounts of arachidonic acid (b) and prostaglandin E_2 (c) in the pseudoamniotic fluid were measured. (From Di Renzo *et al.* 1984b with permission of Geron-X, Inc.)

not act as a β-agonist (Collins & Roberts 1987). Rather, ritodrine acted as a β-antagonist and inhibited (K_i approx. 2 μM) the increase in intracellular cyclic AMP concentration elicited by a β-mimetic, isoproterenol. The tocolytic action of ritodrine, therefore, could also involve inhibition of PGE_2 production by amnion. A function of fetal catecholamines in the initiation of human parturition is also compatible with the importance of the fetal pituitary–adrenal axis in the initiation of parturition because some of the epinephrine in amniotic fluid may originate in the fetal adrenal medulla, where its synthesis is stimulated by cortisol produced in the fetal adrenal cortex (Artal 1980).

Although there is much evidence that the arachidonic acid to support PGE_2 synthesis in amnion is mobilized from amnion lipids, other sources cannot be precluded totally. Niesert *et al.* (1986b) used [^{14}C]arachidonic acid to radiolabel lipids in primary cultures of human amnion cells and, after removal of unincorporated [^{14}C]arachidonic acid, the amnion cells were exposed to [^{3}H]arachidonic acid and stimulated to produce prostaglandins. It was found that, under these conditions, [^{3}H]arachidonic acid was the preferred substrate for PGE_2 synthesis and it was speculated that arachidonic acid used for PGE_2 synthesis by amnion is derived directly from non-esterified arachidonic acid in the extracellular space. The source of much of the arachidonic acid in amniotic fluid, however, is the amnion itself and, prior to the mobilization of arachidonic acid from amnion, the amount of arachidonic acid in amniotic fluid is insufficient to support prostaglandin biosynthesis. On the other hand, it has been reported that fetal urine at term has high activity of a phosphoinositide-specific phospholipase C and that the appearance of this enzyme in amniotic fluid correlates temporally with a decrease in the concentration in amniotic fluid of phosphatidylinositol (which enters the amniotic sac as a component of lung surfactant) (Takahashi *et al.* 1988). It was proposed that in amniotic fluid, as in amnion, phospholipase C catalyses the first reaction in the mobilization of arachidonic acid from phosphatidylinositol. Identification of the other enzymes that are required for mobilization of arachidonic acid from phosphatidylinositol (Fig. 10.5) in amniotic fluid was not reported and it should be noted that the phosphatidylinositol of lung surfactant (relative to phosphatidylinositol in most tissues) is deficient in arachidonic acid. Nevertheless, if phosphatidylinositol in surfactant provides a supply of arachidonic acid that can be used by amnion for prostaglandin synthesis, it is possible that bacterial lipases, which may be found in amniotic fluid during infection, may catalyse mobilization of this arachidonic acid and precipitate preterm labour.

Complementary mechanisms for regulation of prostaglandin production

Amnion tissue that is obtained after labour has commenced has a greater basal rate of production of PGE_2 than does amnion obtained before labour (Mitchell *et al.* 1978a; Okazaki *et al.* 1981a; Olson *et al.* 1983c). This difference persists even in the presence of exogenous arachidonic acid and so probably cannot be attributed to an increase in arachidonic acid availability. Indeed, substances that influence cyclo-oxygenase activity directly have been identified in amniotic fluid. Strickland *et al.* (1983) reported that a substance present in human fetal urine stimulates prostaglandin synthesis by bovine seminal vesicles. Stimulatory activity was greater in urine obtained from neonates delivered at term after labour than in urine of neonates delivered at term by caesarean section before labour. The characteristics of the stimulator (Strickland *et al.* 1983) were indicative that it may be a steroid or other small lipid molecule, but its identification awaits further investigation.

Casey *et al.* (1983b) described a protein in amniotic fluid that produced a delayed but large increase in PGE_2 production by human amnion cells in primary culture. This protein was found in greater concentration in amniotic fluid obtained after labour had commenced than in amniotic fluid obtained before labour. The protein appeared to be synthesized by fetal kidneys and entered the amniotic sac with fetal urine. It was proposed that the protein may be transforming growth factor(s)-α since, like this growth factor, it closely resembled epidermal growth factor (EGF) and its actions on amnion were apparently mediated through EGF receptors. It is possible, however, that this protein has a primary function other than an involvement in the initiation of parturition since it is present in human adult urine, and its renal synthesis is not easily reconciled with the finding that, in pregnancies complicated by Potter's syndrome (fetal bilateral renal agenesis), the onset and course of spontaneous labour is essentially normal (Ratten *et al.* 1973).

EGF is also present in human amniotic fluid in amounts that increase in association with labour (Romero *et al.* 1987b). EGF stimulates PGE_2 efflux from human amnion cells in primary culture (Mitchell 1987) by a mechanism that involves an increase in amounts of immunoprecipitable cyclo-oxygenase (Casey *et al.* 1988). EGF enters the amniotic sac with the fetal urine and the correlation between its concentration in fetal urine and the concentration of creatinine is suggestive of an extrarenal site of synthesis (in contrast to the EGF-like protein discussed above) (Casey *et al.* 1985). Interestingly, the EGF receptor (with ligand) has protein kinase activity and catalyses phosphorylation of a tyrosine residue in lipocortin 1 (Pepinsky & Sinclair 1986). Thus, EGF may potentially increase PGE_2 production in amnion by a dual mechanism: an EGF-induced increase in amounts of cyclo-oxygenase, and an EGF-stimulated phosphorylation of lipocortin 1 that results in disinhibition of phospholipase A_2 and promotion of arachidonic acid mobilization. Other growth factors (e.g. somatomedin and platelet-derived growth factor) are also found in human amniotic fluid, but their involvement, if any, in the initiation of parturition is unknown.

Liggins (1983) has proposed that suppression of prostaglandin production during gestation and the subsequent removal of this suppression at the initiation of parturition are related biochemical events in which the conceptus has dominant functions. Inhibition of prostaglandin release from the endometrium during the luteal phase is essential for the establishment of pregnancy, and associated with the decidualization of the endometrium in early pregnancy is a marked decrease in the prostaglandin content of this tissue (Abel *et al.* 1980). Gurpide and co-workers have investigated extensively the regulation of prostaglandin production in human endometrium (Schatz *et al.* 1984, 1985). Estradiol was found to stimulate $PGF_2\alpha$ production by secretory endometrium *in vitro* whereas either progesterone or dexamethasone inhibited prostaglandin production in both proliferative and secretory endometrium (Gurpide *et al.* 1986). The amounts of lipocortins in endometrium were increased during 48 h of exposure to dexamethasone and this finding is consistent with the inhibition by glucocorticoids of arachidonic acid mobilization in some other tissues (Gurpide *et al.* 1986). Paradoxically, however, the amounts of lipocortins in endometrium were *decreased* during 48 h of exposure to progesterone and, therefore, lipocortins are unlikely to be mediators of the inhibition of endometrial prostaglandin production by progesterone. Importantly, however, secretion of lipocortin by endometrium *in vitro* was observed, and this may afford one mechanism by which the suppression of prostaglandin production by other uterine tissues is maintained. The effects of steroid hormones on prostaglandin production by intrauterine tissues are poorly defined and warrant further investigation.

Inhibitors of prostaglandin synthesis have been detected in amniotic fluid and may be involved in the maintenance of uterine quiescence until term. Wilson *et al.* (1985) described two proteins (approx. M_r 150 000−165 000 and 70 000−80 000) that are present in amniotic fluid obtained late in pregnancy (before labour), and at very low concentration

(10^{-9}M) were able to inhibit PGF$_2\alpha$ production by human endometrial cells in culture. Inhibition was overcome when the endometrial cells were supplied with exogenous arachidonic acid, suggesting that these proteins inhibit mobilization of endogenous arachidonic acid. The proteins inhibited *in vitro* activity of a phospholipase A$_2$ purified from pig pancreas. Release of the smaller inhibitory protein (which is apparently structurally related to the larger protein) was observed from human chorion cells in culture only when the chorion was collected before labour had commenced (Wilson & Liggins 1986). The relationship of these inhibitory proteins to the inhibitor detected in amniotic fluid by Saeed *et al.* (1982) and to the lipocortins is unknown.

Prostaglandin production in several intrauterine tissues is known to be stimulated by physical trauma. Distension or manipulation of the cervix in late pregnancy results in a large increase in the concentration of prostaglandins in maternal plasma and an acceleration of cervical maturation (Mitchell *et al.* 1977; Manabe & Sagawa 1983). This response may involve a neurally mediated reflex release of maternal oxytocin (Theobald 1968; Fuchs & Fuchs 1984a). Similarly, stretching or other trauma of the fetal membranes (e.g. amniotomy, spontaneous rupture of the membranes, chorioamnionitis, irrigation with hyperosmolar solutions) may result in stimulation of prostaglandin synthesis and the initiation of labour (Manabe *et al.* 1983; Guzick & Winn 1985). The mechanism by which membrane stretching stimulates prostaglandin synthesis is not defined but may involve rupture of lysosomes and mobilization of arachidonic acid catalysed by lysosomal lipases (i.e. a process that is different from the mobilization of arachidonic acid discussed earlier). The importance of physical stimulation of prostaglandin production preceding the spontaneous onset of normal labour and any role of the fetus in such a process have not been defined.

Propagation of the signal(s) for parturition

Because an increase in the synthesis of prostaglandins by the amnion is intimately associated with the initiation of parturition, there is reason to suspect that amnion prostaglandins may be involved in the propagation of the signal(s) for parturition to the myometrium. 15-Hydroxyprostaglandin dehydrogenase, an enzyme that catalyses biological inactivation of prostaglandins, is essentially absent from human amnion (Okazaki *et al.* 1981a) and, therefore, prostaglandins produced in amnion are free to diffuse to the amniotic fluid and to the chorion. Nakla *et al.* (1986)

measured the *in vitro* transfer of *exogenous* radiolabelled PGE$_2$ across either amnion alone or intact amnion–chorion–decidua and found that, although the rate of transfer of unmetabolized PGE$_2$ across intact amnion– chorion–decidua was lower than that across amnion alone, it was increased significantly in membranes obtained after the spontaneous onset of labour. McCoshen *et al.* (1987) measured the *in vitro* efflux of *endogenously* synthesized PGE$_2$ on both sides (maternal and fetal) of intact amnion–chorion–decidua and found that, although the efflux of PGE$_2$ to the fetal side was greater in membranes obtained after the onset of labour than before, efflux to the maternal side was reduced. These experiments, however, do not preclude an increased flux of prostaglandins to the maternal side during the initiation of labour, because they provide no information either about the metabolism of PGE$_2$ (to inactive metabolites or other active prostaglandins) or about the availability of arachidonic acid to support prostaglandin synthesis in membranes that were collected after labour is complete (i.e. when stores of esterified arachidonic acid may be depleted). Furthermore, tissues that were obtained after labour were collected vaginally and the associated tissue trauma may impede transfer of prostaglandins in the same manner in which it was proposed that transfer of decidual prolactin may be impeded when contiguity of the fetal membranes is interrupted (McCoshen *et al.* 1982; Tyson *et al.* 1985).

Human chorion has an active 15-hydroxyprostaglandin dehydrogenase (Keirse 1978) that may limit the diffusion of PGE$_2$ from the amnion through the chorion. Suppression of prostaglandin levels in the endometrium during the luteal phase of the menstrual cycle involves a progesterone-induced increase in 15-hydroxyprostaglandin dehydrogenase activity in this tissue (Casey *et al.* 1980). In contrast, the possibility that a decline in progesterone responses at term could result in loss of 15-hydroxyprostaglandin dehydrogenase activity in chorion, and thus lead to increased levels of prostaglandins, is not supported by the finding that 15-hydroxyprostaglandin dehydrogenase activity in chorion obtained at term after labour is similar to that in chorion before labour (Keirse *et al.* 1978).

PGE$_2$ that diffuses from the amnion and reaches the decidua may be either oxidized (inactivated) in a reaction catalysed by 15-hydroxyprostaglandin dehydrogenase or reduced to PGF$_2\alpha$ in a reaction catalysed by 9-ketoreductase. Because the sensitivity of the myometrium to PGF$_2\alpha$ is only about one-tenth of that to PGE$_2$, it has been proposed that the conversion of PGE$_2$ to PGF$_2\alpha$ may be part of a protective mechanism to maintain uterine quiescence in the event of an inappropriate production of PGE_2 by the amnion. The presence of 9-ketoreductase in decidua may also explain the finding that during active labour the prostaglandin metabolite that accumulates in maternal plasma is PGFM, even though the amnion produces largely PGE_2. Niesert *et al.* (1986a), however, concluded that, although the rate of conversion of *endogenous* PGE_2 to $PGF_2\alpha$ in human decidua is significant, the synthesis of $PGF_2\alpha$ from PGE_2 produced in contiguous tissues is low.

PGE_2 produced by amnion may stimulate prostaglandin production by chorion and decidua, presumably by a mechanism that involves PGE_2 receptors and an increase in the intracellular concentration of cyclic AMP (Di Renzo *et al.* 1984b). Thus, the prostaglandins that reach the myometrium may originate from amnion, chorion and decidua. The decidua may also supply the myometrium with arachidonic acid endoperoxides to support myometrial synthesis of prostaglandins (Abel & Kelly 1979). Prostaglandins that act on the myometrium appear to do so through specific receptors (Wendelberger 1987) and may elicit a variety of responses, including qualitative and quantitative alteration of prostaglandin products formed (Casey *et al.* 1985), an increase in sensitivity to oxytocin (Gillespie & Beazley 1972; Novy & Liggins 1980), an enhanced assembly of connexins into gap junctions (Verhoeff & Garfield 1986), and stimulated release of Ca^{2+} from the sarcoplasmic reticulum (Carsten & Miller 1977). Together these actions of prostaglandins promote coordinated contractions of the myometrium and the progression of labour.

Summary

Regulation of the initiation of human parturition is multifarious. Because gestation that is either curtailed or prolonged offers no obvious biological advantage to the mother but may have life-threatening consequences for the fetus, it is reasonable to suspect that the fetus may exert a dominant influence on the timing of parturition. Although there is much clinical evidence in support of an involvement of the fetus in the initiation of parturition, it is apparent that the influence of the fetus is multiple and that no single fetal stimulus is clearly dominant. Perhaps the major contribution of the fetus to the endocrine changes in late gestation is the provision of fetal DHAS for maintenance of the appropriate progesterone–oestrogen status. This fetal contribution requires a functional fetal pituitary–adrenal axis and expression of high activity of sulphatase in the placenta. The latter requirement exemplifies the genetic control of the length of gestation because placental sulphatase deficiency results frequently in prolonged gestation. A variety of other fetal endocrine changes at term promote parturition. Several of these fetal stimuli share the property of increasing prostaglandin production by one or more of the intrauterine tissues. Prostaglandins, therefore, appear to provide one mechanism by which the various maternal and fetal pro-parturitional stimuli are integrated. The earliest changes in prostaglandin production associated with parturition occur in amnion. Amnion tissue is an active producer of prostaglandins and this fetal tissue exhibits several characteristics that are consistent with an involvement in the initiation of parturition. Various substances in amniotic fluid have been found to influence prostaglandin production by the amnion. Prostaglandins produced by the amnion diffuse to neighbouring tissues and, therefore, the amnion may be a component of one mechanism by which fetal signals are communicated to the myometrium. Whereas in sheep fetal cortisol has a major influence on both fetal lung maturation and the initiation of parturition, cortisol does not coordinate these processes in the human. Secretion by human fetal lungs into the amniotic fluid of substances (e.g. PAF) that stimulate prostaglandin production by the amnion may be one mechanism by which fetal lung maturation is coordinated, albeit loosely, with the initiation of parturition.

The regulation of prostaglandin production by intrauterine tissues and the precise functions of prostaglandins in the initiation of parturition are incompletely understood. A complete understanding of the functions of prostaglandins in the initiation of parturition and application of this information to the prevention of preterm labour are important future goals.

References

Abel M.H. & Kelly R.W. (1979) Differential production of prostaglandins within the human uterus. *Prostaglandins*, **18**, 821–8.

Abel M.H., Smith S.K. & Baird D.T. (1980) Suppression of concentration of endometrial prostaglandin in early intra-uterine and ectopic pregnancy in women. *J. Endocrinol.*, **85**, 379–86.

Adlercreutz H. (1974) Analysis of natural and synthetic hormonal steroid in biological fluids by mass fragmentography. In *Mass Spectrometry in Biochemistry and Medicine* (Ed. by A. Frigerio & N. Castagnoli), pp. 165–81. Raven Press, New York.

Amy J.J. & Karim S.M.M. (1974) Intrauterine administration of L-noradrenaline and propranolol during the second trimester of pregnancy. *J. Obstet. Gynaecol. Br. Commonw.*, **81**, 75–83.

Anderson A.B.M., Flint A.P.F. & Turnbull A.C. (1975) Mechanism of action of glucocorticoids in induction of ovine parturition: effect on placental steroid metabolism. *J. Endocrinol.*, **66**, 61–70.

Artal R. (1980) Fetal adrenal medulla. *Clin Obstet. Gynecol.*, **23**, 825–36.

Ballard P.L. (1982) Hormonal aspects of fetal lung development. In *Lung Development: Biological and Clinical Perspectives*, Vol. 2 (Ed. by P.M. Farrell), pp. 205–53. Academic Press, New York.

Ban C., Billah M.M., Truong C.T. & Johnston J.M. (1986) Metabolism of platelet-activating factor (1-0-alkyl-2-acetyl-*sn*-glycero-3-phosphocholine) in human fetal membranes and decidua vera. *Arch. Biochem. Biophys.*, **246**, 9–18.

Barrow S.E., Blair A.I. & Waddell K.A. (1983) Prostacyclin in late pregnancy: analysis of 6-oxo-prostaglandin $F_1\alpha$ in maternal plasma. In *Prostacyclin in Pregnancy* (Ed. by P.J. Lewis, S. Moncada & J. O'Grady), pp. 79–85. Raven Press, New York.

Bigazzi M., Nardi E., Bruni P. & Petrucci F. (1980) Relaxin in human decidua. *J. Clin Endocrinol. Metab.*, **51**, 939–41.

Billah M.M. & Johnston J.M. (1983) Identification of phospholipid platelet-activating factor (1-0-alkyl-2-acetyl-*sn*-glycero-3-phosphocholine) in human amniotic fluid and urine. *Biochem. Biophys. Res. Commun.*, **113**, 51–8.

Billah M.M., Di Renzo G.C., Ban C. *et al.* (1985) Platelet-activating factor metabolism in human amnion and the responses of this tissue to extracellular platelet-activating factor. *Prostaglandins* **30**, 841–50.

Binns W., Lynn J.F., Shupe J.L. & Everett G. (1963) A congenital cyclopian-type malformation in lambs induced by maternal ingestion of a range plant, *Veratrum californicum*. *Am. J. Vet. Res.*, **24**, 1164–75.

Blank M.L., Snyder F., Byers L.W. *et al.* (1979) Antihypertensive activity of an alkyl ether analog of phosphatidylcholine. *Biochem. Biophys. Res. Commun.*, **90**, 1194–200.

Bleasdale J.E. & Johnston J.M. (1984) Prostaglandins and human parturition: regulation of arachidonic acid mobilization. In *Reviews in Perinatal Medicine* (Ed. by E.M. Scarpelli & E.V. Cosmi), pp. 151–91. Alan R. Liss, New York.

Bottari S.P., Guillon G., Goldfien A. & Roberts J.M. (1987) Oxytocin and vasopressin: distinct receptors in human myometrium. *Abstr. Soc. Gynecol. Invest.*, p. 31.

Buster J.E. (1980) Fetal adrenal cortex. *Clin. Obstet. Gynecol.*, **23**, 803–24.

Bygdeman M., Kwon S.U., Mukherjee T. & Miqvist N. (1968) Effect of intravenous infusion of prostaglandin E_1 and E_2 on motility of pregnant human uterus. *Am. J Obstet. Gynecol.*, **102**, 317–26.

Carr B.R. & Simpson E.R. (1981) Lipoprotein utilization and cholesterol synthesis by the human fetal adrenal gland. *Endocr. Rev.*, **2**, 306–26.

Carsten M.E. (1979) Calcium accumulation by human uterine microsomal preparations: effects of progesterone and oxytocin. *Am. J. Obstet. Gynecol.*, **133**, 598–601.

Carsten M.E. & Miller J.D. (1977) Effects of prostaglandin and oxytocin on calcium release from a uterine microsomal fraction. *J. Biol. Chem.*, **252**, 1576–81.

Casey M.L., Hemsell D.L., MacDonald P.C. & Johnston J.M. (1980) NAD^+-dependent 15-hydroxyprostaglandin dehydrogenase activity in human endometrium. *Prostaglandins*, **19**, 115–22.

Casey M.L., Cutrer S. & Mitchell M.D. (1983a) Origin of prostanoids in human amniotic fluid: the fetal kidney as a source of amniotic fluid prostanoids. *Am. J. Obstet. Gynecol.*, **147**, 547–51.

Casey M.L., MacDonald P.C. & Mitchell M.D. (1983b) Stimulation of prostaglandin E_2 production in amnion cells in culture by a substance(s) in human fetal and adult urine. *Biochem. Biophys. Res. Commun.*, **114**, 1056–63.

Casey M.L., Winkel C.A., Porter J.C. & MacDonald P.C. (1983c) Endocrine regulation of the initiation and maintenance of parturition. *Clin. Perinatol.*, **10**, 709–21.

Casey M.L., MacDonald P.C. & Mitchell M.D. (1985) Despite a massive increase in cortisol secretion in women during parturition, there is an equally massive increase in prostaglandin synthesis: a paradox? *J. Clin. Invest.*, **75**, 1852—7.

Casey M.L., Griffin J.E., Korte K. *et al.* (1986) Response of human amnion cells in culture to 1,25-dihydroxycholecalciferol: increased 25-hydroxycholecalciferol 24-hydroxylase activity and prostaglandin E_2 formation. *Am. J. Obstet. Gynecol.*, **155**, 1272—6.

Casey M.L., Korte K. & MacDonald P.C. (1988) Epidermal growth factor stimulation of prostaglandin E_2 biosynthesis in amnion cells. *J. Biol. Chem.*, **263**, 7846—54.

Casper R.F. & Lye S.J. (1987) β-Adrenergic agonist infusion increases plasma PGF levels in pregnant sheep. *Abstr. Soc. Gynecol. Invest.* p. 131.

Castracane V.D. & Jordan V.C. (1975) The effect of estrogen and progesterone on uterine PG biosynthesis in the ovariectomized rat. *Biol. Reprod.*, **13**, 587—97.

Challis J.R.G. & Mitchell B.F. (1981) Hormonal control of preterm and term parturition. *Semin. Perinatol.*, **5**, 192—202.

Challis J.R.G. & Thorburn G.D. (1975) Prenatal endocrine function and the initiation of parturition. *Br. Med. Bull.*, **31**, 57—62.

Challis J.R.G., Manchester E.L., Lye S.J. *et al.* (1983a) The development of the pathway of steroid synthesis. In *Initiation of Parturition: Prevention of Prematurity* (Ed by P.C. MacDonald & J.C. Porter), pp. 11—17. Ross Laboratories, Columbus, OH.

Challis J.R.G., Manchester E.L. & Mitchell B.F. (1983b) Activation of adrenal function in fetal sheep by the infusion of adrenocorticotrophin to the fetus *in utero*. *Biol. Reprod.*, **27**, 1026—32.

Chard T. (1983) The role of the maternal and fetal posterior pituitary gland in parturition. In *Initiation of Parturition: Prevention of Prematurity* (Ed. by P.C. MacDonald & J.C. Porter), pp. 121—6. Ross Laboratories, Columbus, OH.

Clark J.H. & Peck E.J. (1979) *Female Sex Steroid Receptors and Functions*. Monographs on Endocrinology, Springer, Berlin.

Clark J.H., Hsueh A.J.W. & Peck E.J. Jr (1977) Regulation of estrogen receptor replenishment by progesterone. *Ann. NY Acad. Sci.*, **286**, 161—79.

Coceani F., Olley P.M. & Bodach E. (1976) Prostaglandins: a possible regulator of muscle tone in the ductus arteriosus. In *Advances in Prostaglandin and Thromboxane Research*, vol. 1 (Ed. by B. Samuelsson & R. Paoletti), pp. 417—24. Raven Press, New York.

Collins P.L. & Roberts J.M. (1987) Ritodrine acts as an antagonist on the beta$_2$-adrenoreceptors of human amnion. *Abstr. Soc. Gynecol. Invest.*, p. 158.

Creasy R.K. (1983) Implications for treatment of preterm labor. In *Initiation of Parturition: Prevention of Prematurity* (Ed. by P.C. MacDonald & J.C. Porter), pp. 173—6. Ross Laboratories, Columbus, OH.

Dalmaz Y., Peyrin L., Dutruge J. & Sann L. (1980) Neonatal pattern of adrenergic metabolites in urine of small for gestational age and preterm infants. *J. Neural. Transm.*, **49**, 151—65.

Das N.P., Khan-Dawood F.S. & Dawood M.Y. (1985) The effects of steroid hormones and gonadotropins on *in vitro* placental conversion of pregnenolone to progesterone. *J. Steroid Biochem.*, **23**, 517—22.

Davidson F.F., Dennis E.A., Powell M. & Glenney J.R. Jr (1987) Inhibition of phospholipase A_2 by lipocortins and calpactins. An effect of binding to substrate phospholipids. *J. Biol. Chem.*, **262**, 1698—705.

Dawood M.Y. (1983) Neurohypophyseal hormones. In *Endocrinology of Pregnancy* (Ed. by F. Fuchs & A. Klopper), pp. 204—28. Harper & Row, Philadelphia.

Dawood M.Y., Ylikorkala O., Trivedi D. & Fuchs F. (1979) Oxytocin in maternal circulation and amniotic fluid during pregnancy. *J. Clin. Endocrinol. Metab.*, **49**, 429—34.

Demarest K.T., Hahn D.W., Fuchs A.-R. & McGuire J.L. (1987) ORF 22164, an oxytocin antagonist, in animal models of uterine contractility and preterm labor. *Abstr. Soc. Gynecol. Invest.*, p. 28.

Demopoulos C.A., Pinckard R.N. & Hanahan D.J. (1979) Platelet activating factor. *J. Biol. Chem.*, **254**, 9355—8.

DeVane G.W. (1985) Vasopressin levels during pregnancy and labor. *J. Reprod. Med.*, **30**, 324−7.

DeVane G.A. & Porter J.C. (1980) An apparent stress-induced release of arginine vasopressin by human neonates. *J. Clin. Endocrinol. Metab.*, **51**, 1412−16.

Diczfalusy E., Tillinger K.-G., Wiqvist N. *et al.* (1963) Disposition of intra-amniotically administered estriol-16-C^{14} and estrone-16-C^{14} sulfate by women. *J. Clin. Endocrinol. Metab.*, **23**, 503−13.

Di Renzo G.C., Johnston J.M., Okazaki T. *et al.* (1981) Phosphatidylinositol-specific phospholipase C in fetal membranes and uterine decidua. *J. Clin Invest.*, **67**, 847−56.

Di Renzo G.C., Venincasa M.D. & Bleasdale J.E. (1984a) The identification and characterization of β-adrenergic receptors in human amnion tissue. *Am. J. Obstet. Gynecol.*, **148**, 398−405.

Di Renzo G.C., Anceschi M.M. & Bleasdale J.E. (1984b) Beta-adrenergic stimulation of prostaglandin production by human amnion tissue. *Prostaglandins*, **27**, 37−49.

Divers W.A., Wilkes M.M., Babaknia A. & Yen S.S. (1981) An increase in catecholamines and metabolites in the amniotic fluid compartment from middle to late gestation. *Am. J. Obstet. Gynecol.*, **139**, 483−6.

Elsner C.W., Buster J.E., Preston D.L. & Killam A.P. (1979) Interrelationships of circulating maternal steroid concentrations in third trimester pregnancies. III. Effect of intravenous cortisol infusion on maternal concentrations of estriol, 16α-hydroxyprogesterone, 20α-dihydroxyprogesterone, $\triangle^5$-pregnenolone, $\triangle^5$-pregnenolone sulfate, dehydroepiandrosterone sulfate and cortisol. *J. Clin. Endocrinol. Metab.*, **49**, 30−3.

Embrey M.P. & Moir J.C. (1967) A comparison of the oxytocic effects of synthetic vasopressin and oxytocin. *J. Obstet. Gynecol. Br. Commonw.*, **74**, 648−52.

Endo M. & Yosizawa Z. (1973) Hormonal effect on glycoproteins and glycosaminoglycans in rabbit uteri. *Arch. Biochem. Biophys.*, **156**, 397−403.

Fields P.A., Eldridge R.K., Fuchs A.-R. *et al.* (1983) Human placental and bovine luteal oxytocin. *Endocrinology*, **112**, 1544−6.

Flower R.J., Wood J.N. & Parente L. (1984) Macrocortin and the mechanism of action of the glucocorticoids. *Adv. Inflammation Res.*, **7**, 61−9.

France J.T., Seddon R.J. & Liggins G.C. (1973) A study of a pregnancy with low estrogen production due to placental sulfatase deficiency. *J. Clin. Endocrinol. Metab.*, **36**, 1−9.

Fraser D.R. (1980) Regulation of the metabolism of vitamin D. *Physiol. Rev.*, **60**, 551−613.

Fuchs A.R. (1978) Hormonal control of myometrial function during pregnancy and parturition. *Acta Endocrinol. Suppl.*, **221**, 1−69.

Fuchs A.R. & Fuchs F. (1984a) Endocrinology of human parturition: a review. *Br. J. Obstet. Gynaecol.*, **91**, 948−67.

Fuchs A.R. & Fuchs F. (1984b) Endocrinology of term and preterm labor. In *Preterm Birth* (Ed. by F. Fuchs & P.G. Stubblefield), pp. 39−63. Macmillan, London.

Fuchs A.-R., Fuchs F., Husslein P. *et al.* (1982) Oxytocin receptors and human parturition: a dual role for oxytocin in the initiation of labor. *Science*, **215**, 1396−8.

Fuchs A.-R., Goeschen K., Husslein P. *et al.* (1983a) Oxytocin and the initiation of human parturition. III. Plasma concentrations of oxytocin and 13,14-dihydro-15-keto-prostaglandin $F_2\alpha$ in spontaneous and oxytocin-induced labor at term. *Am. J. Obstet. Gynecol.*, **147**, 497−502.

Fuchs A.-R., Periyasami S., Alexandrova M. & Soloff M.S. (1983b) Correlation between oxytocin receptor concentration and responsiveness to oxytocin in pregnant rat myometrium: effect of ovarian studies. *Endocrinology*, **113**, 742−9.

Fuchs F. (1983) Endocrinology of parturition. In *Endocrinology of Pregnancy* (Ed. by F. Fuchs & A. Klopper), pp. 247−70. Harper & Row, Philadelphia.

Fuchs F. & Stakemann G. (1960) Treatment of threatened premature labor with large doses of progesterone. *Am. J. Obstet. Gynecol.*, **79**, 172−6.

Garfield R.E., Baulieu E.E. & Gasc J.M. (1987) Effects of the antiprogesterone RU 486 on preterm birth in the rat. *Abstr. Soc. Gynecol. Invest.*, p. 37.

Gibb W., Lavoie J.-C. & Roux J.F. (1978) 3-β-Hydroxysteroid dehydrogenase activity in human fetal membranes. *Steroids*, **32**, 365−72.

Gillespie A. & Beazley I. (1972) Prostaglandin−oxytocin enhancement and potentiation, and their clinical application. *Br. Med. J.*, **1**, 150−2.

Glickman J.A. & Challis J.R.G. (1980) The changing response pattern of sheep fetal adrenal cells throughout the course of gestation. *Endocrinology.*, **106**, 1371−6.

Golander A., Hurley T., Barrett J. & Handwerger S. (1979) Synthesis of prolactin by human decidua *in vitro. J. Endocrinol.*, **82**, 263−7.

Golichowski A.M. (1986) Biochemical basis of cervical maturation. In *The Physiology and Biochemistry of the Uterus in Pregnancy and Labor* (Ed. by G. Huszar), pp. 261−80. CRC Press, Boca Raton, FL.

Gurpide E., Markiewicz L., Schatz F. & Hirata F. (1986). Lipocortin output by human endometrium *in vitro. J. Clin. Endocrinol. Metab.*, **63**, 162−6.

Gustavii B. (1972) Labour: a delayed menstruation? *Lancet*, **ii**, 1149−50.

Guzick D.S. & Winn K. (1985) The association of chorioamnionitis with preterm delivery. *Obstet. Gynecol.*, **65**, 11−16.

Hamberg M. (1974) Quantitative studies on prostaglandin synthesis in man. III. Excretion of the major urinary metabolites of prostaglandins $F_1\alpha$ and $F_2\alpha$ during pregnancy. *Life Sci.*, **14**, 247−52.

Hillier K. & Wallis R. (1981) Prostaglandins, steroids and the human cervix. In *The Cervix in Pregnancy and Labour* (Ed. by D.A. Ellwood & A.B.M. Anderson), pp. 34−40. Churchill-Livingstone, Edinburgh.

Hirata F. (1981) The regulation of lipomodulin, a phospholipase inhibitory protein, in rabbit neutrophils by phosphorylation. *J. Biol. Chem.*, **256**, 7730−3.

Hoffman D.R., Truong C.T. & Johnston J.M. (1986a) The role of platelet-activating factor in human fetal lung maturation. *Am. J. Obstet. Gynecol.*, **150**, 70−5.

Hoffman D.R., Truong C.T. & Johnston J.M. (1986b) Metabolism and function of platelet-activating factor in fetal rabbit lung development. *Biochim. Biophys. Acta*, **879**, 88−96.

Holm L.W. (1967) Prolonged pregnancy. *Adv. Vet. Sci. Comp. Med.*, **11**, 159−205.

Honnebier W.J. & Swaab D.F. (1973) The influence of anencephaly upon intrauterine growth of fetus and placenta and upon gestation length. *J. Obstet. Gynaecol. Br. Commonw.*, **80**, 577−88.

Hoppenstein J.M., Miltenberger F.W. & Moran W.H. Jr (1968) The increase in blood levels of vasopressin in infants during birth and surgical procedures. *Surg. Gynecol. Obstet.*, **127**, 966−74.

Husslein P., Fuchs A.-R. & Fuchs F. (1981) Oxytocin and the initiation of human parturition. I. Prostaglandin release during induction of labor by oxytocin. *Am. J. Obstet. Gynecol.*, **141**, 688−93.

Huszar G. & Naftolin F. (1984) The myometrium and uterine cervix in normal and preterm labor. *N. Engl. J. Med.*, **311**, 571−81.

Johnston J.M., Bleasdale J.E. & Hoffman D.R. (1987) Functions of PAF in reproduction and development: involvement of PAF in fetal lung maturation and parturition. In *Platelet-activating Factor and Related Lipid Mediators* (Ed. by F. Snyder), pp. 375−402. Plenum Press. New York.

Jolivet A. & Gautray J.P. (1978) Liquide amniotique: aspects hormonaux de la maturation foetale et du déclenchement du travail. In *Endocrinologie Prénatale et Parturition* (Ed. by L. Cédard & C. Sureau), pp. 111−20. INSERM, Paris.

Jung H. (1963) Die Wirkung der ovarial- und der placentar Hormone. In *Pharmacology of Smooth Muscle* (Ed. by E. Bülbring), pp. 113−26. Pergamon Press, Oxford.

Karim S.M.M. (1966) The identification of prostaglandins in human amniotic fluid. *J. Obstet. Gynaecol. Br. Commonw.*, **73**; 903−8.

Karim S.M.M. & Devlin J. (1967) Prostaglandin content of amniotic fluid during pregnancy and labour. *J. Obstet. Gynaecol Br. Commonw.*, **74**, 230–4.

Karim S.M.M. & Filshie G.M. (1970) Therapeutic abortion using prostaglandin F$_2\alpha$. *Lancet*, **i**, 157–9.

Karim S.M.M., Trussell R.R., Patel R.C. & Hillier K. (1968) Response of pregnant human uterus to prostaglandin F$_2\alpha$-induction of labour. *Br. Med. J.*, **4**, 621–3.

Keirse M.J.N.C. (1978) Biosynthesis and metabolism of prostaglandins in the pregnant human uterus. In *Advances in Prostaglandin Thromboxane Research*, vol. 4 (Ed. by F. Coceani & P.M. Olley), pp. 87–102. Raven Press, New York.

Keirse M.J.N.C. (1979) Endogenous prostaglandins in human parturition. In *Human Parturition* (Ed. by M.J.N.C. Kierse, A.B.M. Anderson & J. Bennebroek Gravenhorst), pp. 101–42. Nijhoff, The Hague.

Keirse M.J.N.C., Hicks B.R., Mitchell M.D. & Turnbull A.C. (1977a) Increase of the prostaglandin precursor, arachidonic acid, in amniotic fluid during spontaneous labour. *Br. J. Obstet. Gynaecol.*, **84**, 937–40.

Keirse M.J.N.C., Mitchell M.D. & Turnbull A.C. (1977b) Changes in prostaglandin F and 13,14-dihydro-15-keto-prostaglandin F concentrations in amniotic fluid at the onset of and during labor. *Br. J. Obstet. Gynaecol.*, **8**, 743–6.

Keirse M.J.N.C., Hicks B.R. & Kendall J.Z. (1978) Comparison of intrauterine prostaglandin metabolism during pregnancy in man, sheep, and guinea pig. *Eur. J. Obstet. Gynaecol. Reprod. Biol.*, **8**, 195–203.

Kennedy P.C., Kendrick J.W. & Stormont C. (1957) Adenohypophyseal aplasia, an inherited defect associated with abnormal gestation in Guernsey cattle. *Cornell Vet.*, **47**, 160–78.

Khanna N.C., Tokuda M. & Waisman D.M. (1986) Phosphorylation of lipocortins *in vitro* by protein kinase C. *Biochem. Biophys. Res. Commun.*, **141**, 547–54.

Kirshon B., Moise K.J. Jr & Wasserstrum N. (1987) Prostaglandins play a major role in controlling urinary output in the human fetus. *Abstr. Soc. Gynecol. Invest.*, p. 140.

Kitterman J.A., Liggins G.C., Fewell J.E. *et al.* (1983) Inhibition of breathing movements in fetal sheep by prostaglandins. *J. Appl. Physiol. Resp. Erw. Exer. Physiol.*, **54**, 687–92.

Kurzrok R. & Lieb C.C. (1930) Biochemical studies of human semen. II. The action of semen on the human uterus. *Proc. Soc. Exp. Biol. Med.*, **28**, 268–72.

Lands W.E.M. & Samuelsson B. (1968) Phospholipid precursors of prostaglandins. *Biochim. Biophys. Acta*, **164**, 426–9.

Lanman J.T., Herod L. & Thau R. (1974) Phospholipids and fatty acids in relation to the premature induction of labor in rabbits. *Pediatr. Res.*, **8**, 1–4.

Lazebnik R., Eisenberg Z., Lazebnik N. *et al.* (1983) Vitamin D metabolites in amniotic fluid. *J. Clin. Endocrinol. Metab.*, **56**, 632–4.

Lee T.-C., Malone B., Blank M.L. & Snyder F. (1981) 1-Alkyl-2-acetyl-*sn*-glycero-3-phosphocholine (platelet activating factor) stimulates calcium influx in rabbit platelets. *Biochem. Biophys. Res. Commun.*, **120**, 834–9.

Lehmann W.D. (1974) The influence of prostaglandins and beta-mimetic substances on the aromatization rate in human placentas. *Arch. Gynaekol.*, **217**, 251–61.

Lewis R.B. & Schulman J.D. (1973) Influence of acetylsalicylic acid, an inhibitor of prostaglandin synthesis, on the duration of human gestation and labour. *Lancet*, **ii**, 1159–61.

Liggins G.C. (1969a) The foetal role in the initiation of parturition in the ewe. In *Foetal Anatomy* (Ed. by G.E.W. Wolstenholme & M. O'Connor), pp. 218–31. Churchill Livingstone, London.

Liggins G.C. (1969b) Premature delivery of fetal lambs infused with glucocorticoids. *J. Endocrinol.*, **45**, 515–23.

Liggins G.C. (1976) Adrenocortical-related maturational events in the fetus. *Am. J. Obstet. Gynecol.*, **126**, 931–41.

Liggins G.C. (1983) Initiation of spontaneous labor. *Clin. Obstet. Gynecol.*, **26**, 47−55.

Liggins G.C. & Grieves S.A. (1971) Possible role for prostaglandin F₂α in parturition in sheep. *Nature*, **232**, 629−31.

Liggins G.C., Kennedy P.C. & Holm L.W. (1967) Failure of initiation of parturition after electrocoagulation of the pituitary of the fetal lamb. *Am. J. Obstet. Gynecol.*, **98**, 1080−6.

Liggins G.C., Fairclough R.J., Grieves S.A. *et al.* (1977a) Parturition in sheep. In *The Fetus and Birth* (Ed. by J. Knight & M. O'Connor), pp. 5−25. Elsevier, Amsterdam.

Liggins G.C., Forster C.S., Grieves S.A. & Schwartz A.L. (1977b) Control of parturition in man. *Biol. Reprod.*, **16**, 39−56.

Luukkainen T.U. & Csapo A.I. (1963) Induction of premature labor in the rabbit after pretreatment with phospholipids. *Fertil. Steril.*, **14**, 65−72.

Lytton F.D. & Mitchell M.D. (1988) Phorbol ester-induced stimulation of prostaglandin biosynthesis in human amnion cells. *Biochim. Biophys. Acta*, **959**, 399−401.

McCoshen J.A. (1987) Influence of gestational diabetes on prolactin activity in the amniotic fluid. *Abstr. Soc. Gynecol. Invest.*, p. 244.

McCoshen J.A., Tagger O.Y., Wodzicki A. & Tyson J.E. (1982) Choriodecidual adhesion promotes decidual prolactin transport by human fetal membrane. *Am. J. Physiol.*, **243**, R552−R557.

McCoshen J.A., Johnson K.A., Dubin N.H. & Ghodgaonkar R.B. (1987) Prostaglandin E₂ release on the fetal and maternal sides of the amnion and chorion−decidua before and after term labor. *Am. J. Obstet. Gynecol.*, **156**, 173−8.

MacDonald P.C. (1984) Physiology of labor. In *Williams Obstetrics*, 17th edn (Ed. by J. Pritchard, P.C. MacDonald & N. Gant), pp. 295−321. Appleton-Crofts, Norwalk, CT.

MacDonald P.C. & Porter J.C. (Eds) (1983) *Initiation of Parturition: Prevention of Prematurity*, p. 16. Ross Laboratories, Columbus, OH.

MacDonald P.C., Schultz F.M., Duenhoelter J.H. *et al.* (1974) Initiation of human parturition. I. Mechanism of action of arachidonic acid. *Obstet. Gynecol.*, **44**, 629−36.

MacDonald P.C., Porter J.C., Schwarz B.E. & Johnston J.M. (1978) Initiation of parturition in the human female. *Semin. Perinatol.*, **2**, 273−86.

MacKenzie I.Z., MacLean D.A. & Mitchell M.D. (1980) Prostaglandins in the human fetal circulation in mid-trimester and term pregnancy. *Prostaglandins*, **20**, 649−54.

Manabe Y. & Sagawa N. (1983) Changes in the mechanical forces of cervical distension before and after rupture of the membranes. *Am. J. Obstet. Gynecol.*, **147**, 667−71.

Manabe Y., Okazaki T. & Takahashi A. (1983) Prostaglandins E and F in amniotic fluid during stretch-induced cervical softening and labor at term. *Gynecol. Obstet. Invest.*, **15**, 343−50.

Mati J.K.G., Horrobin D.F. & Bramley P.S. (1973) Induction of labour in sheep and in humans by single doses of corticosteroids. *Br. Med. J.*, **2**, 149−51.

Mercado-Simmen R.C., Bryant-Greenwood G.D. & Greenwood F.C. (1982) Relaxin receptor in the rat myometrium: regulation by estrogen and relaxin. *Endrocrinology*, **110**, 220−6.

Mitchell M.D. (1986) Pathways of arachidonic acid metabolism with specific application to the fetus and mother. *Semin. Perinatol.*, **10**, 242−54.

Mitchell M.D. (1987) Epidermal growth factor actions on arachidonic acid metabolism in human amnion cells. *Biochim. Biophys. Acta*, **928**, 240−2.

Mitchell M.D., Flint A.P.F., Bibby J. *et al.* (1977) Rapid increases in plasma prostaglandin concentrations after vaginal examination and amniotomy. *Br. Med. J.*, **2**, 1183−5.

Mitchell M.D., Bibby J., Hicks B.R. & Turnbull A.C. (1978a) Specific production of prostaglandin E by human amnion *in vitro*. *Prostaglandins*, **15**, 377−82.

Mitchell M.D., Flint A.P.F., Bibby J. *et al.* (1978b) Plasma concentrations of prostaglandins during late human pregnancy: influence of normal and pre-term labor. *J. Clin Endocrinol. Metab.*, **46**, 947−51.

Mitchell M.D., Ebenhack K., Kraemer D.L. *et al.* (1982) A sensitive radioimmunoassay for

11-deoxy-13,14-dihydro-15-keto-11,16-cyclo-prostaglandin E_2: application as an index of prostaglandin E_2 biosynthesis during human pregnancy and parturition. *Prostaglandins Leukotrienes Med.*, **9**, 549−57.

Mitchell M.D., Lytton F.D. & Varticovski L. (1988) Paradoxical stimulation of both lipocortin and prostaglandin production in human amnion cells by dexamethasone. *Biochem. Biophys. Res. Commun.*, **151**, 137−41.

Mochizuki M. & Tojo S. (1980) Effect of dehydroepiandrosterone sulfate on softening and dilatation of the uterine cervix in pregnant women. In *Dilatation of the Uterine Cervix Connective Tissue: Biology and Clinical Management* (Ed. by F. Naftolin & P.G. Stubblefield), pp. 267−86. Raven Press, New York.

Moonen P., Klok G. & Keirse M.J.N.C. (1984) Increase in concentrations of prostaglandin endoperoxide synthase and prostacyclin synthase in human myometrium in late pregnancy. *Prostaglandins*, **28**, 309−21.

Morizaki N., Morizaki J., Hayashi R.H. & Garfield R.E. (1987) Functional and structural study of the innervation of human myometrium. *Abstr. Soc. Gynecol. Invest.*, p. 184.

Murphy B.E.P. (1980) Mechanism of the initiation of labour—a new hypothesis. *Endocrinology*, **106**, Suppl. Abstr. 72.

Murphy B.E.P., Clark S.J., Donald I.R. *et al.* (1974) Conversion of maternal cortisol to cortisone during placental transfer to the human fetus. *Am. J. Obstet. Gynecol.*, **118**, 538−41.

Nakla S., Skinner K., Mitchell B.F. & Challis J.R.G. (1986) Changes in prostaglandin transfer across human fetal membranes obtained after spontaneous labor. *Am. J. Obstet. Gynecol.*, **155**, 1337−41.

Nathanielsz P.W., Abel M. & Smith G.W. (1973) Hormonal factors in parturition in the rabbit. In *Foetal and Neonatal Physiology* (Ed. by K.S. Comline, K.W. Cross & G.S. Dawes), pp. 594−601. Cambridge University Press, Cambridge.

Niesert S., Christopherson W., Korte K. *et al.* (1986a) Prostaglandin E_2 9-ketoreductase activity in human decidua vera tissue. *Am. J. Obstet. Gynecol.*, **155**, 1348−52.

Niesert S., Mitchell M.D., MacDonald P.C. & Casey M.L. (1986b) The effect of fetal urine on arachidonic acid metabolism in human amnion cells in monolayer culture. *Am. J. Obstet. Gynecol.*, **155**, 1310−16.

Nishihira J., Ishibashi T., Mai Y. & Muramatsu T. (1984) Mass spectrometric evidence for the presence of platelet activating factor (1-0-alkyl-2-acetyl-*sn*-glycero-3-phosphocholine) in human amniotic fluid during labor. *Lipids*, **19**, 907−10.

Nishizuka Y. (1984) The role of protein kinase C in cell surface signal transduction and tumor promotion. *Nature*, **308**, 693−8.

Nissenson R., Flouret G. & Hechter O. (1978) Opposing effects of estradiol and progesterone on oxytocin receptors in rabbit uterus. *Proc. Natl. Acad. Sci. USA*, **75**, 2044−8.

Novy M.J. & Liggins G.C. (1980) Role of prostaglandins, prostacyclin, and thromboxanes in the physiologic control of the uterus and in parturition. *Semin. Perinatol.*, **4**, 45−66.

O'Donohoe N.V. & Holland P.D.J. (1968) Familial congenital adrenal hypoplasia. *Arch. Dis. Child.*, **43**, 717−23.

Okazaki T., Okita J.R., MacDonald P.C. & Johnston J.M. (1978) Initiation of human parturition: X. Substrate specificity of phospholipase A_2 in human fetal membranes. *Am. J. Obstet. Gynecol.*, **130**, 432−8.

Okazaki T., Casey M.L., Okita J.R. *et al.* (1981a) Initiation of human parturition: XII. Biosynthesis and metabolism of prostaglandins in human fetal membranes and uterine decidua. *Am. J. Obstet. Gynecol.*, **139**, 373−81.

Okazaki T., Sagawa N., Okita J.R. *et al.* (1981b) Diacylglycerol metabolism and arachidonic acid release in human fetal membranes and decidua vera. *J. Biol. Chem.*, **256**, 7316−21.

Okazaki T., Sagawa N., Bleasdale J.E. *et al.* (1981c) Initiation of parturition: XIII. Phospholipase C, phospholipase A_2, and diacylglycerol lipase activities in fetal membranes and decidua vera tissues from early and late gestation. *Biol. Reprod.*, **25**, 103−9.

Okita J.R., MacDonald P.C. & Johnston J.M. (1982a) Mobilization of arachidonic acid from specific glycerophospholipids of human fetal membranes during early labor. *J. Biol. Chem.*, **257**, 14029−34.

Okita J.R., MacDonald P.C. & Johnston J.M. (1982b) Initiation of parturition: XIV. Increase in the diacylglycerol content of amnion during parturition. *Am. J. Obstet. Gynecol.*, **142**, 432−5.

Olson D.M., Opavsky M.A. & Challis J.R.G. (1983a) Prostaglandin synthesis by human amnion is dependent upon extracellular calcium. *Can. J. Physiol. Pharmacol.*, **61**, 1089−92.

Olson D.M., Skinner K. & Challis J.R.G. (1983b) Estradiol-17β and 2-hydroxyestradiol-17β-induced differential production of prostaglandins by cells dispersed from human intrauterine tissues at parturition. *Prostaglandins*, **25**, 639−51.

Olson D.M., Skinner K. & Challis J.R.G. (1983c) Prostaglandin output in relation to parturition by cells dispersed from human intrauterine tissues. *J. Clin Endocrinol. Metab.*, **57**, 694−9.

Ovlisen B. & Iversen J. (1963) Treatment of threatened premature labor with 6α-methyl-17α-acetoprogesterone. *Am. J. Obstet. Gynecol.*, **86**, 291−5.

Parker C.R. Jr, Leveno K.J., Carr B.R. *et al.* (1982) Umbilical cord plasma levels of dehydroepiandrosterone sulfate during human gestation. *J. Clin. Endocrinol. Metab.*, **54**, 1216−20.

Pepinsky R.B. & Sinclair L.K. (1986) Epidermal growth factor-dependent phosphorylation of lipocortin. *Nature*, **321**, 81−4.

Philippe M. (1983) Fetal catecholamines. *Am. J. Obstet. Gynecol.*, **146**, 840−55.

Philippe M. & Ryan K.J. (1981) Catecholamines in human amniotic fluid. *Am. J. Obstet. Gynecol.*, **146**, 840−55.

Posner B.I., Kelly P.A., Shiu R.P.C. & Friesen H.G. (1974) Studies of insulin, growth hormone, and prolactin binding: tissue distribution, species variation and characterization. *Endocrinology*, **95**, 521−31.

Price H.V., Cone B.A. & Keogh M. (1971) Length of gestation in congenital adrenal hyperplasia. *J. Obstet. Gynaecol. Br. Commonw.*, **78**, 430−4.

Ratten G.J., Beischer N.A. & Fortune D.W. (1973) Obstetric complications when the fetus has Potter's syndrome. I. Clinical considerations. *Am. J. Obstet. Gynecol.*, **115**, 890−6.

Roberts J.M., Insel P.A. & Goldfien A. (1981) Regulation of myometrial adrenoreceptors and adrenergic response by sex steroids. *Mol. Pharmacol.*, **20**, 52−8.

Romero R., Wan M., Hobbins J.C., & Mitchell M.D. (1987a) Amniotic fluid levels of lipoxygenase products are increased during spontaneous human labor. *Abstr. Soc. Gynecol. Invest.*, p. 134.

Romero R., Wu Y.K., Hobbins J.C. & Mitchell M.D. (1987b) Is there a role for epidermal growth factor in the onset of labor? *Abstr. Soc. Gynecol. Invest.*, p. 134.

Saarikoski S. (1974) Fate of noradrenaline in the human foetoplacental unit. *Acta Physiol. Scand. Suppl.*, **421**, 1−82.

Saeed S.A., Strickland D.M., Young D.C. *et al.* (1982) Inhibition of prostaglandin synthesis by human amniotic fluid: acute reduction in inhibitory activity of amniotic fluid obtained during labor. *J. Clin. Endocrinol. Metab.*, **55**, 801−3.

Sagawa N., Bleasdale J.E. & Di Renzo G.C. (1983) The effects of polyamines and aminoglycosides on phosphatidylinositol-specific phospholipase C from human amnion. *Biochim. Biophys. Acta*, **752**, 153−61.

Sanborn B.M. (1986) The role of relaxin in uterine function. In *The Physiology and Biochemistry of the Uterus in Pregnancy and Labor* (Ed. by G. Huszar), pp. 225−38. CRC Press, Boca Raton, FL.

Sanborn B.M., Heindel J.J. & Robinson G.A. (1980) The role of cyclic nucleotides in reproductive processes. *Annu. Rev. Physiol.*, **42**, 37−57.

Schatz F., Markiewicz L. & Gurpide E. (1984) Effects of estriol on PGF₂α output by cultures of human endometrium and endometrial cells. *J. Steroid Biochem.*, **20**, 999–1003.

Schatz F., Markiewicz L., Barg P. & Gurpide E. (1985) *In vitro* effects of ovarian steroids on prostaglandin $F_2\alpha$ output by human endometrium and endometrial epithelial cells. *J. Clin. Endocrinol. Metab.*, **61**, 361–7.

Schwarz B.E., Milewich L., Gant N.F. *et al.* (1977) Progesterone binding and metabolism in human fetal membranes. *Ann. NY Acad. Sci.*, **286**, 304–10.

Shaughnessy E.A., Khan-Dawood F.S. & Dawood M.Y. (1983) *In vitro* conversion of pregnenolone to progesterone, progesterone receptors and hormone levels in term human placenta and fetal membranes. *Clin. Res.*, **31**, 817A.

Siiteri P.K. & MacDonald P.C. (1966) Placental estrogen biosynthesis during human pregnancy. *J. Clin. Endocrinol. Metab.*, **26**, 751–61.

Siiteri P.K. & Séron-Ferré M. (1981) Some new thoughts on fetoplacental unit and parturition in primates. In *Fetal Endocrinology* (Ed. by M.J. Novy & J.A. Resko), pp. 1–19. Academic Press, New York.

Skinner K.A. & Challis J.R.G. (1985) Changes in the synthesis and metabolism of prostaglandins by human fetal membranes and decidua at labor. *Am. J. Obstet. Gynecol.*, **151**, 519–23.

Soloff M.S. (1975) Uterine receptor for oxytocin: effects of estrogen. *Biochem. Biophys. Res. Commun.*, **65**, 205–12.

Steele P.A., Flint A.P.F. & Turnbull A.C. (1976) Activity of steroid C-17,20 lyase in the ovine placenta: effect of exposure to foetal glucocorticoid. *J. Endocrinol.*, **69**, 239–46.

Strickland D.M., Kraemer D.L. & Mitchell M.D. (1982) Production of prostaglandins by human intrauterine tissues: influence of oxytocin. *IRCS Med. Sci.*, **10**, 102–3.

Strickland D.M., Saeed S.A., Casey M.L. & Mitchell M.D. (1983) Stimulation of prostaglandin biosynthesis by urine of the human fetus may serve as a trigger for parturition. *Science*, **220**, 521–2.

Szlachter B.N., Quagliarello J., Jewelewicz R. *et al.* (1982) Relaxin in normal and pathogenic pregnancies. *Obstet. Gynecol.*, **59**, 167–70.

Takahashi H., Murata M. & Maki M. (1988) Phospholipase C activity and phosphatidylinositol in amniotic fluid. *Gynecol. Obstet. Invest.*, **25**, 25–30.

Theobald G.W. (1968) Nervous control of uterine activity. *Clin. Obstet. Gynecol.*, **11**, 15–33.

Thorburn G.D. (1983) Past and present concepts on the initiation of parturition. In *Initiation of Parturition: Prevention of Prematurity* (Ed. by P.C. MacDonald & J.C. Porter), pp. 2–8. Ross Laboratories, Columbus, OH.

Tomasi A., Bangalore S. & Phillippe M. (1987) Myometrial contractile and inositolphosphate response to oxytocin. *Abstr. Soc. Gynecol. Invest.*, p. 213.

Tomita K., McCoshen J.A., Fernandez C.S. & Tyson J.E. (1982) Immunologic and biologic characteristics of human decidua prolactin. *Am. J. Obstet. Gynecol.*, **142**, 420–6.

Tulchinsky D. (1973) Placental secretion of unconjugated estrone, estradiol, and estriol into the maternal and fetal circulation. *J. Clin. Endocrinol. Metab.*, **36**, 1079–87.

Tulchinsky D., Hobel C.J., Yeager E. & Marshall J.R. (1972) Plasma estrone, estradiol, estriol, progesterone and 17-OH-progesterone in human pregnancy. *Am. J. Obstet. Gynecol.*, **112**, 1095–100.

Tuvemo T., Strandberg K. & Hamberg M. (1976) Maintenance of the tone of human umbilical artery by prostaglandin and thromboxane formation. In *Advances in Prostaglandin and Thromboxane Research*, vol. 1 (Ed. by B. Samuelsson & R. Paoletti), pp. 425–8. Raven Press, New York.

Tyson J.E., McCoshen J.A. & Dubin N.H. (1985) Inhibition of fetal membrane prostaglandin production by prolactin: relative importance in the inhibition of labor. *Am. J. Obstet. Gynecol.*, **151**, 1032–8.

Van Lierde M. & Thomas K. (1982) Ritodrine concentrations in maternal and fetal serum and amniotic fluid. *J. Perinat. Med.*, **10**, 119–24.

Verhoeff A. & Garfield R.E. (1986) Ultrastructure of the myometrium and the role of gap junctions in myometrial function. In *The Physiology and Biochemistry of the Uterus in Pregnancy and Labor* (Ed. by G. Huszar), pp. 73–91. CRC Press, Boca Raton, FL.

Von Euler U.S. (1935) Über die spezifische blutdrucksenkende Substanz des menschlichen Prostata- und Samenblasensekretes. *Klin. Wochenschr.*, **14**, 1182–3.

Vonkeman H. & van Dorp D.A. (1968) The action of prostaglandin synthetase on 2-arachidonyl-lecithin. *Biochim. Biophys. Acta*, **164**, 430–2.

Wakeling A.E. & Wyngarden L.J. (1974) Prostaglandin receptors in the human, monkey and hamster uterus. *Endocrinology*, **95**, 55–64.

Walsh S.W., Stanczyk F.Z. & Novy M.J. (1984) Daily hormonal changes in the maternal, fetal and amniotic fluid compartments before parturition in a primate species. *J. Clin. Endocrinol. Metab.*, **58**, 629–39.

Waltman R., Tricomi V. & Palav A.B. (1972) Mid-trimester hypertonic saline-induced abortion: effect of indomethacin on induction/abortion time. *Am. J. Obstet. Gynecol.*, **114**, 829–31.

Ward S.M., Caritis S.N. & Moore J.J. (1987) Dexamethasone reverses beta agonist induced myometrial desensitization. *Abstr. Soc. Gynecol. Invest.*, p. 53.

Weisman Y., Harrell A., Edelstein S. *et al.* (1979) 1α, 25-dihydroxyvitamin D_3 and 24,25-dihydroxyvitamin D_3 *in vitro* synthesis by human decidua and placenta. *Nature*, **281**, 317–21.

Weiss G., O'Byrne M., Hochman J.A. *et al.* (1977) Secretion of progesterone and relaxin by the corpus luteum at midpregnancy and at term. *Obstet. Gynecol.*, **50**, 679–81.

Wendelberger K.J. (1987) Prostaglandin and leukotriene receptors in pulmonary, vascular, and uterine smooth muscle. *Semin. Perinatol.*, **11**, 1–11.

Willcox D.L., Yovich J.L., McColm S.C. and Phillips J.M. (1985) Progesterone, cortisol and estradiol-17β in the initiation of human parturition: partitioning between free and bound hormone in plasma. *Br. J. Obstet. Gynaecol.*, **92**, 65–71.

Wilson T. & Liggins G.C. (1986) Isolation of an inhibitor of phospholipase A_2 from human chorion. *Abstr. Sixth Int'l. Conf. Prostaglandins*, p. 133.

Wilson T., Liggins G.C., Aimer G.P. & Skinner S.J.M. (1985) Partial purification and characterization of two compounds from amniotic fluid which inhibit phospholipase activity in human endometrial cells. *Biochem. Biophys. Res. Commun.*, **131**, 22–9.

Winters A.J., Colston C., MacDonald P.C. & Porter J.C. (1975) Fetal plasma prolactin levels. *J. Clin. Endocrinol. Metab.*, **41**, 626–9.

Wintour E.M., Brown E.H., Denton R.A. *et al.* (1975) The ontogeny and regulation of corticosteroid secretion by the ovine adrenal gland. *Acta Endocrinol.* **79**, 301–316.

Witter F.R. & Niebyl J.R. (1986) Inhibition of arachidonic acid metabolism in the perinatal period: pharmacology, clinical application, and potential adverse effects. *Semin. Perinatol.*, **10**, 316–33.

Ylikorkala O. & Viinikka L. (1980) Thromboxane A_2 in pregnancy and puerperium. *Br. Med. J.*, **281**, 1601–2.

11

Somatic Gene Therapy

D.J. WEATHERALL

The advent of recombinant DNA technology, with its potential for providing unlimited quantities of cloned genes, has raised the expectation that within a few years if may be possible to replace defective genes in patients with inherited diseases. While this may turn out to be the case for at least a few of these conditions, and much progress has been made in the study of gene transfer, there is still a long way to go before gene therapy becomes part of routine clinical practice.

In this short review I shall consider current research directed towards the development of gene therapy. But before discussing this complex problem it might be helpful to outline the structure of normal genes and what is known about their regulation. This topic will not be considered in detail and readers who wish to learn more about recombinant DNA technology in general, and gene regulation in particular, are referred to several monographs and reviews written for the non-specialist (Watson *et al.* 1983; Emery 1984; Weatherall 1985).

Normal gene structure and regulation

The products of genes are peptide chains. The information that directs the order of amino acids in peptide chains is contained in DNA in the order of bases in its two homologous strands. It is stored as a triplet code, i.e. three bases constitute the codeword for a particular amino acid. The latter do not interact directly with DNA, which stays in the cell nucleus directing operations. When a gene is to be transcribed one of its strands is copied by an enzyme called RNA polymerase into a mirror image molecule called messenger RNA which travels from the nucleus to the cytoplasm where it acts as a template on which peptide chains are synthesized. Amino acids are brought to the appropriate place on messenger RNA by molecules called transfer RNAs, each of which has three nucleotides, called anticodons, that find their appropriate partners on the messenger RNA. In this way amino acids are put together in the correct order as directed by the sequence of messenger RNA bases. This is not a random process but starts at one end of the messenger RNA and proceeds sequentially to the other. The growing chains, together with transfer RNAs, are held together in an appropriate steric arrangement on the messenger RNA by the ribosomal subunits. The messenger RNA has codons to indicate where to start and terminate chain synthesis.

Thus the flow of genetic information from nucleus to cytoplasm can be represented as transcription → translation → peptide chain (Fig. 11.1).

Gene structure and function

The structure of a typical mammalian gene and the way in which its primary transcript is modified and transported to the cell cytoplasm to act as a template for protein synthesis is summarized in Fig. 11.1. Most mammalian genes consist of coding regions, or exons, and non-coding inserts called intervening sequences (IVS) or introns. Comparisons of the sequences of introns from many different genes reveal only a few common features, most notably in those immediately adjacent to and around the coding sequences that they interrupt, and a sequence 20–40 bases from the 3' end, which is probably involved in the formation of a branched splicing intermediate. In every case the dinucleotides GT and AG are found at the 5' and 3' intron/exon junctions respectively. As we shall see later, these sequences, and the sequences that immediately surround them, are critical for the correct excision of introns and splicing of exons during the processing of messenger RNA.

The regions flanking the coding sequences contain a number of conserved sequences that are necessary for correct expression of the genes (Fig. 11.1). The first is the ATA box, which serves to locate the site of transcription initiation at the so-called CAP site (see below), usually about 30 bases downstream, and which also appears to influence the level of transcription. Seventy or 80 base pairs upstream, there is a second conserved sequence, the CCAAT box; this is also involved in regulating the rate of transcription. Finally, approximately 80–100 base pairs from the CAP site, there is a GC-rich region with the general structure GGGGTG or CACCCC, which can also appear in an inverted orientation and which may be duplicated. Again these sequences are thought to be involved in the optimal transcription of structural genes. There is another highly conserved sequence at the 3' end of all mammalian

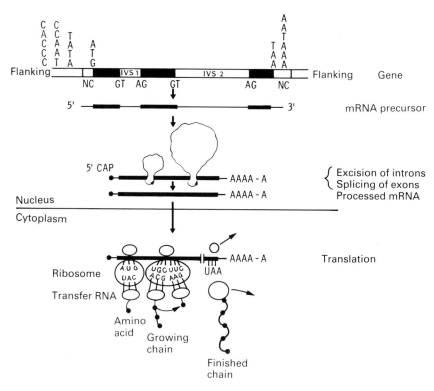

Fig. 11.1. The genetic control of protein synthesis (see text).

genes, AATAAA, which is the signal site for polyadenylation of messenger RNA (see below).

When a structural gene is transcribed, the entire sequence is copied to form a long primary transcript that contains both intron and exon sequences. While in the nucleus, this large messenger RNA precursor molecule undergoes considerable modification. The introns are cut out and the exons spliced together in a complex two-stage process. First, the precursor is cut at the 5′ splice site to generate two intermediates, a linear first exon and a branched lariat-form containing the intron and second exon. In the second step, the 3′ splice site is cleaved, the lariat intron released, and the two exons spliced together. In this way, the introns are removed in a sequential manner until the mature messenger RNA is produced. In addition, there is a chemical modification of the 5′ end of the messenger RNA, so-called capping, and the 3′ end is also processed by the addition of a string of A residues (Fig. 11.1).

The processed messenger RNA is now transported from the nucleus to the cytoplasm, where it acts as a template for peptide chain synthesis. This involves interaction of the ribosomes, the transfer RNAs and the initiation codon with the formation of an initiation complex. Amino acids are added sequentially to a growing peptide chain until the ribosomes reach the termination codon, at which time the completed chain is released and the ribosomes recycled for further protein synthesis. These steps are shown diagrammatically in Fig. 11.1.

Regulation

One of the main difficulties in developing gene therapy is that so little is known about how mammalian genes are regulated. Mechanisms must exist that ensure that genes are switched on in the right tissues at the appropriate stage of development and that, once activated, they are transcribed at an appropriate rate. Some genes only function at specific developmental stages and many require very precise setting of their rates of transcription. Others, so-called housekeeping genes, are transcribed at a fairly constant rate in most cells and at all phases of development. Furthermore, in understanding how a gene is regulated, we have to consider not only the control of the gene itself but also how its activity is coordinated with other batteries of genes, the concerted expression of which is required for a variety of cellular functions.

We have already seen that conserved sequences at the 5′ end of all mammalian genes are involved in setting their rates of transcription. These include the ATA box and the so-called upstream promoter elements (UPEs). Taken together, these sequences are involved in defining the rates of transcription of their structural genes. Their importance in this role in human gene regulation is reflected by the finding that single base mutations in these regions, such as those found in some forms of thalassaemia, can drastically reduce the rate of transcription of the associated structural genes.

There is another class of regulatory elements called enhancer sequences (Maniatis *et al.* 1987). Unlike the promoter sequences, these may lie at a considerable distance from their structural genes, although they may become opposed to them by changes in chromosomal configuration. At least some enhancer sequences have been found to be important for tissue specific gene expression. Both UPEs and enhancer sequences can interact with regulatory proteins. It has been found that transcription can be stimulated by interactions between protein bound to both types of regulatory elements, with looping out of the intervening DNA.

Finally, it is clear that genes may be activated or repressed by so-called *trans*-activating factors, that is proteins that are produced at a distance from the structural gene and which are involved in their regulation, presumably by interaction with chromatin.

Genes in cells are not there in the form of simple strands of DNA, but are complexed with histones and other proteins in chromatin. One of the consequences of this sophisticated packaging is that the transcriptional activity of the genes may be quite limited. For example, in erythroid cells only a few per cent of the total DNA sequences are capable of being expressed. Undoubtedly, some of this variability in expression is achieved by major alterations in chromatin structure that can be demonstrated experimentally by increased sensitivity to a variety of nucleases such as DNAse I. There is increased sensitivity to these enzymes affecting a considerable region of DNA surrounding an active gene, which appears to signify that a specific region is capable of being expressed. In addition, there are more specific regions of much higher sensitivity to nucleases that correlate with active transcription. Increased sensitivity to these enzymes appears to be related to the binding of a group of non-histone proteins to active genes. It is also clear that the methylation state of a gene has an important influence on expression; by and large actively transcribed genes are usually hypomethylated, and vice versa. For example, in human tissues globin genes are found to be extensively methylated in non-erythroid organs, and to be relatively undermethylated when they are being expressed in erythroid tissue. Clearly, the conformation of chromatin and the methylation state of DNA are important indicators of the activity of genes. But how these different states are regulated is not known; presumably in some cases they reflect the results of the interaction of DNA with regulatory proteins.

It should be remembered that many genes are activated by external regulatory signals, such as growth factors and hormones. This involves a complex series of interactions in which these molecules bind to and activate specific receptors that generate second messengers, usually cyclic adenosine monophosphate. The latter triggers a chain of intracellular reactions that involve the phosphorylation of effector enzymes by protein kinases. These changes may, in turn, activate a series of genes which have to work as an orchestrated whole to promote normal cellular function. Presumably coordination of this type is mediated through the activity of interactions of *trans* regulatory transcription factors, that is, molecules that act on both pairs of homologous structural genes, although how these activate or repress structural genes is still unknown.

In summary, most mammalian genes have promoter sequences that are involved in regulating their rates of transcription, and enhancer elements that may also be involved in specificity of transcription in particular tissues. They are also controlled by a number of *trans* regulatory molecules. Although changes in gene activity are reflected by alterations in their methylation state and in the configuration of chromatin, there is very little information about how these physical alterations are mediated.

The molecular pathology of single gene disorders

The availability of methods for cloning and sequencing genes from patients with single gene disorders has led to the elucidation of the molecular pathology of a number of these conditions (Caskey 1987; Davies & Robson 1987). In the majority of cases, they result from point mutations that give rise to premature termination codons in exons or an alteration in the reading frame of the genetic code. Others are caused by single base changes that interfere with the processing of messenger RNA. Some diseases are caused by deletions of part or the whole of the particular structural gene. All these molecular defects should be amenable to treatment by gene replacement therapy.

It is becoming apparent, however, that some genetic disorders result from lesions at some distance from structural genes. For example, a form of α-thalassaemia has been described recently in which the structural genes are intact but in which there is a long deletion at a considerable distance from them (Nicholls *et al.* 1987). Quite clearly this type of defect will not be amenable to direct gene replacement and, until we know more about how these 'distant' lesions modify gene expression, it will not be possible to correct them.

Requisites for successful gene transfer

The requisites for successful gene therapy are discussed in detail by Anderson & Fletcher (1980), Anderson (1984) and Weatherall (1985), and will only be outlined here.

In designing a strategy for successful gene transfer, we shall have to overcome a number of technical problems. The first question is how to transfer genes into a foreign cell. As we shall see later, methods for the direct transfer of DNA are relatively inefficient and we may well have to develop specific carriers or vectors to allow us to transfer our genes into a sufficient number of cells. Another important question is: how do we define our target cell? Consider the genetic blood disorders for example.

It would be no good transferring genes into committed erythroid or white cell progenitors since, once in the appropriate differentiation compartment of the marrow, these cells undergo maturation and, after release into the blood, have a limited lifespan. Thus, our target cell would have to be a haemopoietic stem cell that is capable of self-renewal. But these cells only make up a tiny percentage of the total marrow population and hence we would be unable to transfect enough of them unless we were able to develop methods for their isolation. While these problems seem formidable, they pale into insignificance compared with the difficulty of transferring genes into large numbers of cells in a solid organ such as the liver or brain.

And so, even if we are successful in transferring our genes into, say, haemopoietic stem cells, it is unlikely that we are going to transfect more than a small proportion of them. Unfortunately, there is no reason why putting a 'good' gene into these cells would give them any proliferative advantage over their defective fellows, unless the genes are expressed at the stem cell stage of maturation. For example, in the case of the haemoglobin disorders such as sickle cell anaemia or thalassaemia, the genetic defect is only important once stem cells have differentiated into the erythroid compartment; pluripotential cells containing the normal globin genes would have no proliferative advantage over their fellows. Thus, as well as transferring our genes for correcting a genetic defect, we might, at least in some cases, have to try to transfer other genes that could be used for *in vivo* selection of the cells that we had treated. For example, we might incorporate a gene for methotrexate resistance together with the gene that we wish to replace so that we could select for our treated population by the administration of methotrexate.

But the most formidable problems for gene transfer therapy are in regulation. Unless we can direct our genes into precisely the right place in the genome, we do not know whether they will function normally. This brings us back to the questions posed in the introductory section. We know that many genes require enhancer elements for their appropriate expression in the right tissues and that these sequences may be at a considerable distance from the genes that they regulate. And so we must find out exactly how much of the flanking regions of structural genes is required for their regulation, particularly in an inappropriate part of the genome.

The degree to which 'tight' regulation is important may depend on the type of gene that we are trying to replace. For example, the so-called housekeeping genes, which are expressed at a relatively low level in most cells and at all stages of development, will not require as precise control as, say, the globin genes, which must be expressed at appropriate stages of development at a very precisely regulated level.

And, finally, we shall have to determine whether the insertion of foreign genes in any particular regions of the genome will cause deleterious effects on the expression of adjacent genes. Could gene therapy cause inappropriate activation of oncogenes, for example, and result in a malignant phenotype? Or, if we were embarking on gene therapy early in fetal life, could we modify the action of important developmental loci with our inserted genes? And, as will become apparent from the next section, since it may be impossible to insert genes without the use of potentially dangerous carriers such as retroviruses, there is always the possibility that we could produce serious side-effects, including cancer, with our viral vectors.

Potential methods for gene transfer

The transfer of genes into foreign cells may be achieved either directly or using a form of delivery system. In this section, we shall consider the pros and cons of each of the different approaches that have been attempted to date.

Direct insertion

There are a variety of ways in which DNA can be inserted into another cell (Anderson 1984). One of the earliest methods is based on the principle of the uptake of calcium microprecipitates of DNA, which can be used to insert cloned genes. Although very selective, it is relatively inefficient and the rate of stable transfection is probably only about one cell in 10^5. A number of variations on this theme have been attempted, including transfection of cells in suspension or following their treatment with dimethylsulphoxide (DMSO), glycerol, chloroquine or sodium butyrate. Unfortunately, the efficiency of transfection by these techniques varies widely between different cell lines and is often unacceptably low. Furthermore, when a better level of efficiency is achieved, it is often confined to a specific cell line and hence is not generally applicable. By and large, these techniques seem unlikely to be suitable for use in human gene therapy.

Another direct approach is to microinject DNA directly into the nucleus of cells. This requires considerable expertise and, because it involves treating one cell at a time, is unlikely to have any practical application in gene therapy. A more recent method involves the exposure of cells to a pulsed electric field, a technique called electroporation. It is believed that cells treated in this way open up pores in their plasma membranes. Although when it was first developed this approach also gave a low efficiency of transfection, there have been some improvements. A modification has been described recently that has resulted in more than 1% of the viable cells showing stable expression of a selectable marker gene (Chu *et al.* 1987). To date, there is no information about the long-term viability of cells that have been treated in this way or about the possibility of genetic damage caused by exposure to a strong electrical field.

Finally, Tao *et al.* (1987) have described a relatively efficient method of DNA transfer using laser micropuncture to cell membranes.

RNA viruses (retroviruses)

Retroviruses are adapted by evolution for the efficient delivery of their genome into cells, with integration into the host genome and a high level of expression of their internal sequences. At the time of writing, the use of retroviral vectors seems to be the most promising approach to gene therapy (Anderson 1984; Anderson *et al.* 1986; Miller *et al.* 1986; Williams & Orkin 1986; Yee *et al.* 1986; Nichols 1988).

Retroviruses have a complicated life style (Fig. 11.2(a)). The virion particle contains a dimer of viral RNA within a protein coat surrounded by a lipid bilayer that contains viral-specific glycoproteins, which attach themselves to cells during infection. The virion contains the virus-coded enzyme, reverse transcriptase. After it has entered cells, the coat is shed and the RNA genome is copied into DNA by reverse transcriptase. A double-stranded DNA circle is formed and specific retroviral sequences direct the integration of viral DNA into the host genome. After integration, viral sequences transcribe full-length and spliced RNAs. The spliced RNAs are translated to generate glycoproteins while the full-length RNA is either translated into internal structural proteins of the virion core and reverse transcriptase or packaged into virion particles as new genomic RNA. The subsequent assembly and budding of virion particles from infected cells is non-lytic.

The central features of the genome of a typical retrovirus are shown in Fig. 11.2(b). By some ingenious genetic engineering, a variety of recombinant retrovirus vectors have been constructed; the viral genome

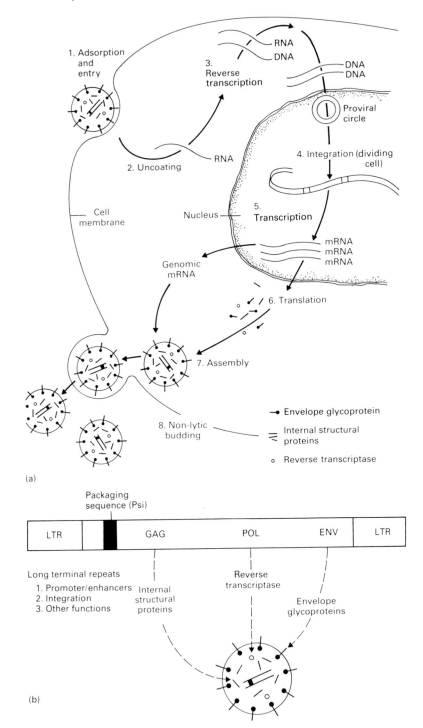

(a)

(b)

needed for the infection, integration and transcriptional control of the genome, which is all contained in the long terminal repeat sequences (LTRs), is preserved, but viral sequences, the function of which can be supplied in *trans*, are deleted. Thus the *gag* sequences, which encode internal structural proteins of the virion core, *pol* genes, which encode reverse transcriptase, and *env* genes, which encode the envelope glyco-proteins, are all deleted and are replaced by a dominant selectable marker and a restriction enzyme site into which the sequence that is to be transferred, that is, the gene we wish to insert, can be cloned.

The recombinant and now defective retroviral genome, in the form of plasmid DNA, is then introduced by transfection into murine fibro-blasts to generate cell lines that produce the recombinant retrovirus. Simultaneous infection with wild-type helper viruses can provide the required packaging proteins, although it is now possible to achieve the same result by the use of specialized packaging cell lines. Virus particles are shed into the surrounding medium, which can then be harvested and used to infect the recipient cells, or the latter can be incubated directly with the cells budding off the viral particles.

Experiments using recombinant retroviruses of this type have demon-strated that gene transfer can be achieved. For example, murine bone marrow has been cultivated with packaging cell lines that produce recombinant retrovirus, collected, and injected into lethally irradiated recipient mice (Williams *et al.* 1986). Since injected stem cells colonize the spleen, it is possible to follow the fate of the transfected genes by analysis of the DNA of colonies formed in the spleen of the irradiated mice. Studies of this kind have shown that genes have been transferred into pluripotential haemopoietic stem cells and that the transfected cells appear to be long-lived, at least up to four months after transplantation. Furthermore, they are totipotential, i.e. they give rise to both lymphoid and myeloid progeny.

Fig. 11.2(*facing page*). Retroviruses. (a) The lifecycle of wild-type retrovirus. The steps in the cycle include (1) adsorption and entry; (2) uncoating of the virion particle; (3) a DNA copy of the viral genome by reverse transcriptase; (4) integration of provirus after its entry into the nucleus; (5) transcription of new genome; (6) translation of messenger RNA into new glycoprotein, etc.; (7) non-lytic budding of new particles. (b) Genome of wild-type virus. LTR indicates long terminal repeats which include the viral promoter, enhancers and integration sequences. Psi are the packaging sequences required for packaging of genomic RNA into virion particles. The other abbreviations are described in the text. (From Williams & Orkin 1986, with permission.)

A variety of genes have been transferred into intact mice using retroviral vectors, including G418 (a neomycin-resistant gene), hypo-xanthine phosphoribosyl transferase (HPRT), dihydrofolate reductase (DHFR) and human adenosine deaminase (ADA). In addition to murine stem cells, retrovirus-mediated transfer and expression of drug-resistance genes have also been carried out using human haemopoietic progenitors in culture (Miller *et al.* 1986). And the human ADA gene has been transferred into and expressed in diploid skin fibroblasts obtained from an ADA-deficient human (Willis *et al.* 1984).

While these results are encouraging, the level of expression of many of these transferred genes has been extremely variable. Retrovirus-mediated transfer of genes into cultured haemopoietic cells has often resulted in their expression at levels similar to or even higher than that of the endogenous genes. For example, a homozygous Lesch−Nyhan lymphoblast line, deficient in HPRT, was used to determine whether the defect could be corrected by a retroviral vector containing a functional HPRT gene. This turned out to be the case, and the metabolic derange-ments associated with HPRT deficiency were almost completely corrected (Willis *et al.* 1984). On the other hand, transplantation of transfected haemopoietic cells into mice often results in low or almost undetectable expression of the inserted genes. Similarly, although expression of human ADA or neomycin-resistant genes has been demonstrated in monkeys after transfection of their bone marrow, the expression was confined to a very small proportion of peripheral blood white cells (Anderson *et al.* 1986).

It is not yet clear why the expression of transferred genes is so low in these *in vivo* experiments. It is possible that the genes may be inactivated or rearranged during haemopoietic differentiation. In this context, it has been possible to obtain expression of the genes for factor VIII and HPRT in human skin fibroblasts. It will be interesting to see whether these cells are able to maintain more persistent expression of transferred genes, particularly as they undergo very little differentiation after engraftment (Anson *et al.* 1987).

It is clear that many problems remain, in particular the efficiency of transfection and level of expression using retroviral vectors for gene transfer. A number of ingenious attempts have been made to improve the level of expression (reviewed by Anderson 1984). For example, some encouraging results have been obtained by inserting the sequence for rat growth hormone, together with 237 bases of genomic 5′ flanking sequence, into a retroviral vector. The growth hormone genes were regulated in fibroblasts by their own promoter and regulatory sequences, as evidenced by stimulation by glucocorticoid and thyroid hormones. But there are still enormous problems concerning the level and stability of expression to be overcome using retroviral vector systems. Whether it will be possible to improve the situation by the incorporation of enhancer sequences into these vectors remains to be seen. Retroviruses have their own enhancers immediately upstream from their promoters in the LTR. But the species and tissue specificity of enhancers, as mentioned earlier, may be of particular importance in determining the appropriate expression of inserted genes.

Finally, as mentioned earlier, it should be emphasized that very little is known about the safety of retroviral delivery systems. There is no doubt that they can rearrange their own structure as well as exchange sequences with other retroviruses. There is still a distinct possibility that a retroviral vector might recombine with an endogenous viral sequence to produce an infectious recombinant virus. Although the properties of a virus of this type are difficult to anticipate, the outside possibility remains that they might be oncogenic.

Targeted modification of human genes

Targeted modification of genes by exogenous DNA has been possible in yeast for many years. However, it is only recently that preliminary studies of this approach to the alteration of the human genome have been attempted (Gregg & Smithies 1986; Thomas & Capecchi 1986).

In principle, this approach to the replacement of defective genes has many attractions. In particular, it is site-directed and hence should not cause the problems of random integration. The idea is that the exogenous DNA should contain a region with the same nucleotide sequence as the target gene, so that homologous recombination can occur between the regions of sequence identity. In other words, the method uses nature's way of gene mixing. Depending on the arrangement of the incoming sequences relative to the target, the recombination event could either introduce new sequences into the recipient chromosome by a single crossover or substitute sequences by gene conversion or double crossover events.

Several ingenious attempts at targeted gene modification have been made recently. Plasmids have been linearized with restriction enzymes to produce a double-strand break within the region homologous to the gene target. These have tended to be much more efficient than closed circular molecules, which are also capable of generating recombination. It is presumed that the ends of the DNA molecules are more active in recombination. Although there have been some spectacular successes with this approach, many problems remain. In particular, the efficiency is low and there is a worrying tendency to induce new mutations after recombination with the 'foreign' DNA. However, because of its specificity it is very important to continue work to develop this method.

Specific correction of genetic defects with suppressor tRNA genes

Several forms of thalassaemia result from so-called nonsense mutations. These are single base changes that produce premature stop codons in the middle of exons and hence make it impossible for the affected genes to produce full-length protein products. It is possible to correct these defects by the use of so-called suppressor transfer RNAs, i.e. transfer RNAs which will insert amino acids into the altered codons (see Ho *et al.* 1986).

Recent work has suggested that functional suppressor genes of this type can be constructed by site-specific mutagenesis. Unfortunately, however, these molecules mediate only low levels of suppression. Thus, a major problem is whether it would be possible to achieve a level of suppression at which the appropriate genes could function in such a way as to produce adequate amounts of gene product. Current work in this field is directed towards constructing retrovirus vectors that contain the suppressor transfer RNA genes so that they can be inserted with high efficiency into bone marrow cells.

Again, there is a long way to go before this equally ingenious approach to gene therapy could have practical application. However, this method should be developed further because it also has the advantage of being a precise site-directed approach to gene therapy.

Transgenic approaches

The experimental introduction of DNA into fertilized eggs and subsequent integration into both somatic cells and germ cells have been achieved successfully in a variety of species. These experiments have been carried out with the object of developing the transgenic animal system as a model for studying gene regulation. DNA has been injected directly into fertilized eggs, and genes have also been transferred using retroviral vectors.

There is no doubt that foreign DNA introduced either by microinjection or retroviral transfection integrates into chromosomal DNA and is carried in germ cells and then transmitted to subsequent generations (see Palmiter & Brinster 1985); some remarkable results have been obtained. For example, the introduction of metallothionein/growth hormone fusion genes into mice stimulates the production of growth hormone in tissues that normally synthesize metallothionein. Suitable induction of the metallothionein genes with metals has caused treated mice to grow to about twice their normal size. Tissue-specific expression of a variety of genes has been obtained and a number of genetic diseases of mice have been corrected. This model is also extremely useful for studying the effects of oncogene expression and for the analysis of defective embryonic development by insertional mutagenesis.

Likely candidate diseases for gene therapy

As mentioned earlier, it seems likely that the best candidates for gene therapy for the immediate future are disorders like Lesch−Nyhan disease, purine nucleoside phosphorylase deficiency, and ADA deficiency. All three conditions are severely disabling and it is hoped that a low level expression of inserted genes into deficient cells might correct at least some of their functional abnormalities. The limited *in vitro* experience with HPRT deficiency suggests that this is the case. However, even in these disorders, there are enormous difficulties to be overcome. In particular, although the defect in each of these conditions is expressed in cells of bone marrow origin, at least in the case of the Lesch−Nyhan syndrome there is deficiency of HPRT in brain cells, which could probably not be corrected by current technology. If it proves possible to obtain prolonged and relatively high levels of production of factor IX in skin fibroblasts, Christmas disease might be another condition for early consideration for gene therapy of this type (see Anson *et al.* 1987).

Other single gene disorders will be even more difficult to correct in this way. For example, although a great deal is known about the molecular defects in thalassaemia and some of the structural haemoglobin disorders, it seems unlikely that it will be possible to insert normal globin genes in the immediate future. These genes have to be under extremely tight regulation; for example, it would be no good inserting a β-globin gene into the haemopoietic stem cells of a patient with β-thalassaemia only to see it overexpressed in their progeny, with the production of the clinical phenotype of α-thalassaemia!

One encouraging fact for the future of gene therapy is that ADA deficiency can be corrected by bone marrow transplantation, as can a number of other single gene disorders that affect haemopoietic stem cells, β-thalassaemia for example (see Thomas 1987). Hence, there is no reason why these conditions should not be cured by somatic gene therapy, once the difficulties of transfection and expression are overcome. But, until it becomes possible to transfect a sufficient number of stem cells, it may still be necessary to attempt to provide the treated population with some form of selective advantage; cells must be in cycle to be infected with retroviruses and since the majority of haemopoietic stem cells are out of cycle the efficiency of transfection will remain a serious problem. However, it is conceivable that, by the use of the recently purified haemopoietic growth factors, it may be possible to encourage a greater number of stem cells into cycle.

The future; ethical issues

It is becoming clear that it may be possible to replace at least a few defective genes within the next few years. In considering the clinical applications of this new technology, it is very important to make a clear distinction between somatic and germline gene therapy. The replacement of a gene into somatic cells raises no fundamentally new ethical issues. In a sense, it is no different from organ transplantation or, for that matter, blood transfusion. On the other hand, germline therapy, that is, injecting genes into fertilized eggs so that they become incorporated into both somatic and germline genes, is quite a different matter. These genes would be handed on to the progeny and this would open up a completely new chapter in human genetics. Nobody is contemplating transgenic therapy in man and there is no reason why they ever should. As techniques for the identification of genetic disorders improve, it should be possible to diagnose single gene disorders in tissue obtained from fertilized ova. The use of *in vitro* fertilization would then make it possible to sort through a number of fertilized ova and to discard those that carried a single gene defect and implant those that were normal in this respect. Thus there is no reason why germline therapy should ever be considered as an option in man.

It will be very important to develop guidelines for early attempts at gene therapy. Efforts to develop a sensible code of practice for this field are currently being made in both Europe and the USA. These include careful measures to ensure the safety of the procedure and strict criteria for selection of cases.

It seems likely that, as this field develops, it will start to have major impacts in the whole area of fetal medicine. Although it may be possible to carry out gene therapy in the early years of life for a number of single gene disorders, those that involve early development, particularly of the nervous system, may not be amenable to treatment except during fetal life. This may require considerable ingenuity in fetal surgery. And here we may well run into much more difficult ethical issues. While all this is for the future, it is something that obstetricians should be considering carefully as we make our first faltering steps into somatic gene therapy for disorders that can be corrected in postnatal life.

References

Anderson W.F. (1984) Prospects for human gene therapy. *Science*, **226**, 401–9.

Anderson W.F. & Fletcher J.C. (1980) Gene therapy in human beings: when is it ethical to begin? *N. Engl. J. Med.*, **303**, 1293–7.

Anderson W.F., Kantoff P., Eglitis M. *et al.* (1986) Gene transfer and expression in nonhuman primates using retroviral vectors. *Cold Spring Harbor Symp. Quant. Biol.*, **51**, 1073–81.

Anson D.S., Hock R.A., Austen D. *et al.* (1987) Towards gene therapy for hemophilia B. *Mol. Biol. Med.*, **4**, 11–20.

Caskey C.T. (1987) Disease diagnosis by recombinant DNA methods. *Science*, **236**, 1223–7.

Chu G., Hayakawa H. & Berg P. (1987) Electroporation for the efficient transfection of mammalian cells with DNA. *Nucleic Acids Symp. Ser.*, **15**, 1311–26.

Davies K.E. & Robson K.J.H. (1987) Molecular analysis of human monogenic disease. *Bioessays*, **6**, 247–53.

Emery A.E.H. (1984) *An Introduction to Recombinant DNA*. Wiley, Chichester.

Gregg R.G. & Smithies O. (1986) Targeted modification of human chromosomal genes. *Cold Spring Harbor Symp. Quant. Biol.*, **51**, 1093–100.

Ho T-S., Norton G.P., Palese P., Dozy A.M. & Kan Y.W. (1986) Expression and function of suppressor tRNA genes in mammalian cells. *Cold Spring Harbor Symp. Quant. Biol.*, **51**, 1033–40.

Maniatis T., Goodbourn S. & Fischer J.A. (1987) Regulation of inducible and tissue-specific gene expression. *Science*, **236**, 1237–45.

Miller A.D., Palmer T.D. & Hock R.A. (1986) Transfer of genes into human somatic cells using retrovirus vectors. *Cold Spring Harbor Symp. Quant. Biol.*, **51**, 1013–20.

Nicholls R.D., Fischel-Ghodsian N. & Higgs D.R. (1987) Recombination at the human α-globin gene cluster: sequence features and topological constraints. *Cell*, **49**, 369–78.

Nichols E.K. (1988) *Human Gene Therapy*. Harvard University Press, Cambridge, Mass.

Palmiter R.D. & Brinster R.L. (1985) Transgenic mice. *Cell*, **41**, 343–5.

Tao W., Wilkinson J., Stanbridge E.J. & Berns M.W. (1987) Direct gene transfer into human cultured cells facilitated by laser micropuncture of the cell membrane. *Proc. Natl. Acad. Sci. USA*, **84**, 4180–4.

Thomas E.D. (1986) Marrow transplantation and gene transfer as therapy for hematopoietic diseases. *Cold Spring Harbor Symp. Quant. Biol.*, **51**, 1009–12.

Thomas K.R. & Capecchi M.R. (1986) Targeting of genes to specific sites in the mammalian genome. *Cold Spring Harbor Symp. Quant. Biol.*, **51**, 1101–14.

Watson J.D., Tooze J. & Kurtz D.T. (1983) *Recombinant DNA: a Short Course*. Scientific American Books, New York.

306   *Chapter 11*

Weatherall D.J. (1985) *The New Genetics and Clinical Practice*, 2nd edn. Oxford University Press, Oxford.

Williams D.A. & Orkin S.H. (1986) Somatic gene therapy. Current status and future prospects. *J. Clin. Invest.*, **77**, 1053−6.

Williams D.A., Orkin S.H. & Mulligan R.C. (1986) Retrovirus-mediated transfer of human adenosine deaminase gene sequences into cells in culture and into murine hematopoietic cells *in vivo*. *Proc. Natl. Acad. Sci. USA*, **83**, 2566−70.

Willis R.C., Jolly D.J., Miller A.D. *et al.* (1984) Partial phenotypic correction of human Lesch−Nyhan (hypoxanthine-guanine phosphoribosyltransferase-deficient) lymphoblasts with a transmissible retroviral vector. *J. Biol. Chem.*, **259**, 7842−9.

Yee J-K., Jolly D.J., Moores J.C., Respess J.D. & Friedman T. (1986) Gene expression from a transcriptionally disabled retroviral vector. *Cold Spring Harbor Symp. Quant. Biol.*, **51**, 1021−6.

Index

The following abbreviations are used in the index:
ATP = autoimmune thrombocytopenic purpura;
IUGR = intrauterine growth retardation;
SLE = systemic lupus erythematosus.
Page numbers in italic refer to illustrations. Illustrations may also be found within textual references.

abnormalities *see* malformations
abortion
  iatrogenic 38
  recurrent 40−1
    causes 48−9
    paternal cell immunization for 47−56
  spontaneous 26−46
    in anticardiolipin patients 217−18
    associations with 31−8
    in ATP 213
    in diabetic mothers 182
    in lupus anticoagulant patients 217
    mechanisms and pathology 38−40
    natural history 26−30
    in SLE 223
acetylcholine receptor antibodies 226
acetyltransferase activity in fetal organs 265−6
acid−base parameters, fetal 57−89
acidaemia, methylmalonic 154−5
ACTH role in parturition 246−7
adenosine deaminase expression 300, 303−4
adipose tissue excess in macrosomia 189
adrenal
  hyperplasia, congenital 155
  role in parturition 245, 246
age, maternal, effects on spontaneous abortion 33−5
albumin infusion in hydrops fetalis 157
alcohol effects on spontaneous abortion 36
alloxan-induced diabetes, malformations in 180

alphafetoprotein levels, myasthenia gravis and 227
amino acids
  defects in, macrosomia and 190−1
  organization of 289−90
aminopterin
  effects on spontaneous abortion 37
  toxicity 15
amiodarone for fetal tachyarrhythmias 166, 168, 170−1
amniocentesis for blood gas studies 69−70
amnion tissue
  cAMP levels in 269, *271*
  beta-adrenergic receptors in 269, *270*
  levels of prostaglandins 261, 262, 265
amniotic fluid
  levels of bilirubin pigments 123
  levels of insulin and C peptide in diabetic mothers 190−1
  levels of prostaglandins at parturition 261, 265
  volume determination 136−7
cAMP role in arachidonic acid metabolism 269, *271*
anaemia
  fetal 65
    pathophysiology 74−7
  maternal, megaloblastic, birth defects following 16
anaesthetic effects on spontaneous abortion 37
anencephaly
  aminopterin causing 15
  dietary factors in 9
animal models
  for diabetes mellitus 180−1
  for fetal blood gas and acid−base status 61−6
  for malformations 90−118, 133−4
  for parturition 243−6
antibodies 207−8, *209*
  see also specific antibodies
anticardiolipin 216−20
  antibodies, recurrent abortion and 50
  in SLE 225
anti-D antibodies in recurrent abortion 50−1